D1278855

ECOLOGICAL VALIDITY OF NEUROPSYCHOLOGICAL TESTING

Edited by
Robert J. Sbordone
Charles J. Long

GR Press/St. Lucie Press
Delray Beach, Florida

Direct all inquiries to:
    St. Lucie Press, Inc.
    100 E. Linton Blvd., Suite 403B
    Delray Beach, Florida, 33483.
    Phone: (407) 274-9906
    Fax: (407) 274-9927

GR Press/St. Lucie Press
Delray Beach, Florida

DEDICATION

This book is dedicated to Nelson Butters, Ph.D.

TABLE OF CONTENTS

ABOUT THE EDITORS

Robert J. Sbordone, Ph.D., A.B.C.N., A.B.P.N., A.B.A.P.

Dr. Sbordone received his doctorate from U.C.L.A. and was a National institute of Health Postdoctoral Fellow at the U.C.L.A. Neuropsychiatric and Brain Research Institutes. He has been awarded a Diplomate in clinical neuropsychology from both the American Board of Professional Psychology and the American Board of Professional Neuropsychology. He is also a Diplomate at the American Board of Assessment Psychology. He is a Fellow of the National Academy of Neuropsychology and has authored over 90 books, chapters, and publications, including Neuropsychology for the Attorney, and Disorders of Executive Functions: Civil and Criminal Law Applications (with Harold V. Hall, Ph.D.). He also served as the editor of The Neuropsychological Analysis of Problem Solving that was written by Luria and Tsvetkova.

Dr. Sbordone maintains a private practice in Irvine, California and is a Clinical Assistant Professor in the Departments of Neurosurgery, Physical Medicine and Rehabilitation at the University of California at Irvine College of Medicine. He has consulted to many of the leading head trauma programs in the United States, and served on the Editorial Advisory Board of the International Journal of Clinical Neuropsychology, Journal of Head Trauma Rehabilitation, The Journal of Head Injury, JMA Bulletin and Neurolaw.

Charles J. Long, Ph.D.

Charles J. Long is associated with the University of Memphis as both a professor and the Director of the Clinical Neuropsychology Training Program. Dr. Long earned his B.S. and M.A. degrees at Memphis State University and his Ph.D. at Vanderbilt University. He has published 64 articles in professional journals, 18 book chapters, and four books. A frequent workshop and conference speaker, Dr. Long is nationally known for his major contributions to the fields of clinical neuropsychology and head trauma. Since 1992, Dr. Long has acted as a consultant to the FAA, and has served on the editorial board of *Archives of Clinical Neuropsychology* since 1986. In the past, he also served on the editorial boards for the *International Journal of Clinical Neuropsychology* (1984-1992) and *Child and Adolescent Psychotherapy* (1984-1992); he was Medical Editor for *The Journal of Head Injury: A search for understanding* (1990-1992). Honors include: Diplomate (1984), Vice-President (1988) and President (1993) of the American Board of Professional Neuropsychology; Fellow (1986) and Treasurer (1986) of the National Academy of Neuropsychologists; and Fellow (1990) of the American Psychological Society.

CONTRIBUTING AUTHORS

Chapter 1
Charles J. Long, Ph.D.

Chapter 2
Robert J. Sbordone, Ph.D., A.B.C.N., A.B.P.N.

Chapter 3
Andrew W. Siegal, Ph.D.
Private Practice, Albany, NY

Chapter 4
Gerald Goldstein, Ph.D., ABPP in Clinical Neuropsychology
Research Career Scientist, DVA Medical Center, Pittsburgh, PA
Professor of Psychiatry and Psychology, University of Pittsburgh

Chapter 5
Michael D. Franzen, Ph.D.
Associate Professor, Medical College of Pennsylvania, Hahnemann
University School of Medicine, Philadelphia, PA
Director, Neuropsychology, Allegheny Neuropsychiatric Institute

Karen L. Wilhelm, Ph.D.
Department of Psychology, Wake Rehabilitation Institute, Raleigh, NC

Chapter 6
David E. Hartman, Ph.D., A.B.P.N.
Director of Neuropsychology, Isaac Ray Center, Rush Human Performance
Laboratory, Rush Presbyterian St. Lukes Hospital
Adjunct Professor, Chicago Medical School

Chapter 7
J. Michael Williams, Ph.D.
Associate Professor, Hahnemann University, Philadelphia, PA

Chapter 8
Kimberly A. Kerns, Ph.D.
Assistant Professor, Department of Psychology, University of Victoria, Victoria, BC, Canada

Catherine A. Mateer, Ph.D., A.B.P.P., A.B.C.N.
Professor and Director of Clinical Training, Department of Psychology, University of Victoria, Victoria, BC, Canada

Chapter 9
Lloyd I. Cripe, Ph.D., A.B.P.P.
Private Practice, Seattle, WA

Chapter 10
Barbara Ann Cubic, Ph.D.
Assistant Professor, Departments of Psychiatry/Behavioral Sciences and Family and Community Medicine, Eastern Virginia Medical School, Norfolk, VA

William Drew Gouvier, Ph.D.
Associate Professor of Psychology, Louisiana State University, Baton Rouge, LA

Chapter 11
Glenn J. Larrabee, Ph.D., A.B.C.N., A.B.P.P.
Department of Psychiatry, Sarasota Memorial Hospital
Faculty Associate, The Center for Neuropsychological Studies, University of Florida

Thomas H. Crook III, Ph.D.
President, Memory Assessment Clinics, Inc., Bethesda, MD

Chapter 12
Bruce Crosson, Ph.D.
Department of Clinical and Health Psychology, University of Florida, Gainesville, FL

Chapter 13
Linas A. Bieliauskas, Ph.D., A.B.P.P., Cl, Cn
Staff Psychologist, Veterans Administration Medical Center
Associate Professor, Psychiatry, University of Michigan, Ann Arbor, MI

Chapter 14
Patricia Perez-Arce, Ph.D.
San Francisco General Hospital

Antonio E. Puente, Ph.D.
University of North Carolina at Wilmington

Chapter 15
Lawrence C. Hartlage, Ph.D.
Augusta Neuropsychology Center

Donald I. Templer, Ph.D.
California School of Professional Psychology

Chapter 16
Tedd Judd, Ph.D., A.B.P.P., A.B.C.N.
Department of Psychology, University of Costa Rica, San Pedro, Costa Rica

David Fordyce, Ph.D.
Virginia Mason Clinic, Seattle, WA

Chapter 17
Arthur M. Horton, Jr., Ed.D, A.B.P.P.(CL), A.B.P.N.
Psych Associates, Towson, MD

Chapter 18
Brian T. McMahon, Ph.D., C.R.C.
Professor, Educational Psychology Department, University of Wisconsin Milwaukee

Linda R. Shaw, Ph.D., C.R.C.
Assistant Professor, Department of Rehabilitation Counseling Health Science Center, University of Florida, Gainesville, FL

Chapter 19

Thomas J. Guilmette, Ph.D., A.B.P.P.
Director, Neuropsychology, Rhode Island Hospital
Clinical Assistant Professor, Department of Psychiatry and Human
Behavior Brown University, Providence, RI

Marianna Pinchot Kastner, M.A.
Doctoral Candidate, Clinical Psychology, University of Rhode Island
Kingston, RI

Chapter 20

Barbara A. Wilson, M. Phil., Ph.D., F.B.Ps.S.
Senior Scientist, Medical Research Council, Applied Psychology Unit
Cambridge, England
Honorary Clinical Psychologist, Addenbrookes Hospital, Cambridge,
England

Appendix

Andrew W. Siegal, Ph.D.
Private Practice, Albany, NY

Marshall D. Schecter, M.D.
Professor Emeritus & Former Program Head, Division of Child &
Adolescent Psychiatry, School of Medicine, University of Pennsylvania

Sidney P. Diamond, M.D.
Professor, Department of Neurology, Mt. Sinai School of Medicine, New
York, NY

PREFACE

Although the field of neuropsychology has enjoyed three decades of unparalleled growth, it has recently been undergoing a transition from its primary role of contributing to diagnostic decisions in psychiatric, neurological, and neurosurgical cases to that of addressing a broad range of questions regarding the relationship between neuropsychological test data and the patient's level of functioning in real-world settings. This shifting emphasis is, in part, due to a combination of advances in neurodiagnostic imaging and change in the referral questions. For example, neuropsychologists, particularly those in rehabilitation and forensic settings, have been asked to deal with the issue of predicting how brain-damaged patients would be expected to perform when they return to school, work, home, and the community, even though actuarial data to support their opinions are not yet available and the ecological validity of many of our widely used tests and batteries has not yet been established.

Neuropsychologists working in the field of rehabilitation are frequently asked by referral sources to provide opinions regarding functional skills, treatment options, rehabilitation potential, and optimal living arrangements. They are also being asked to identify patients who would most likely benefit from specific rehabilitation or training experiences, as well as provide information regarding whether or not a particular patient can return to work or school. To provide effective answers to such complex issues, neuropsychologists must identify the cognitive processes required, select the appropriate tests to evaluate such processes, adequately assess emotional and psychosocial factors which are involved, and assess the demand characteristics of the patient's job. In conducting the needed ecological research, several points of focus appear necessary. First, it is essential that the neuropsychologist understand the relationship between the various cognitive functions and the specific behavior(s) in question. Second, it is important to further investigate and clarify the relationship between the identified cognitive functions and specific test scores and/or patterns of test scores. Third, the neuropsychologist must assess the demand characteristics of the patient's environment by consulting with vocational specialists, the patient's employer, co-workers, and significant others. Finally, the fourth requirement is that the neuropsychologist must establish the relationship between the patient's performance on neuropsychological testing and the target level of behavioral functioning necessary to successfully return to work.

Neuropsychologists who are involved in forensic cases are frequently asked by attorneys and/or the Court for opinions about whether a particular patient can return to work and/or live independently. While the neuropsychologist may discuss his or her numerous test scores and make specific statements in Court as to the cognitive strengths and weaknesses of the individual in question, this information may be of little value in assisting the Court or the tryer-of-fact if it is not supported by empirical research specifically linking it to these issues. In the event a neuropsychologist renders an opinion that the individual is not able to work, the Court may seek to determine the extent of assumed loss related to the reduction of income and/or related factors. Until very recently, physicians were placed in this position and had to generalize from their medical tests and brief encounters with the patient as to the patient's ability to function in the real world. Neuropsychologists, who generally spend considerably more time with patients than physicians, may have a distinct advantage, particularly if they are able to base their opinions about the patient's ability to function if their neuropsychological test data is supported by empirical research. Thus, it is clear that the acquisition of data regarding the ecological validity of our tests will serve to significantly enhance the credibility of the neuropsychologist's testimony in court as an expert witness.

While neuropsychology has made a major contribution in our understanding of the functional consequences of neurological damage, future and perhaps even greater contributions may well come from a better understanding of the relationship between assessed cognitive functioning and predicted future performance in real-world settings. Investigation of the ecological validity of neuropsychological tests appears to offer a new and important direction for the field of neuropsychology since it is unlikely that the patient's ability to function within his or her environment will be determined solely by neuroradiological tests.

This book presents the views of many highly respected and prominent neuropsychologists regarding the history and changing emphasis of neuropsychology and raises what the authors consider to be significant ecological issues confronting neuropsychologists today. Included within these issues are a critical examination of many of our widely held assumptions regarding neuropsychological testing, as well as the methods many neuropsychologists currently utilize, which may actually handicap them in addressing the issue of ecological validity. Specific focus has been directed to issues involving the evaluation of specific functions (e.g., attention, memory, and executive functions), as well as previous research which has been conducted on the ecological validity of our neuropsychological and psychological tests. Finally, directions for future research are discussed to enhance our understanding of the ecological validity.

Robert J. Sbordone, Ph.D.
Laguna Beach, California

Charles J. Long, Ph.D.
Memphis, Tennessee

1995

ACKNOWLEDGEMENTS

The editors wish to acknowledge the following individuals for their contributions in the development of this book:

Richard Balvin, who recognized the issue of ecological validity over 30 years ago. John Garcia, who was one of the first psychologists to recognize the difference between an organism's behavior in a laboratory setting and its behavior in a naturalistic setting. Irving Maltzman, for his recognition that our current methodologies for generalizing behavior seen in the laboratory to real-world settings were inadequate. Frank Ervin and Michael McGuire for their courage to disregard traditional psychiatric methodologies and replace them with ecological and observational methodologies in the study of psychiatric disorders. Finally, Michael Howard and Arnold Purisch for their invaluable insights and feedback, which helped make this book possible.

The editors would also like to thank Drs. M. Spica, J.B. Orange, J.R. Julian, and M.B. Spina for their critical readings of earlier drafts of this manuscript and for their helpful suggestions.

GENERAL OVERVIEW

Chapter 1 through 3 outline the changing emphasis of neuropsychology and raise what the authors consider to be significant issues confronting neuropsychologists today. The chapters present evidence that neuropsychology is undergoing radical changes. The major impetus for such change evolves from changes in both health care delivery and management and will significantly affect the future of neuropsychology. It is hoped that readers will share the view of the authors and editors, that effective changes place neuropsychology and neuropsychologists in a crucial position to have a very positive impact on comprehensive rehabilitation as well as vocational and educational planning.

The chapters in this first section describe some of the critical issues in neuropsychology, including the difficulty generalizing from current test data to real world situations, to faulty assumptions sometimes held by neuropsychologists. This section lays the groundwork for future research and development by outlining basic problem areas and identifying some of the needs for further development. Finally, it presents a detailed approach to the history as the essential first step in organizing an approach to the problem.

GENERAL ISSUES

As discussed in chapters in chapters 4 through 7, it is clear that the role of neuropsychology is changing from the assessment of cognitive functions to aid in diagnosis to the use of such data to predict outcome, outline treatment needs, and provide data of value in assisting neurologically impaired individuals in dealing effectively with their environment. While neuropsychologists appear to have recognized this need, they have attempted to work in the area of ecological validity without adequate training or experience. Not only is there a need for a shift in emphasis, but there is an even greater need for the development of relevant normative data. This might include job analysis or functional analysis, modification of the tests and/or the testing environment, and a more conservative use of data.

Neuropsychological data were not designed to be ecologically valid and attempts to use such data in this capacity are fraught with pitfalls. Correlation of scores with outcome measures and the development of new measures is clearly needed.

The authors present several different views of ecological validity in neuropsychological assessment. Some argue that we have neglected the issue of ecological validity due to the historical focus on diagnosis, others argue that neuropsychology is founded in ecological validity and that it is simply undergoing change in the process. All agree that there is much room for improvement and we should either reevaluate our existing tests or develop new tests. The development of new measures should include consideration of the similarity of the task to the predictive behaviors and the extent to which test results predict such behavior. Clearly, the target behavior must be identified (e.g., by job description). Assessment should consider the extent to which compensatory mechanisms are available and utilized; something that is largely eliminated in existing batteries due to restrictions in methods which may be employed to perform a task.

Chapter 7 discusses the everyday skill movement and suggests that this movement emphasizes the fact that many of our tests are abstract and not clearly related to ecological issues. There appears to be a need to construct specific everyday skill measures and to relate neuropsychological data to everyday skills; including activities of daily living, employment status, and other miscellaneous skills.

SPECIFIC FUNCTIONS

Chapters 8 through 17 deal with more specific cognitive processes and discuss strategies for assessment. Cognitive research has served to assist neuropsychological research by outlining a more effective taxonomy of behavior. Several of the cognitive constructs (e.g., attention) can be approached from one or more of the hierarchical models available. While various brain regions have specialized roles, these cognitive processes directly relate to real world behaviors. The cognitive constructs of attention, perception, working memory, language, and executive functioning are covered in detail in the following section. There is also consideration given to the assessment of special populations including children, minorities, substance abusers, the elderly, and emotionally disturbed neurologic populations.

VOCATIONAL FUNCTIONING

Chapters 18 through 20 focus the ability of neuropsychology to predict return to work and the ability to resume activities of daily living. In order to understand the process of returning to work after brain injury, a better understanding of vocational rehabilitation is needed. Chapter 18 focuses on the vocational rehabilitation and its role in the rehabilitation process. It also provides an interpretation of the philosophical orientation of vocational rehabilitation including the need to focus holistically on the individual in a natural environment. Limitations of neuropsychology in terms of its lack of exposure to vocational issues and lack of specific treatment recommendations are discussed.

Chapter 19 provides insight into the ability of neuropsychological assessment to predict vocational functioning. Neuropsychology's previous focus was on determination of the presence of brain damage and its location. Now the focus is on the capacity of the individual to function in the everyday environment. Prediction of work behavior is the second most frequent reason for neuropsychological evaluation. The problem is we are bound by the limits of our tests which were developed to answer other questions. Neuropsychological assessment is also limited by lack of norms based on job types. We need different norms for the various occupations to enhance our accuracy in predicting return to work. There is also the need to know the skills required by the job in order to measure them during the assessment. Four approaches used in attempting to predict work ability from neuropsychological data are discussed. It was found that the Halstead-Reitan Average Impairment Index is better at predicting unemployment than successful employment. Psychosocial measures, such as the MMPI, are better predictors of success on the job. The need to incorporate psychosocial measures into neuropsychological assessment is also discussed.

Another primary question is how much information about everyday functioning can be gained from neuropsychological tests. In rehabilitation, neuropsychologists must predict how problems resulting from brain injury will affect activities of daily living and plan rehabilitation programs to deal with deficits as expressed in real life activities. However, neuropsychological assessment is often of little direct assistance to therapists involved in treatment. Test items are not analogous to tasks encountered in everyday situations. Neuropsychological tests need to be more ecologically valid; we must devise tests that map directly onto everyday behaviors. An example offered is the Rivermead Behavioral Memory Test. The Rivermead Behavioral Memory Test correlates highly with traditional memory tests, is a test of everyday memory, and has research which shows it correlates with memory failures during daily rehabilitation. Chapter 20 discusses other tests which measure aspects of cognitive functioning found in real world.

1

NEUROPSYCHOLOGICAL TESTS:
A Look at Our Past and the Impact that Ecological Issues May Have on Our Future

Charles J. Long, Ph.D.

PERCEPTIONS OF THE HISTORY OF US NEUROPSYCHOLOGY

Like many other disciplines, neuropsychology (or the study of brain-behavior relationships) developed from a coalition of data, procedures, and concepts garnered from other areas. Early research on brain-behavior relationships by physiologists and treatment by neurologically oriented anatomists and physicians helped further define neuropsychology—even though the available technology was limited at that time. In this century, physiological psychologists, neurologists, neurosurgeons, psychologists, and neuroscientists have expanded and refined our understanding of brain-behavior relationships.

The actual term *neuropsychology* has been in existence since the early days of basic animal-lesion research (Beach, Hebb, Morgan, & Nissen, 1960). *Clinical neuropsychology* evolved from the application of basic findings regarding brain-behavior relationships in both animals and humans (i.e., information gathered in the experimental setting began to be used in the assessment of neurological and neurosurgical patients). The development of clinical neuropsychology was greatly influenced by the clinical application of behavioral techniques by individuals such as Kurt Goldstein. In the 1940s, much of his study involved the behavioral consequences of combat injuries. Aleksandr Luria also made major contributions and provided a basic theoretical foundation for the study of brain-behavior relationships. Ward Halstead (1947) focused on the study of human brain-behavior relationships and attempted to evaluate the biological basis of

intelligence. While there were many researchers focusing on the clinical application of behavioral tests, Ralph Reitan's organization and modification of
Halstead's developing test battery in the 1950s played a key role in launching
clinical neuropsychology as a viable clinical entity. His extensive research regarding human brain-behavior relationships contributed to the credibility of
the Halstead-Reitan Battery and resulted in escalating demands for neuropsychological assessments by neurologists and neurosurgeons.

During the days of its initial application (and for many years to come), the
neuropsychological test battery provided a valuable alternative to the
pneumoencephalograph and/or the early brain scan. These crude neurological
procedures provided poor resolution and allowed the detection of only very
large lesions. The pneumoencephalograph, in particular, was an invasive procedure with many associated risks and much discomfort for the patient. In contrast, the neuropsychological assessment provided a non-invasive procedure for
investigating cognitive processes and correlating observed weaknesses with central nervous system (CNS) deficits. As the use of this procedure expanded,
considerable research was directed at understanding the relationship between
cognitive processes and various structures, or functional systems, in the brain.
As a result of such studies, it was strongly demonstrated that this procedure was
effective in detecting the presence of cerebral dysfunction. Further research
supported the application of this process to the determination of laterality. Some
studies even related specific patterns of cognitive deficit with focal lesions.

CHANGE IN NEUROPSYCHOLOGY

In addition to making statements about the presence, laterality, and extent
of brain damage, neuropsychologists have provided the unique dimension of
describing the functional consequences of cerebral damage (i.e., establishing
brain-behavior relationships). This led to an emphasis on describing cognitive
strengths and weaknesses. Obtaining this specific information about the
individual's intelligence, memory, and other cognitive functions is extremely
important because it indicates educational and occupational potential as well as
ability to manage personal affairs. In addition, this information may be of significant value in assisting the individual to develop realistic vocational goals
and to obtain needed and appropriate rehabilitation. Finally, information regarding the individual's emotional adjustment will clarify the above and identify potential barriers to recovery that can be effectively minimized with early
intervention. The shifting emphasis in neuropsychology, as outlined above,
doesn't necessarily require a radical change in assessment procedures but does

require a shift in emphasis in both the application and interpretation of neuropsychological test findings.

Neuropsychological assessment remains the primary tool for evaluating the functional consequences of neurological impairment; yet, as previously indicated, the role of neuropsychology is changing. In the 1970s, more advanced neuroradiological techniques (e.g., the CT scan) became available. This has been followed by a seemingly endless supply of more sophisticated devices with greater resolution (e.g., CT, MRI, PET, SPECT) which are quick and effective for certain diagnostic purposes, such as verifying the presence of space occupying lesions, aneurysms, or strokes. As a result, neuroradiological tests have subsumed much of the initial diagnostic role in neurosurgery and neurology— even though they provide no information about the functional consequences of the brain damage.

The preferred use of neuroradiological techniques for diagnostic purposes may, in the final analysis, be related to economics. These neuroradiological instruments are owned by hospitals and generate considerable revenue. Of equal importance is the changing impact of economics on health care delivery. Insurance companies are tending to shift more to brief, essential, medical intervention with less concern on outcome or broader rehabilitation issues. Thus, while neuropsychological assessments may provide important information regarding the functional consequences of neurological injury and its effect on the individual's ability to function in society, this is viewed more as a social (rather than a medical) issue.

Because of the changing role of neuropsychological assessment, the nature of referral questions has also changed, and new areas must now be addressed. For instance, with the increased emphasis on cognitive retraining and the development of compensatory strategies, neuropsychologists are now being asked to make statements regarding functional skills, treatment options, rehabilitation potential, and optimal living arrangements (Henrichs, 1990). Clinical judgment and experience in neuropsychological assessment issues is obviously useful in making such evaluations; but it is not enough. To relate test findings to new and/or different external criteria, we must: (a) understand our area of competency as well as our limitations; (b) operate from a foundation based on past research; (c) conduct research to extend our foundation; and (d) develop tests which are adequate in answering such questions. The future face of clinical neuropsychological assessment is, therefore, still being defined.

In spite of this shifted emphasis, the diagnostic usefulness of neuropsychological assessment has not been totally eliminated. Although neuroradiological procedures are quick to identify focal structural defects in the brain, these tests are generally less effective in the detection of more diffuse damage. Progress is being made in this area, however. For example, neuroradiological procedures are now being used to identify demyelenization in multiple sclerosis. But current technology still is unable to detect many subtle, diffuse forms of neurological damage. In addition, there is still no one-to-one correlation between specific structural deficits and behavioral changes (i.e., there may be focal deficits without corresponding, detectable behavioral deficits and vice versa). For example, in cases of head trauma, electrical shock, chemical exposure, and early stage dementia, there may be significant behavioral deficits without corresponding detectable structural changes. For these reasons, there remain a number of areas where the neuroradiological procedures are of less value than the neuropsychological test findings. In fact, not only are the neuroradiological techniques of limited value in such cases, but they can also be misleading if their limitations are not properly understood. In addition, the primary strength of the neuropsychological assessment is identifying the functional consequences of neurological damage. Therefore, neuropsychological tests provide valuable information which can augment the findings of other diagnostic procedures which focus more on structural integrity.

A comprehensive neuropsychological assessment also serves another important function. While neuropsychological tests are sensitive to brain functioning, they are known to be influenced by, or to interact with, non-organic factors as well (e.g., age, education, occupation, emotional adjustment, situational stress. The neuropsychologist must evaluate cognitive, emotional, and situational factors because of the impact of non-neurological factors on cognitive functions. The comprehensive neuropsychological evaluation is thus designed to evaluate the relative contribution of neurological, emotional, and situational symptoms to the patient's functional problems. This is essential for developing a clear understanding of the etiology and consequences of brain disease (or injury) in that particular individual and for developing an effective treatment plan. Neuroradiological measures do not provide this broader perspective.

Another factor worthy of consideration relates to what the neuropsychological assessment measures and what questions are to be addressed. As previously mentioned, these questions have shifted from basic diagnostic issues to the evaluation of present cognitive functioning and relating this measure to an unknown premorbid level of functioning or to future performance. This latter issue suggests a potential new emphasis for neuropsychology and serves as the focus for this book. Of course, many competent neuropsychologists have, through years of experience, gained much information in this area. Their clinical judgment has developed to the point that they are able to make useful suggestions and knowledgeable predictions about the person's likelihood of being able to function adequately in certain vocational environments. However, there is currently little or no empirical foundation for such predictions.

This problem needs to be resolved. Research is needed to establish the relationship between the neuropsychological tests we administer and specific jobs and/or courses in school. What is the expected range of variability for individuals who can function successfully versus those who can't? How do our tests relate to existing areas of vocational assessment, school psychology, industrial psychology, etc.? In short, what is the ecological validity of neuropsychological tests?

These are certainly issues that need addressing, and further understanding may well pave the way for the future development of neuropsychology. In raising these issues, we may have come full circle: ecological validity was also of concern in Halstead's early research.

> As Halstead studied brain-damaged persons in their typical everyday living situations, he observed that most of them seemed to have difficulties in understanding the essential nature of complex problem-situations, in analyzing the circumstances that they had observed, and in reaching meaningful conclusions about the situations they faced in everyday life. (Reitan & Wolfson, 1993)

CRITICAL VARIABLES AND/OR PROCEDURES IN STUDYING BRAIN-BEHAVIOR RELATIONSHIPS

THE MEDICAL MODEL

In evaluating medical patients and either addressing diagnostic issues or brain-behavior relationships, neuropsychology has followed a medical model. Patients with apparent neurological symptoms are evaluated using behavioral tests; strengths and weaknesses are measured, and inferences are made as to possible underlying neurological pathology and etiology. Years of research have yielded strong support for conclusions obtained in this manner. Nevertheless, there are many methodological problems that must be addressed in conducting such research.

The selection of relatively homogeneous samples of patients is a major source of variance which should receive careful consideration in neuropsychological research. There is almost always bias in subject selection. Only certain patients are available and willing to participate in research. Even with clinical referrals, neuropsychologists see only patients who perceive symptoms sufficient to seek medical attention. For example, in the study of head injury, patients with severe brain injury are often evaluated because of continued cognitive deficits whereas patients with mild brain injury may be referred because of consistent post-concussion symptoms (reflecting more emotional distress than neurological damage). Both groups may reveal deficits but for entirely different reasons, and the underlying factors may play a large role in determining outcome.

Neurological tests (e.g., EEG, MRI, PET) and neuropsychological tests are not equivalent. Each is maximally sensitive to different conditions, and group composition will be affected by the particular method used for subject selection. Neuropsychological research is also affected by many potentially significant intervening variables. In the case of head injury research, for instance, numerous critical variables must be considered: severity and nature of the injury, time since injury, age, education, and socioeconomic status. In addition, the modality involved, the material presented, and the measurement procedure all influence research findings.

ECOLOGICAL ISSUES

In contrast to the traditional medical model, where the focus is on the relationship of cognitive functions to brain integrity and diagnosis of underlying neuropathology, neuropsychologists are increasingly being asked to address a different set of questions. Seldom is the referral source interested in the individual's cognitive functioning on a particular day. Rather, the referral questions require the comparison of the neuropsychological test data to some unknown. For instance, the neuropsychologist may be asked to estimate the extent of decline in cognitive functioning due to some injury or neurological disease. In other cases, the question relates to expected future performance on the job or in school, for example. In neither of these instances are neurpsychologists able to utilize specific criterion measures or empirical data; and, as a result, are often drawn away from their data base and led into making judgments or predictions they cannot back with research.

The first situation described is less of a problem. With a careful history addressing the important demographic, psychological, and neurological questions, neuropsychologists can arrive at fairly accurate statements regarding decline in function from some estimated premorbid level (see Chapter 3 by Siegal). Though the research in this area is far from perfect or complete, there is sufficient foundation for certain types of inferences. In the case of predicting future behavior, however, the problem is much more difficult. In such cases, the neuropsychologist must draw on known relationships of change in cognitive functioning and subsequent recovery in other groups of patients with similar etiology and time since injury. This requires having an empirical foundation from which to work. The problem is relatively easy in cases where the dysfunction is either profound or nonexistent, but it becomes very difficult between these two extremes. It is imperative that neuropsychologists be aware of existing data and not go beyond it; or, if they do, they should be careful to communicate the decreased probability of their decisions.

Wedding and Faust (1989) raise issues that become even more salient when dealing with judgment and decisions regarding ability to predict future behavior in the environment. They argue for the development of an actuarial base and suggest the awareness of a number of corrective procedures. Some of these are: (a) know the literature on human judgment, (b) start with the most valid information, (c) collect appropriate norms, and (d) make a deliberate effort to obtain feedback. Faust's statements have been the subject of varying interpretation and concern to neuropsychologists. Certainly the point that one should communicate both the prediction, the foundation for such predictions, and the confidence in such predictions is sound advice.

Not only do neuropsychologists need to make sure they do not go beyond their data by making unsupported claims without prefacing them as such, but they also must be careful to include and consider all relevant data sources when making an evaluation. Many individuals (especially those who attempt to do neuropsychological assessments without the benefit of extensive pre- or post-doctoral training in these methods) mistakenly assume that test scores can be interpreted in isolation. This simply is not the case. In addition to cognitive measures, a thorough neuropsychological evaluation must include: (1) a detailed description of the course of illness or injury (including details of loss of consciousness, post-traumatic amnesia, related surgeries and hospitalizations, and subsequent treatment in rehabilitation facilities); (2) symptoms at the time of the illness/injury and at time of assessment; (3) personal, psychological, and medical history; (4) situational factors that may be negatively affecting the recovery process; (5) intellectual assessment; and (6) personality assessment. It is only in the context of all of the above information that neuropsychological test scores can be properly interpreted. Confidence in any conclusions about level of cognitive function and confidence in predictions about future performance will necessarily decline in proportion to the extent that any of the above factors are ignored.

MODEL OF PREDICTION

Confirmation of the *presence* of brain damage is important because cognitive deficits will affect the individual's ability to understand and successfully deal with environmental demands. However, the *degree or severity* of the damage determines the extent to which an individual will be impaired. Therefore, ecological validity is highly related to both the individual's current level of cognitive functioning and to the type of measure used to evaluate this.

LEVEL OF FUNCTIONING

When the overall level of functioning is markedly impaired or is well above average, the prediction of behavior is more accurate. As the individual's cognitive abilities increase or decrease (i.e., approach the mean), the ability to predict behavior is reduced and is more likely to be influenced by other factors. The neuropsychologist's prediction of abilities can be stated with a high degree of confidence for patients whose IQ falls below 55 and above 145 since less than 99% of the population will fall outside this range by chance. Considerable confidence (95%) may also be obtained in cases where the IQ is below 70 or above 130; however, this only applies to 4.56% of the population. The remaining 95.44% fall closer to the mean; and confidence, therefore, declines substantially with the majority of the population. In addition, the neuropsychologist must next consider the relationship between IQ (or any other cognitive measure) and the behavior being predicted. Ecological validity suggests that the accuracy of prediction of future behavior is further influenced by the extent to which the test score relates to the behavior to be predicted. This latter point raises new issues that are the topic of this book.

TYPE OF MEASURE TAKEN

There are numerous ways of obtaining information about an individual's level of functioning. Direct behavioral measures (e.g., performance on the job or in class) may be available. Such measures are accurate and reflect the external criteria to be predicted in some cases. When available, they may provide important information as to behavior in similar situations. The confidence here is related to the confidence we have in the similarity. Surprisingly, the neuropsychologist is occasionally asked to evaluate a patient and predict behavior at work (or school) when the patient is already at work (or school), data are available, and no problems are reported. Obviously, in such cases, no neuropsychological test will answer this question better than the direct measure of performance. In contrast, when problems have been noted in the work or school setting, neuropsychological data help identify underlying cognitive weaknesses which should be considered in modifying the job or seeking remediation.

Less direct measures, such as simulation tests, structured interviews with the patient and significant others, questionnaires, and quality of performance, all provide important information useful in making predictions about everyday performance capabilities. While such measures provide a less direct measure, they do give reasonably accurate information about the specific performance in question. Indirect tests or behavioral observations obtained in a clinical assessment, but with a known relationship to job or school performance, are even further removed from the real-life abilities being evaluated.

The most indirect method of obtaining information regarding real-world behavior is psychometric tests; yet they represent the major source of information for many neuropsychological evaluations. This is unfortunate. Psychometric tests represent samples of behavior in a reasonably controlled situation which may have a relationship to daily behaviors in other situations. However, in almost all cases, it is a sample that only represents a part of the criteria behavior to be predicted.

If we are to be accurate in our predictions of future performance, we must: (1) understand what cognitive skills are required for a task, (2) use enough tests to measure these skills, and (3) study the relationship between test scores and the cognitive skill in question. As the measure moves further from direct performance, the relationship becomes weaker and prediction is more difficult. Likewise, as the level of function increases, the ability to predict future performance decreases. Furthermore, other variables may increase in their importance with changes in the level of cognitive functioning.

While neuropsychological tests are primarily designed to assess higher cognitive processes, each test invariably measures a number of broad constructs such as attention, perception, memory, and language skills. In addition, higher cognitive processes influence other functions and vice versa. For example, a memory assessment instrument might measure some aspects of memory; but memory itself may be influenced by attention, depression, motivation, language function, etc. Likewise, deficits in memory will undoubtedly affect performance in these other cognitive domains.

This problem is confounded by the fact that our tests, no matter how selective, measure all of these psychological constructs to a greater or lesser extent. We don't have a test that only measures one construct. All tests are influenced by many different factors, although to varying degrees. For this reason, strict interpretation of individual test scores is of limited value in making statements about specific cognitive processes. However, interpretation of the overall pattern of test scores makes it possible to identify particular areas of weakness.

Further understanding is offered by cognitive research which attempts to explain complex global (e.g., memory or attention) by subdividing them into functional units. Perhaps, with more refined definitions, more specific tests can be constructed to augment our understanding. In addition, the neuropsychologist needs to be knowledgeable regarding the extent to which impaired perception, attention, memory, language skills, or motivation might effect test performance. The influence of depression or other emotional factors on test performance must also be understood and considered. And, finally, the ability to provide meaningful answers to specific referral questions depends upon our knowledge of how physical ability, social support, and socioeconomic status will affect the individual's cognitive and emotional status.

THE PROCESS OF RECOVERY: RECOVERY VS. COMPENSATION

Initial recovery from neurological injury appears to involve reorganization, recovery, or other internal neurological processes which are not clearly understood. Neuropsychological tests appear to reflect this recovery rather well. However, later stage recovery appears to be more reflective of awareness of deficit (or weakness) and the use of compensatory strategies. Neuropsychological tests do not measure and do not reflect this aspect of recovery. Thus, if the intent of an assessment is to relate present performance to future functional ability in some specific capacity, predictions must be adjusted to include the possibility of effective compensatory skills and the likelihood that the patient will be both able and willing to develop and use them.

Research by Wilson (1993) suggests that while neuropsychological tests do not actually measure the effects of compensatory strategies, they do provide some idea as to compensatory ability. Thus, measurement of intelligence, memory, etc., provides important information regarding the individual's ability to acquire compensatory skills.

REHABILITATION-RELATED ASSESSMENT

Neuropsychologists have, in recent years, played a predominant role in rehabilitation programs designed for individuals with cognitive impairment. In rehabilitation-related assessment, the focus has already been shifted away from diagnosis to ecological factors. Such treatment focuses on behaviors and has less of a problem with ecological validity; however, the major limitation here, too, relates to difficulty in generalizing to other situations what has been learned. Recent research indicates that neuropsychological assessments were highly accurate (77%) in predicting whether subjects would successfully complete a vocational evaluation (Ryan, Sautter, Capps, Meneese, & Barth, 1992). The best predictors were reading comprehension, immediate and delayed verbal memory, depression, and dysphasic symptomatology. As discussed earlier, these findings indicate that basic cognitive functions and emotional adjustment serve as good predictors of ability to function in a vocational assessment setting.

Further research in this area will provide valuable data regarding the ecological validity of various cognitive tests and the factors that will improve the generalizability of associated predictions. There is also a need to focus on both validity and utility. Heinrichs (1990) differentiates between these two: validity refers to *accuracy* of inferences; utility, on the other hand, involved the actual *benefit* of these inferences to the patient. Much like the difference between statistical and clinical significance, validity relates to statistical procedures, whereas utility refers to the value that a particular test or tests have in predicting rehabilitation potential or outcome.

In addition to investigating the relationship of existing tests to real-world behaviors, other assessment strategies may also be of value. One promising area is the assessment of speed of information processing. Most cognitive measures focus on capacity (or ability), and speed of information processing is only indirectly measured. Yet, research reveals that speed of processing (as measured on reaction time tasks) is very sensitive to cognitive weaknesses and represents a dimension that should be measured in a comprehensive battery.

NEW DIRECTIONS

There are many potential new directions which should be investigated and many overlap with areas of assessment already in existence. For example, using neuropsychological assessment data to make predictions about a person's ability to function adequately in prospective work settings overlaps with the areas of vocational evaluation and industrial-organizational psychology. Making probability statements about future school performance extends into the areas normally associated with school psychology. The question is this: By making the changes proposed in this chapter, will we merely be replicating the work of others, or can neuropsychology provide new information which can both supplement and complement what is already being done in these other specialty areas? Certainly there are indications that assessment of basic cognitive functions offers insight as to the individual's ability to acquire compensatory skills and to function adequately in other assessment settings. It also appears to provide important information about rehabilitation, vocational, and academic potential. While we currently can make predictions with a reasonable level of confidence about the more extreme scores, future research investigating the predictive accuracy of various cognitive tests can serve only to expand the range and accuracy of our prediction.

ASSESSMENT OF ECOLOGICAL FUNCTION

Investigation of the ecological function of neuropsychological testing appears to offer new and important directions to neuropsychology. Certainly, assessment of the individuals' ability to interact with their environment will not likely be accomplished by neuroradiological techniques. While the understanding of functional consequences of neurological damage remains a major contribution of neuropsychology, greater future contributions may well come from the relationship of cognitive function at time of assessment to expected future performance.

In conducting the needed ecological research, several points of focus appear necessary. First, it is essential to understand the relationship between various cognitive functions and the specific behavior in question. Second, it is important to investigate and clarify further the relationship between individual cognitive functions and specific test scores and patterns of test scores. Closely associated with this is a third requirement: establishing the relationship between test scores and the behaviors to be predicted.

A good beginning point for achieving the above goals would be to evaluate existing neuropsychological tests, both from the standpoint of the cognitive functions measured and their relationship to predicted behaviors. Once this foundation is obtained, research can then be extended to focus on developing new or more ecologically valid tests.

In addition to the above, it may also be advantageous to study the relationship between neuropsychological and vocational assessment devices. Neuropsychological tests provide information regarding cognitive functions and brain-behavior relationships. Vocational tests, in comparison, provide information regarding the individual's ability to perform Activities of Daily Living (ADL) skills and/or function on a specific job. Therefore, by correlating neuropsychological and vocational tests findings, the relationship between brain function and/or cognitive function and vocational performance can be better understood. While the correlations of existing tests may not be high, they will certainly provide an important foundation.

In keeping with this point, we investigated the relationship of the Halstead-Reitan Battery with the GATBY. This provided important information of the type outlined above. Unfortunately, the GATBY is no longer used, and more current data should be obtained from the Valpar or other vocational instruments.

SUMMARY

In the beginning, neuropsychology apparently focused on the differences between the daily behavior of brain-damaged patients and controls. This interest led to the development of behavioral measures to assess these weaknesses. These advances were widely received by neurologists and neurosurgeons, leading to clinical applications while neuropsychology was still in its infancy.

With the advent of neuroradiological procedures, the focus of neurological and neurosurgical referrals has shifted. Neuropsychologists are not usually consulted for strictly diagnostic questions. Rather, they tend to be contacted when there is a question as to how much change has been produced by the damage and what treatment procedures are required to maximize recovery. In addition, questions are often asked as to expected extent of and time for recovery and what future social and professional roles the individual will be able to adequately perform.

In attempting to move into this area of need, neuropsychologists again find themselves searching for answers. These answers relate to the ecological validity of the test findings. While research will continue to investigate brain-behavior relationships and further evolve a taxonomy of behavior, applications of these findings will undoubtedly be directed toward the use of behavioral measures to effectively plan and implement treatment. This will involve learning the relationship between existing tests and external performance measures. Newer, more ecologically valid, tests also need to be developed.

Neuropsychology will venture into areas closely aligned with other disciplines. With effective communication within these disciplines, it is hoped that more effective applications of behavioral measures are obtained.

REFERENCES

Beach, F. A., Hebb, D. O., Morgan, C. T., & Nissen, H. W. (1960). *The neuropsychology of Lashley.* New York: McGraw-Hill Book Company, Inc.

Halstead, W. C. (1947). *Brain and intelligence: A quantitative study of the frontal lobes.* Chicago: University of Chicago Press.

Henrichs, R. W. (1990). Current and emergent applications of neuropsychological assessment: Problems of validity and utility. *Professional Psychology: Research and Practice, 21*, 3, 171-176.

Reitan, R. M., & Wolfson, D. (1993). *Theoretical, methodological and validational bases of the Halstead-Reitan Neuropsychological Test Battery.* Tucson, Arizona: Reitan Neuropsychology Laboratory.

Ryan, T. V., Sautter, S. W., Capps, C. F., Meneese, & Barth, J. T. (1992). Utilizing neuropsychological measures to predict vocational outcome in a head trauma population. *Brain Injury, 6*, 2, 175-182.

Wedding, D., and Faust, D. (1989). Clinical judgment and decision making in neuropsychology. *Archives of Clinical Neuropsychology*, (4), 233-265.

Wilson, B. A. (1993). Ecological validity of neuropsychological assessment: Do neuropsychological indexes predict performance in everyday activities? *Applied & Preventive Psychology, 2*, 209-215.

2

ECOLOGICAL VALIDITY:
Some Critical Issues for the Neuropsychologist

Robert J. Sbordone, Ph.D., A.B.C.N., A.B.P.N., A.B.A.P.

INTRODUCTION

The increasing use of neuropsychological tests in the courtroom over the past several years has forced neuropsychologists to critically examine many of their widely held beliefs and assumptions stemming from the published professional and scientific literature (Matarazzo, 1990). For example, the relationship between scores or level of performance on neuropsychological tests and/or batteries and the patient's present and future functioning in real-world settings has frequently been challenged by attorneys in the courtroom. The neuropsychologist who attempts to infer the patient's present and future functioning in real-world settings solely on the basis of test data typically does so with little or no experimental support and usually relies on a number of experimentally unexamined and often faulty assumptions regarding which elements of cognition or behavior are essential for specific adaptive tasks in real-world settings (Bach, 1993). The neuropsychologist, in caparison, who tries to search for empirically demonstrated relationships between neuropsychological test scores and specific vocationally related behaviors, often finds that such empirical evidence is "embarrassing limited" (Brown, Baird, & Shatz, 1986).

As a result of the enormous pressure being placed on neuropsychologists within the medi-legal arena, the issues of reliability and validity, which are inherent within most of the frequently used neuropsychological tests, have been replaced by the issue of ecological validity. Thus, the neuropsychologist's claims of high test reliability and validity are overshadowed by the fact that many of these tests lack ecological validity in the sense that the particular scores derived from such tests may have little bearing on the patient's ability to function in his or her environment or society (Sbordone, 1988, 1991). The purpose of this chapter is to critically evaluate some of the issues facing neuropsychologists with respect to the topic of ecological validity. This chapter also examines several of the assumptions widely held by many neuropsychologists, and introduces a theoretical model to obtain an operational estimate of the ecological validity of neuropsychological test data, using a vector analysis approach.

DEFINITION OF ECOLOGICAL VALIDITY

Ecological validity can be defined as the functional and predictive relationship between the patient's performance on a set of neuropsychological tests and the patient's behavior in a variety of real-world settings (e.g., at home, work, school, community). This definition also assumes that demand characteristics within these various settings are idiosyncratic and fluctuate as a result of their specific nature, purpose, and goals. The interface between the demand characteristics of these settings and the patient's functional, cognitive strengths, goals and objectives, premorbid skills and abilities, and biological systems, may either compensate for the patient's cognitive and/or behavioral impairments, or exacerbate such impairments, resulting in secondary psychological disorders.

Implicit within this above definition is the notion that the neuropsychologist's choice of tests administered to the patient, assess cognitive and behavioral functions that are germane to the demand characteristics of the various real-world settings the patient currently functions within, or is considering returning to, or expects to be functioning within in the future. Since these various settings are idiosyncratic, it is essential that the neuropsychologist gather information about the demand characteristics of these various settings from the patient, the patient's family, friends, co-workers, and significant others, as well as vocational and occupational therapy specialists. Such information will provide the neuropsychologist with valuable insights about the various demands each of these particular settings make upon the patient's cognitive strengths, goals and objectives, premorbid skills and abilities, and biological systems (e.g., medical condition, health). Unfortunately, it has been the experience of this writer that such information is rarely obtained by neuropsychologists prior to the administration of neuropsychological tests (with the possible exception of Workers' Compensation cases where such information may be contained within the patient's medical records).

The predictive relationship between the patient's performance on a set of neuropsychological tests and the patient's behavior in real-world settings is clearly one which has often been ignored by neuropsychologists, particularly those who seem more interested in localizing brain damage. However, in the absence of a clear understanding of the demand characteristics of the various settings in which the patient functions, or is likely to function in the future, such predictions, based solely on the neuropsychological test data, are likely to be viewed as "sheer speculation" in the courtroom where such issues are of paramount importance. Finally, it should be recognized that all environments are not alike, and that the demands made within a particular setting may fluctuate considerably for a variety of different reasons, based on the setting's specific nature, purpose and goals. For example, in many work settings, the amount of work a particular job requires may fluctuate according to various economic conditions or certain times of the year (e.g., Christmas, tax season). The demand characteristics inherent in the patient's workplace may fluctuate considerably as a function of economic factors, absenteeism, sickness, organizational or administrative changes, competition from other companies, changes in equipment, marketing goals and/or strategies, etc. Furthermore, the issue of prediction is most likely to be more problematic when the neuropsychological tests show cognitive impairments of overall moderate severity, since patients who test as having deficits on both sides of the continuum of severity (e.g., minimal-slight and severe-profound) are likely to be either capable or incapable of functioning effectively in these settings.

Depending on the particular interface between the patient's functional cognitive strengths and the demand characteristics of the particular setting in which the patient finds him- or herself, the latter may serve to either compensate for the patient's cognitive and/or behavioral impairments, or exacerbate such impairments. This is likely to result in secondary psychological disorders (e.g., generalized anxiety reaction, adjustment reaction with depressed mood, or major depression). Should any of these problems occur, the cognitive functioning of the brain-injured patient is likely to diminish significantly, according to the principle of a conditional neurological lesion (Sbordone, 1987, 1988, 1991). This principle argues that the behavioral manifestations of a neurological insult, such as a brain injury, are a function of the degree to which the individual is under stress, fatigue, emotional distress, or excessive metabolic demands. This principle predicts that the cognitive and behavioral functioning of the brain-injured patient is likely to diminish when they become depressed, anxious, or exposed to stress. For example, a number of authors have reported that depression can exaggerate, or even introduce cognitive impairments on a variety of neuropsychological tests (e.g., Fisher, Sweet, & Pfalzer-Smith, 1986). For example (Sbordone, 1987) described a 51-year-old male who had sustained a closed head injury that resulted in three days of coma and post-traumatic amnesia for 12 days. When this patient was tested six months post injury, he obtained a full-scale WAIS IQ of 97. When re-tested one year post injury, his full scale IQ had dropped to 90. When Sbordone interviewed the patient's family, employer, and co-workers, it was discovered that the patient, who had been an attorney prior to his accident, returned to work shortly after he was initially examined. Unfortunately, the patient returned to the same job he held prior to his injury and was exposed to the same demands that had been placed on him prior to his brain injury. As a result of his brain injury, he was unable to cope with these demands and became significantly depressed. For example, his profile on the MMPI (Hathaway & McKinley, 1951) revealed considerably more depression and anxiety at one year post injury than when he was initially tested at six months post injury. Thus, it is essential that the neuropsychologist make every effort to understand the demand characteristics of the patient's environment.

SOME CRITICAL ISSUES FOR NEUROPSYCHOLOGISTS WITH RESPECT TO THE ISSUE OF ECOLOGICAL VALIDITY

1. The physical conditions and circumstances present during the time the neuropsychological test data is collected may significantly weaken any generalizations about the patient's behavior in real-world settings.

Neuropsychologists typically test brain-damaged patients in quiet environments, which are relatively free of extraneous stimulation. For example, Lezak recommended that the neuropsychological examination should be conducted in what she describes as a "sterile environment" in that the examining room should be relatively soundproof and decorated in quiet colors, with no bright or distracting objects in sight. She also pointed out that the examiner's clothing, too, can be an unwitting source of distraction (Lezak, 1976). She further recommends that the examining table be kept bare, except for materials needed for the test at hand, and that when one test is completed the material should be cleared away and placed out of the patient's sight before the next materials are brought in. She also stressed that clocks should be quiet and out of sight, even when the test instructions include references to timing. While these particular conditions are likely to optimize the patient's performance on neuropsychological tests, particularly tests which require a high level of attention and concentration, the issue is how can we generalize our neuropsychological test data under such conditions to the patient's home, workplace, or community, when such conditions may be quite noisy, contain numerous extraneous stimuli, and are highly dissimilar to the conditions under which testing occurred.

2. The type and scope of the neuropsychological tests administered under such conditions may be inappropriate, inadequate, and generate inaccurate or unrealistic expectations of the patient's behavior in real-world settings.

Sbordone (1991) noted that many psychologists assume that complex processes such as attention-concentration skills are adequately assessed by administering one or two tests to the brain-damaged patient. Such tests often include the Digit Span (Wechsler, 1981), Trail Making (Parts A and B) (Reitan, 1958), or Symbol Digit Modalities Test (Smith, 1968). "Normal" scores on these tests, however, may not rule out that a particular patient has attentional impairments, since these tests may only be sensitive to certain aspects of attention and concentration and relatively insensitive to others. For example, attention-concentration skills can be broken down into the following:

1. Alertness, which is defined as the general state of readiness of the individual to respond to the environment.
2. Stimulus selectivity, which is defined as the patient's ability to select specific stimuli from the environment.
3. The ability to maintain a particular attentional set.
4. Freedom from distraction: The ability to inhibit inappropriate shifting or loss of a mental set.
5. Vigilance: The ability to detect small changes in stimulus input.
6. Flexibility: The ability to initiate the shifting or discarding of mental sets.
7. Capacity: The amount of information which can be effectively processed by a particular individual at any one time.
8. Speed of processing: The speed at which attentional tasks can be processed.
9. Resistance to fatigue: The ability to prevent set deterioration.
10. Resistance to emotional factors: The ability to maintain a particular attentional set in the presence of emotional factors.
11. Resistance to interference from stimulus overload: The ability to preserve a particular attentional set under conditions of stimulus overload.
12. Resistance to contiguous stimuli: The ability to maintain a particular attentional set when presented with contiguous stimuli.

Thus, normal scores on these above tests, may result in the neuropsychologist concluding that the patient's attention and concentration skills are intact and recommend that the patient return to his or her job (e.g., as a commodities trader at the Chicago Stock Exchange). Thus, the combination of the neuropsychologist's "sterile" testing environment and the limited tests which are administered to the patient under such conditions, are likely to create an inaccurate or unrealistic expectation of how this particular patient is likely to function at work.

3. The interactions between the examiner and patient immediately prior to and during the administration of neuropsychological testing may actually mask the patient's cognitive and behavioral impairments.

It has been generally accepted that neuropsychologists frequently engage in what Lezak (1976) terms "necessary embellishments to the standard instructions" when testing brain-injured patients. In fact, Lezak has advocated giving the brain-damaged patient more flexibility and looseness when interpreting standard instructions or procedures to them. In fact, she has stressed that the examiner should attempt to obtain the patient's optimal level of performance during testing by modifying the testing procedures, instructions, and interaction with the patient, to insure that the patient's level of performance is at optimal levels. Unfortunately, while many neuropsychologists employ such modifications when evaluating brain-damaged patients, particularly patients who are severely impaired, relatively few of these psychologists carefully record the specific modifications of the testing protocol and/or their compensatory interventions during the testing process.

For example, a 28-year-old female, who sustained a severe traumatic brain injury approximately one year earlier as a result of a motor vehicle accident, was tested by Dr. X in a very small, soundproof room, which was devoid of any pictures and contained only a desk and two chairs. Dr. X, who spoke in a calm, soothing, and gentle manner, explained that he was going to give the patient a test which required her to concentrate. He then placed the Trail Making Test directly in front of her and carefully explained, in a slow manner, what the test tried to accomplish, and provide the patient with several examples of how to perform this particular test. However, the patient seemed puzzled, even after Dr. X's clear instructions. Dr. X then repeated the test instructions several times, in a gentle and patient manner, and had the patient practice the test several times. He also noticed that the patient seemed somewhat anxious just prior to administering the actual test. He then informed the patient, in a very gentle and calm manner, that he expected that she would have little or no difficulty on this test and that if the patient did well, he would permit her to take an early lunch. As the patient began the actual test, she became confused and connected the circles incorrectly. Upon discovering this, Dr. X stated, in a calm manner, "You should have gone to the circle containing the letter A, instead of the circle containing the number 2." He also repeated the test instructions and informed the patient that they were going to try the test again from the beginning, but before he began he wanted to make sure that she understood the test instructions. After spending approximately 10 minutes practicing and rehearsing for the test, Dr. X finally proceeded to administer the actual test to the patient. During testing, Dr. X provided the patient with gentle prompts, such as "What letter comes after E?," or "The last number you connected was 7." As a consequence, the patient was able to complete the test.

While her quantitative test score placed her within the mildly impaired range with respect to normative data for persons of her age, sex, and educational background, Dr. X made no mention, in his report, of the amount of practice, number of rehearsals, cues or prompts he administered to this patient prior and during testing, nor of any of the modifications he made in the test protocol. Unfortunately, Dr. X's modifications and interventions most likely compensated for the patient's problems of attention and concentration, recent memory, task orientation, initiation, and motivation and problem-solving skills. The real question is what would this patient's performance have been like if a different neuropsychologist (Dr. Y) had administered the same test without any of the above modifications or "prompts"?

Since such modifications occur more frequently when brain-injured patients are tested, neuropsychologists should recognize this issue, which can be termed "conditionality" and be defined as specific modifications of the testing protocol and/or compensatory interventions employed by the examiner and/or patient during testing which are effective in permitting the patient to ignore the distracting effects of extraneous stimuli, attend to the examiner, comprehend and recall the test instructions, perform according to the test requirements, minimize the influence of negative emotional or psychological states or attitudes, maintain an optimal level of motivation, compensate for the patient's problems of initiation and organization, and insure that the patient performs at an optimal level.

Examples of conditionality include:

1. Quiet environment.
2. Few, if any, distracting stimuli.
3. One-on-one communication between the patient and examiner.
4. Modification and/or simplification of the test instructions.

5. Repetition and clarification of task instructions.
6. Practice and rehearsal.
7. Cues and prompts.
8. Cognitive strategies suggested by the examiner.
9. Cognitive and/or compensatory strategies utilized by the patient.
10. Praise or encouragement.
11. Redirection by examiner.
12. Error recognition by examiner.
13. Reminders.
14. Rest breaks.
15. Breaking up testing over several sessions.
16. Use of psychotherapeutic devices or techniques.
17. Use of external incentives or rewards.

Recognizing conditionality permits the neuropsychologist to identify the various compensatory interventions furnished by the examiner (while serving in the functional capacity of an "ancillary cortex") that may mask many of the patient's cognitive and behavioral impairments. Conditionality was recognized by Plato (1952), in his Dialogues, when he discussed how Socrates convinced Meno that all knowledge was innate by demonstrating that an illiterate slave knew the principles of geometry. Socrates demonstrated this by stating, "Attend now to the questions which I ask him and observe whether he learns of me or only remembers," to which Meno replied, "I will." Socrates then asked the slave boy, "Tell me, boy, do you know that a figure like this is a square?," to which the slave boy replied, "I do." Socrates then asked, "And you know that a square figure has these four lines equal?," to which the slave boy replied, "Certainly." Socrates then asked, "And these lines which I have drawn through the middle of the square are also equal?," to which the slave boy stated, "Yes." Socrates then went on to ask, "A square may be of any size?," and then proceeded to convince Meno (by his leading questions) that this slave boy innately knew the principles of geometry. Unfortunately, in a neuropsychological setting the failure to recognize conditionality can result in inaccurate or unrealistic expectations and predictions of the patient's behavior in real-world settings.

4. The nature and extent of the protocols used during neuropsychological testing may not permit the patient to exhibit the pathognomic behavior expected for a particular brain insult.

Since the brain-injured patient is typically tested in a quiet, highly structured setting, many of the brain-injured patient's cognitive and behavioral impairments may not be manifested under such conditions. This is particularly true in the case of patients with frontal lobe pathology involving the orbital frontal lobes. For example, the gentle and calm manner of the examiner, combined with deliberate efforts to avoid getting the patient fatigued or upset, often results in the patient failing to display poor frustration tolerance, irritability, aggressive outbursts, and poor regulation of their behavior and emotions. Thus, the neuropsychologist and/or examiner will often report that the patient's test performance on a standardized neuropsychological test battery either fell into the normal range, or was only slightly impaired. The neuropsychologist, based on these test findings, combined with his or her failure to interview significant others (e.g., the patient's family, spouse, significant other), will often be unaware that the patient's major problem is an inability to regulate his or her emotions and behavior, which is more likely to be seen in a relatively unstructured home environment, or within the community. Thus, the neuropsychologist may recommend that the patient return to work, not realizing, of course, that it is typical for such patients to return to work and be fired within a relatively short time because of their explosive tempers, impulsivity, and poor frustration tolerance. The neuropsychologist, of course, may also fail to recognize that his or her recommendation (that the patient return to work) is likely to result in a highly stressful and traumatic (failure) experience for the patient, and their family, which may exacerbate the patient's cognitive and behavioral difficulties according to the principle of a conditional neurological lesion.

5. The patient's performance during neuropsychological testing may be adversely affected by a variety of factors (e.g., medications, peripheral neuropathies, pain, anxiety, sensory impairments, orthopedic problems, emotional issues) and result in an inaccurate and misleading assessment of the patient's cognitive and behavioral functioning.

A variety of factors can adversely effect a patient's performance on a neuropsychological test or battery. These factors may include the failure of the patient to understand the test instructions, sensory difficulties, peripheral neurological difficulties, poor motivation, fatigue, anxiety, depression, psychotic behavior, medications (e.g., anticonvulsant, antipsychotic or antidepressant medications), medical diseases (e.g., hypothyroidism), litigation, alcoholism, substance abuse, antagonism toward the examiner, time of day (e.g., testing at 9:00 a.m., whereas the patient typically does not awaken until 1:00 or 2:00 P.M. low blood sugar level, previous assessment history (e.g., the patient may have taken this particular test several times previously), pain, patient age (e.g., elderly patients may not appreciate the tests which are administered to them and thus may not take them seriously), ethnic background of patient, cultural background of patient (e.g., some cultures feel that it is more important to please the examiner than to do well on a particular test), premorbid IQ, pre-existing history of learning difficulties, concentration difficulties secondary to non-neurological factors (e.g., pain, high levels of anxiety, paranoia, depression), the background and experience of the examiner, and recent emotional stressors (e.g., recent divorce, loss of significant relationship, getting fired from work, argument with spouse the morning of the examination).

The neuropsychologist's failure to critically address the potential impact of one or more of these above factors is likely to result in an inaccurate and misleading assessment of the patient's cognitive and behavioral functioning. For example, this writer vividly recalls reviewing a neuropsychological report which concluded that a 56-year-old female patient displayed evidence of severe cognitive impairments as a result of a motor vehicle accident which occurred several years earlier (even though the patient had sustained only a slight concussion). When this patient was later interviewed by this writer, she indicated that she had had a chronic history of hypothyroidism and had not been consistent in taking her medications. She also reported that she had fallen three weeks prior to her previous neuropsychological examination and had sustained a rather severe low back injury, which made it extremely difficult for her to sleep at night. As a consequence, she had been taking large amounts of pain medications, as well as a variety of other medications which were well known to produce deleterious cognitive effects. She also indicated that she had forgotten to wear reading glasses when she was previously tested, and that on the date of previous testing her 65-year-old husband was undergoing open heart surgery. As a consequence, she found it particularly difficult to concentrate on that day. Unfortunately, the neuropsychologist did not take an adequate history and was unaware of these factors and stressors. He appeared to base his conclusions and opinions entirely on her level of test performance. As a consequence, his conclusions resulted in an inaccurate and misleading assessment of her cognitive and behavioral functioning stemming from her head injury. Furthermore, he informed her that she was not capable of working and that her condition would most likely not improve. As a consequence, the patient confessed to this writer that she felt very depressed and entertained serious thoughts of committing suicide.

6. Over-reliance on neuropsychological test data, combined with strict adherence to a number of faulty assumptions about the practice of neuropsychology,

can lead to distorted perceptions and inaccurate expectations of the patient's behavior in real-world settings.

This writer has put together a list of 25 widely held assumptions in the field of Clinical Neuropsychology. These assumptions are as follows:

1. It is not necessary to take a detailed clinical history, since such information may bias test interpretation.
2. It is not necessary to interview collateral sources, since such information may bias test interpretation.
3. Defective performances on neuropsychological tests are indicative of cognitive dysfunction and/or brain damage.
4. Defective performances on certain neuropsychological tests are indicative of dysfunction or damage to specific areas of the brain.
5. It is not essential that the neuropsychologist actually test or interview a particular patient if the neuropsychologist has access to the patient's raw test data.
6. Collecting reliable test data is the primary goal of the neuropsychologist and/or psychological assistant.
7. Careful interpretation of test data using appropriate norms is essential in arriving at accurate opinions about the patient's cognitive impairments and/or the localization of brain dysfunction.
8. It is essential that standardized tests and/or batteries are utilized to arrive at meaningful conclusions about the presence or absence of cognitive dysfunction and/or brain damage.
9. Changes in cognitive functioning are best determined by careful examination of the serial neuropsychological test data.
10. It is unwise to continue testing a brain-injured patient if they become fatigued, since the test data will become unreliable.
11. It is essential to test brain-damaged patients in relatively quiet settings that are free from distraction or extraneous stimuli.
12. The neuropsychologist's primary responsibility is to record the patient's specific responses to specific test stimuli during testing.
13. It is not essential to record the amount and type of practice, cues, prompts, or various strategies given to or utilized by the patient during testing, since the raw test data is sufficient to determine the patient's cognitive impairments.
14. Test data can accurately be interpreted in the absence of information from other sources (e.g., historical information, medical records)

15. Interpretations, based on test data alone, can predict the patient's ability to function in the workplace, school, at home, or in real-world settings.

16. Patients who sustain traumatic brain damage will make most of their recovery during the first six months and continue to recover for up to two years post injury.

17. It is not essential to observe the patient function outside of the testing (laboratory) environment, since careful interpretation of the test data will provide us with a sufficient basis to predict how the patient is likely to respond in real-world settings (e.g., work, community, school).

18. Intact performance on a standardized neuropsychological test battery (e.g., WAIS-R, HRNB, LNNB) rules out the likelihood that the patient has cognitive deficits or sustained a brain insult.

19. It is not essential for the neuropsychologist to review the patient's medical chart if the neuropsychologist is trying to determine whether the patient has sustained a brain injury, since this can be determined by a careful review of the test data.

20. It is not necessary to review the patient's educational, vocational, or medical records if the neuropsychological test data shows strong indications of brain damage.

21. Neuropsychological test reports need only contain a brief description of the reason for referral, identifying information about the patient, the names of the tests administered, the raw test data, and an interpretation of the test data.

22. Neuropsychological tests are sensitive to brain damage and can reliably be used to identify such damage if it is present.

23. Rather than wasting valuable time taking a history from the patient, the neuropsychologist can simply rely on the patient's medical records to arrive at an understanding of the types of injuries the patient has sustained.

24. Intact performances on a variety of neuropsychological tests (e.g., Category, Wisconsin Card Sorting, and Trail Making), known to be sensitive to frontal lobe damage, rules out frontal lobe pathology.

25. The results of neuropsychological testing should be consistent with the patient's complaints.

Unfortunately, each of these widely held assumptions is faulty. For example, while Reitan and his associates (Reitan & Wolfson, 1993), had previously emphasized that obtaining a detailed clinical history prior to interpreting the raw test data would bias test interpretation. Reitan recently stressed that it is extremely important to take a detailed clinical history when the patient is seen for clinical purposes (see Siegal, Chapter 3). Reitan stressed that his prior admonitions about not taking a detailed clinical history only applied to research studies in which the Halstead-Reitan Neuropsychological Test Battery was being evaluated in terms of its ability to discriminate between brain-damaged and non-brain-damaged controls. He stated at that time that he felt that the inclusion of such information would most likely have biased his scientific objectivity and conclusions and as a consequence recommended a policy of "blind interpretations" in an attempt to make the field of Clinical Neuropsychology a rigorous scientific discipline.

It is extremely important to interview collateral sources, since many patients who sustain traumatic brain injuries are unreliable historians. Thus, it is essential that the patient be accompanied by a family member or significant other during neuropsychological assessment, who can rectify the patient's faulty recollections of past events, furnish details of the patient's childhood, such as birth weight, childhood illnesses, or prior history of neurological disorders (e.g., history of hyperactivity). Significant traumatic events, which the patient may deny or repress, may be reported by another informant. The informant may also clarify specific information furnished by the patient, such as why the patient repeated the second grade or was taken to a psychiatrist during his or her childhood. Obtaining careful background information will frequently uncover a history of pre-existing neurological disease, psychological problems, a history of prior head trauma, drowning episodes, seizures, hyperactivity, dyslexia, left-handedness, stuttering, history of sexual molestation and rape, alcoholism, criminal behavior, poor academic performance, or drug abuse. This information should assist the neuropsychologist in interpreting the results of the neuropsychological test data, particularly with respect to determining whether the test data reflect a pre-existing insult or problem and/or recent injury.

Sbordone (1991) provides an example of the importance of obtaining a highly detailed clinical and background history from the patient with the assistance of collateral sources. He reported a case involving a 52-year-old electrician, who had reportedly fallen 20 feet from a telephone pole while installing new equipment, and fractured both legs. He was seen by a neuropsychologist, whose neuropsychological test data demonstrated strong evidence of diffuse brain damage, which was attributed to the fall. When the patient was later examined by another neuropsychologist, who obtained a careful clinical and background history, it was learned that this patient had been struck by an automobile when he was 10 years old, and was rendered comatose for one week. When the patient was 17, he had become a professional boxer and had fought in 25 bouts and had been knocked out 10 times. Six months prior to the patient's accident, he noticed that he had been dropping objects and had been experiencing balance and coordination difficulties. He described them as "drop attacks". He was then seen by a neurologist, who diagnosed his condition as vertebrobasilar artery insufficiency syndrome. The patient was prescribed a vasodilator, to alleviate this condition, which he did not take because it interfered with his consumption of 12 to 18 beers a day (a habit he admitted he had had for the past 30 years). He also admitted that he had consumed 12 beers at lunch prior to his fall, and that approximately three days after he was hospitalized, he began seeing "little green men under his bed" (which was diagnosed as delirium tremens).

Defective performances on neuropsychological tests can be due to a variety of different factors, including brain damage. However, it is essential that the neuropsychologist rule out the contaminating effect of these factors by obtaining a careful and complete history, reviewing the patient's medical records, and interview the patient's significant others. In medi-legal cases, poor performances can be a result of hysteria, a major depressive disorder, psychosis, malingering, or a variety of different etiologies. Poor performances on neuropsychological tests should be consistent with the patient's medical records, the number of complaints the patient is spontaneously able to provide (e.g., patients with severe traumatic brain injuries rarely provide more than one or two complaints), with results of various neurodiagnostic tests (e.g., CT, MRI, topographical brain mapping, PET or SPECT scans). They should also be consistent with the behavioral observations of the patient and the observations of significant others.

The question the neuropsychologist should be asking is whether or not this patient behaves like he or she is brain-damaged. In other words, does the patient exhibit behaviors inside and outside of the examiner's office that are generally consistent with brain-injured patients? For example, a patient who had been referred for neuropsychological testing by the patient's treating physician was taken to a neuropsychologist by his wife. When the patient was asked whether he had any problems or difficulties, the patient stated, "No, I don't think so." The patient also appeared confused and bewildered and did not know the correct day of the week or month. The patient appeared to be a poor historian in that his memory for events which had occurred since his accident was very spotty and fragmented. The patient denied any recollection of the accident, which was supported by a review of his medical records which indicated that he was rendered comatose for 14 days. An interview with the patient's wife revealed that she had observed a dramatic change in her husband's behavior since his accident in that he had become absent-minded, irritable, appeared oblivious to what was going on around him at home, and displayed impulsive behavior and poor judgment whenever they went shopping. During neuropsychological testing, this patient appeared to perform poorly on tests which are particularly sensitive to frontal lobe pathology, but performed well on tests which are generally sensitive to posterior cerebral pathology. The examiner also observed that after the patient went to the bathroom, he was found wandering up and down the hallway and appeared confused and bewildered. His wife then explained to him that she had to leave to pick up their children from school. Later, when the patient was asked, "When did you last see your wife?," he indicated, "Yesterday." During neuropsychological testing, he exhibited severe recent memory impairment for recent events and confabulation. He also demonstrated impulsivity, distractibility, and perseveration during testing. Whenever he was informed that he had made an error during testing, he did not become upset and instead appeared indifferent. His affect was flat. He was also observed to speak in an almost robotic-like fashion.

Failing to interview a particular patient suspected of having sustained a traumatic brain injury is a grave error and unfortunately one that is too often made by neuropsychologists who are "test bound." In other words, while the patient's performance on neuropsychological testing may actually fall within the normal range, the patient may exhibit evidence of pathognomic behavior during the interview, particularly when he or she is asked broad open-ended questions. In such cases, the patient may exhibit tangential and/or circumstantial thinking and/or lose his or her train of thought, whereas the patient's performance in a more highly structured testing environment may be generally intact.

The importance of collecting reliable test data has been over-emphasized. Such an approach often ignores the conditionality of the testing environment, as well as a variety of previously discussed factors, which can seriously bias interpretation of the test data (even though it may be reliable in the sense that the patient can obtain similar test scores one week later). However, this faulty assumption may result in the neuropsychologist noticing a few trees, without realizing that he or she is actually lost in the forest.

The comparison group, to which the patient's scores are compared, may not be representative of the patient's background skills or abilities. For example, if a Hispanic patient, who has only completed three years of formal education and speaks little English, is given the Categories Test and achieves a score of 55 (which exceeds the norms which Reitan developed to categorize individuals as either brain-damaged or normal), then the psychologist must either find appropriate norms to fit this particular individual, or utilize conventional norms. While it is generally assumed that the means and standard deviations for normal controls are representative of that population, this assumption has been challenged by Fromm-Auch and Yeudall (1983), who found that the means and standard deviations for normal controls, based on a number of validation studies of the Halstead-Reitan Battery, showed a wide range of variability. Thus, one psychologist using one set of norms and analyzing test data could conclude that a particular patient's score on one of the Halstead-Reitan tests was impaired, while another, using a different set of norms, might conclude that there was no impairment in the patient's cognitive functioning, as determined by this particular test. Whatever norms the neuropsychologist utilizes, the neuropsychologist should be able to justify his or her choice for using a particular set of norms in terms of how well the particular patient "fits" the normative control group in terms of such attributes as: sex, age, occupation, educational achievements, intellectual functioning, cultural and linguistic background, etc. When a particular patient does not fit a particular normative group, then the use of "normative data" to judge whether a particular patient is impaired, is likely to result in spurious conclusions about the patient's cognitive impairments and/or the localization of brain dysfunction.

A more important question, which has often been avoided by neuropsychologists, is what a particular score on a neuropsychological test really tells us about the patient's functioning in real-world settings. Too often, it has been fallaciously assumed that the scores themselves can predict how the patient is likely to function in a variety of real-world settings (irrespective of the demand characteristics of such environments). For example, Acker (1986) reviewed most of the studies completed up to that time, which had examined the relationship between neuropsychological test scores following traumatic brain injury, and vocational or occupational achievement. While she reported that the number of such studies was small and raised some concerns about their methodology, such studies only revealed a modest correlation between some neuropsychological test scores and vocational outcome. As Bach (1993) states, "One would only reasonably expect a modest significant correlation between neuropsychological test scores and vocational outcome, given the wide variety of behavioral demands included across a broad range of jobs ... one reason for the modest correlations between neuropsychological test scores and daily functioning following traumatic brain injury is the broad variability of factors impinging on successful functioning for which no single factor or subset of variables can account in various jobs, living situations, and patients" (Page 137).

While it has been commonly assumed that standardized tests and/or batteries must be utilized in order to arrive at meaningful conclusions about the presence or absence of cognitive dysfunction and brain damage, it should be recognized that many notable individuals in the field, including Luria and Kaplan, were able to make highly accurate and meaningful statements about cognitive impairments and precisely localize brain damage, without relying on standardized tests and/or batteries. It should be recalled that Goldstein (1942) strongly argued that only quantitative evaluations were valid and that quantitative assessments only confused the issue, since while a brain-damaged patient and a normal subject might obtain the same quantitative score, they differed qualitatively in the manner in which they obtained such a score. Goldstein emphasized that it was imperative for the examiner to observe the brain-damaged patient's performance in order to determine whether the brain damage has imposed any limitations on the patient's cognitive functioning.

Luria (1966, 1969, 1990) felt that little, if anything, could be gained by relying on normative data to arrive at meaningful conclusions about the patient's brain-dysfunction. He felt that it was essential for the neuropsychologist to observe the particular qualitative aspects of the patient's performance in order to gain an understanding of brain-behavior relationships. Similarly, the work of the Boston Group, consisting primarily of Edith Kaplan, Harold Goodglass, and Nelson Butters, has emphasized that an understanding of the patient's brain behavioral relationships requires a careful understanding of the qualitative aspects of the patient's behavior, as well as the strategies the patient adopts during testing. They also pointed out that patients with superficially similar neuropsychological deficits may reflect different underlying pathological processes (Jones & Butters, 1983).

The majority of neuropsychologists have been reported to utilize what has been described as "flexible batteries" to evaluate patients who have been referred for neuropsychological assessment. For example, Sweet and Moberg (1990) examined the types of neuropsychological tests and batteries used by Diplomates of the American Board of Clinical Neuropsychology and non-board-certified neuropsychologists, and found that a flexible neuropsychological approach was utilized approximately four times as often as standardized neuropsychological batteries such as the Halstead-Reitan, or Luria-Nebraska. The use of such batteries is particularly suitable for elderly patients, minorities, or patients with many problems (e.g., visually impaired, deaf, unable to speak, motor paralysis) and for specific types of neurological disorders (e.g., dementia, stroke, hypoxic encephalopathy, traumatic brain injury), since it permits the neuro- psychologist to select the most appropriate and/or sensitive neuropsychological tests to evaluate the patient's cognitive and behavioral functioning (Sbordone, 1991).

It has often been fallaciously assumed by many neuropsychologists that intact performance on "tests of frontal lobe pathology," such as the Category, Wisconsin Card Sorting and Trail Making Tests, would rule out the likelihood that the patient had frontal lobe pathology. This writer has reviewed numerous neuropsychological reports which concluded that there was no evidence of frontal lobe pathology, based on the patient's intact performance on these tests. However, it should be recalled that Damasio (1979) noted that since the frontal lobes are not anatomically homogeneous structures, there is no such thing as a "single frontal lobe syndrome" identical across patients. Similarly, Stuss (1989) stated that the frontal lobes were likely to serve multiple discrete, but highly interconnected functions. In addition, Benson (1989) has stressed that frontal lobe pathology is rarely discrete or focal, particularly as a consequence of head trauma, since the variability of physical factors that occur during a traumatic brain injury are likely to result in widespread tissue destruction and thereby produce a variety of clinical syndromes. In fact, Damasio (1985) stated that the signs and symptoms of frontal lobe dysfunction do not lend themselves easily to quantitative measurement and that neuropsychological tests simply are not adequate to address these disturbances. He emphasized that frontal lobe dysfunction was more readily described as changes in quality, particularly subtle changes in alertness, affect, emotional response, and appropriate control of regulatory behaviors. He also reported a case where the CT scan showed clear evidence of bilateral damage of the frontal lobes (e.g., the orbital frontal surface and the frontal polar cortex of both hemispheres were almost entirely missing as a consequence of an extensive ablation necessary to remove the patient's tumor). However, he noted that the patient's neuropsychological test performances were almost "completely normal".

Similarly, Luria (1990), while examining the problem-solving difficulties in patients with lesions of the frontal lobes, noted that while many of these patients did fairly well on many neuropsychological tests, they approached problem-solving tasks quite differently, in that they were generally unable to draw up the solution plan necessary to solve the problem when the problem required preliminary analysis of the problem statement. It should be recalled that earlier, Zangwill (1966) pointed out that patients with frontal lobe injuries may still perform at average levels of intelligence and that intelligence tests were unlikely to address the type of cognitive abilities which have been compromised by patients with frontal lobe damage. Finally, Cummings (1985) noted that patients who sustained primarily orbital frontal lobe damage frequently did not exhibit any deficits on neuropsychological tests, but were significantly impaired with respect to their ability to regulate their emotions and behavior in relatively unstructured settings (e.g., at home, community).

Many neuropsychologists have erroneously assumed that the results of the patient's performance on neuropsychological tests should correlate highly with the patient's complaints. Unfortunately, in the case of traumatic brain injuries, Sbordone (1991) has reported an inverse correlation between the patient's spontaneously generated complaints and the severity of their traumatic brain injury. He found, however, a high correlation between the discrepancy between the patient's complaints in comparison to the complaints of significant others (about the patient's behavior) and the severity of the patient's brain injury. For example, patients who sustained severe traumatic brain injuries would often deny or minimize their cognitive or behavioral problems. On the other hand, their spouse or family members would report as many as 30-35 problems. With respect to the issue of malingering, Sbordone (1991) has found a high correlation between the number of complaints given by malingerers and poor performance during neuropsychological testing. In the majority of cases, it should also be noted that malingerers tend to have more complaints of cognitive dysfunction than their spouses or any collateral source.

It has been widely assumed by both neuropsychologists and a variety of different medical specialists (e.g., neurosurgeons, neurologists, psychiatrists) that most of the recovery following head trauma occurs within the first six months and that virtually all of their recovery occurs within the first year or two post injury. This assumption appears to be primarily based on the studies of Bond (1975) and Bond and Brooks (1976), who assessed the recovery of patients with severe head injuries. Bond grouped his patients according to their duration of post-traumatic amnesia and time since injury. He then compared the WAIS IQ scores of these groups (since he did not actually perform serial testing). He found that these patient groups had approximately the same IQ scores when he compared the duration of time since injury. Therefore, he argued that the most rapid recovery occurred within the first six months, followed by a slow rate of improvement which continued steadily and reached a maximum of 24 months post injury. However, it should be noted that Bond did not perform any serial testing, nor did he study any patients who were more than two years post injury. In addition, he did not compare the patients' scores to their premorbid level of intellectual functioning, nor did he utilize any suitable control groups and ignored the possible influence in IQ of such factors as age, sex, education, employment status, medications, physical disabilities, or emotional factors (Sbordone, 1987). In a second study (Bond & Brooks, 1976), 40 of the patients from the previous study were serially administered the WAIS at intervals of approximately three months, after grouping these patients according to their duration of post-traumatic amnesia. They reported that most of the improvement in the WAIS IQ scores occurred during the first six months, and noticed little change from six months to two years. However, their study can be questioned for the same reasons the first study was questioned. More importantly, they failed to consider the influence of confounding emotional factors that typically evolve over the course of recovery from brain injury, such as the effects of depression and anxiety, which generally begin between six and 12 months post injury. Such patients (Sbordone, 1987) typically develop emotional problems during this stage of recovery which inhibit their cognitive functioning. Thus, the results of the Bond and Brooks (1976) study are confounded by their failure to recognize the disruptive effects of secondary emotional factors during the course of the patient's recovery. Unfortunately, these investigators made no effort to evaluate the patient's emotional functioning, either clinically or psychometrically, during the course of their study.

Sbordone, Liter, and Pettler-Jennings (1995) carefully examined a group of 20 patients who had sustained severe traumatic brain injuries (based on their period of post-traumatic amnesia and duration of coma) approximately 20 years earlier. Rather than utilizing psychological tests, these investigators utilized a modified version of the Portland Adaptability Scale and interviewed each of these patients' significant others to evaluate the patients' functioning at one year, two years, five years, and an average of 10.3 years post injury. The investigators found that these patients made significant improvements in their cognitive functioning between two and five years post injury and also between five and 10 years post injury. Their findings were consistent with previous studies. For example, Klonoff, Low, and Clark (1977) reported that 76.3% of head-injured children and adolescents made a marked recovery during a five-year post injury follow-up period. These investigators also reported significant improvement between years four and five post injury. Miller and Stern (1965) followed 100 consecutive cases of severe head injury, whose mean duration of post-traumatic amnesia was 13 days. Ninety-two survivors were re-examined at an average of 11 years post injury. Only 10 of the 92 survivors showed evidence of persistent dementia, and only five of the 92 were unemployed. Despite the severity of their initial injury, half of these patients had returned to their previous occupations. They also reported that 73.7% had returned back to work, even though their physicians who evaluated them on an average of three years post injury had expressed serious doubts that these patients would ever be able to work again. Similarly, Thomsen (1981) reported a case involving a 44-year-old male who sustained a profound head trauma, which resulted in a severe global aphasia. She noted that at eight months post injury, the patient exhibited signs of marked frontal lobe dysfunction and disinhibition, severe rigidity, and perseveratory behavior. At two years post injury, the patient continued to exhibit signs of marked cognitive impairment. However, when the patient was seen again at 14 years post injury, he was found to have only mild residual cognitive impairment.

7. Such assumptions can create a state of cognitive dissonance about the purpose and goals of neuropsychological testing and result in a tendency for neuropsychologists to ignore the issue of ecological validity in their practice.

For many neuropsychologists, the cognitive dissonance between these widely held assumptions and the issue of ecological validity is likely to create an unpleasant state of tension, which may cause the neuropsychologist to consciously or unconsciously avoid the issue of ecological validity within his or her practice. This appears to be corroborated by the relatively small number of studies conducted by neuropsychologists on the issue of ecological validity.

8. The lack of accurate and timely feedback about the patient's behavior in real-world settings is likely to reinforce the neuropsychologist's faulty assumptions and strict reliance on the test data, as well as the continued use of tests and/or batteries which are either ineffective or inappropriate.

The relative dearth of studies attempting to correlate the patient's behavior on neuropsychological tests and the patient's behavior in real-world settings caused Hart and Hayden (1986) to conclude, after summarizing the research in this area, that "Our systems for classifying and describing (i.e., measuring) the behaviors related to brain injury do have predictive power for localizing an injury, but apparently less for understanding its effects on adaptive functioning." Unfortunately, many neuropsychologists who have been called into the courtroom, or who have been referred Workers' Compensation cases, have been forced to deal head-on with this issue, as well as the rather harsh criticisms of neuropsychologists put forth by Ziskin and Faust (1988). Under such rigorous assault in the courtroom, in which the neuropsychologist is usually a relative neophyte, combined with little or no formal training in forensic neuropsychology, the neuropsychologist's testimony frequently results in scorn and ridicule, as well as embarrassment. Under such circumstances, many neuropsychologists will usually rely on their faulty neuropsychological assumptions and place strict reliance in their test data, since it is the "only rock they can hide behind" in the courtroom. Unfortunately, the tryers of fact (i.e., the judge or jury) are often unimpressed and rule in favor of the opposing party. Such humiliating experiences may cause the neuropsychologist to make one of three choices: (1) to avoid any further involvement in medi-legal cases, (2) to seek out more appropriative norms and/or use more widely accepted standardized tests, (3) or face the issue of ecological validity by critically examining the widely held assumptions about neuropsychological testing and modifying their method of neuropsychological assessment so that it can better predict the relationship between the patient's performance on a set of neuropsychological tests and their behavior in a variety of real-world settings. With respect to this last alternative, the writer proposes the following model to derive an operational estimate of the ecological validity of the neuropsychological test data.

AN OPERATIONAL ESTIMATE OF THE ECOLOGICAL VALIDITY OF NEUROPSYCHOLOGICAL TEST DATA

With respect to ecological validity, the issue is not whether quantitative or qualitative neuropsychological approaches should be utilized, or whether one particular approach is more important or valid to our understanding of brain-behavior relationships. It is the degree to which the data obtained from either of both approaches is consistent with data from other sources (e.g., clinical history, patient's complaints, observations of significant others, the patient's academic, vocational, and medical records, neurodiagnostic tests [e.g., CT, MRI, EEG, PET, SPECT] and behavioral observations), since the degree of consistency among these data and the neuropsychological test data can provide us with an operational estimate of the ecological validity of such data. Thus, the neuropsychological test data, which is generally inconsistent with data from other sources, would most likely have little ecological validity, while neuropsychological data which is highly consistent with other data, would most likely have high ecological validity.

This writer also proposes the use of a vector analysis approach to determine the ecological validity of the test data. With this approach, each data source can be represented by a vector. Thus, when all of the various data sources are reviewed, the vector represented by the neuropsychological test data should be consistent with the vectors from the other data sources.

Table 1 presents a series of vectors resulting from the various data sources, with respect to the issue of whether the patient has sustained brain damage (an issue which is of paramount importance within the medi-legal arena or courtroom setting). For the neuropsychologist to conclude that his or her neuropsychological test data has a high degree of ecological validity, the vector generated by the neuropsychological test data should be generally consistent with the vectors from other data sources. For purposes of illustration, two case examples are used to demonstrate the difference between neuropsychological test data which has high vs. low ecological validity.

TABLE 1
VECTOR ANALYSIS APPROACH TO EVALUATE THE ECOLOGICAL VALIDITY OF
NEUROPSYCHOLOGICAL TEST DATA

History of Injury >>>>>>>>>>>>>>
Complaints of Patient >>>>>>>>>>
Complaints of Family
   and Significant Others >>>>>>>>>
Academic/Vocational Records >>>>   Brain Damage?
Medical Records >>>>>>>>>>>>>>
Neurodiagnostic Tests >>>>>>>>>>
Behavioral Observations >>>>>>>>
Neuropsychological Testing >>>>>>

HIGH ECOLOGICAL VALIDITY

The patient, a 36-year-old, right-handed Caucasian male, was referred for neuropsychological testing by his attorney. The patient was involved in a motor vehicle accident approximately one year earlier, in which he was rendered comatose for two days. Initial CT and MRI scans revealed evidence of bilateral frontal lobe contusions. The patient was hospitalized for 10 days and was referred to an inpatient cognitive rehabilitation program for three months. The patient attempted to return to work as a service manager at an automobile dealership. Unfortunately, the patient was fired within a month of returning to work for shouting obscenities at the customers, showing poor judgment, and displaying poor work habits and inappropriate behavior. While he was able to find work at another dealership in a similar capacity approximately two months later, he only lasted two weeks before he was fired for physically assaulting one of the customers and shouting obscenities at several others. When the patient was seen for neuropsychological assessment, he denied any cognitive, behavioral, or emotional difficulties. Comparatively, his wife (in a separate interview), described a dramatic change in her husband's behavior and personality since his accident. She indicated that while he had been a very calm and patient individual prior to his accident, he had now become egocentric, impatient, irritable, argumentative, and prone to sudden outbursts of violence. She also observed that he had virtually lost all of his friends, used coarse and crude language in front of their children, and often refused to bathe or comb his hair. During a lengthy interview with the patient, the neuropsychologist observed evidence of tangential and circumstantial thinking, perseverations, impulsivity, emotional liability, use of inappropriate language (verbal dysdecorum), and a flat affect.

Neuropsychological testing included a flexible neuropsychological battery, combined with careful notes and observations of the patient's behavior prior to, during, and following testing. These latter observations revealed that the patient required a great deal of structure and organization (e.g., conditionality) before he was able to even begin taking the neuropsychological tests which he was administered. In addition, the patient had to be frequently redirected back to the test, as he tended to be easily distracted. He also required frequent cues and prompts, since he tended to lose his train of thought or attentional set easily. The patient's scores placed him within the markedly impaired range, based on appropriate norms, based on the patient's sex, age, and educational background. The neuropsychologist also utilized a qualitative process approach while examining the patient, which revealed severe impairment with respect to this patient's ability to plan, organize, initiate, and regulate his behavior. The neuropsychologist also interviewed, via telephone, the patient's two prior employers, who corroborated the patient's problems with executive functions within the workplace. The neuropsychologist also interviewed many of the patient's family members and close friends, who corroborated that the patient's behavior had changed dramatically, in that he was no longer the same calm and patient individual he once was, and that his behavior was now impulsive, irrational, argumentative, and often unpredictable. The neuropsychologist carefully reviewed the patient's prior academic, vocational, and medical records, and concluded that there had been no evidence of such problems in this patient's past. He therefore concluded that his neuropsychological test findings were consistent with the patient's functioning in a variety of real-world settings, based on the observations of the patient's spouse, family members, friends, employers, and co-workers. He also stated that his neuropsychological observations and test findings were consistent with the information obtained from the patient's medical records, neurodiagnostic tests, vocational records, the patient's complaints, the observations of significant others, and the patient's functioning at home, work, and in the community.

LOW ECOLOGICAL VALIDITY

A 45-year-old construction worker was referred for neuropsychological testing by his attorney after the patient had complained of severe headaches, memory difficulties, and an inability to work, after he had slipped and fallen on an apparently wet floor while shopping in a supermarket. The patient arrived for his scheduled appointment approximately 30 minutes late, stating that there had been a major accident on the freeway, involving several cars, which kept traffic backed up for 30 minutes. He appeared well-groomed and spoke clearly in an articulate manner. His thinking was observed to be logical and goal-oriented. Even though he complained of having severe problems with his recent memory, he was able to provide the examiner with several examples of these difficulties. He was also able to provide the examiner with a very careful and detailed history of his fall, including his recollection of his head striking the ground. He indicated that he had been rendered unconscious for approximately 10 minutes as a result of his fall (this was not supported by any of his medical records, which noted him to be alert and oriented in all spheres when he was seen within a few minutes of his fall). During the interview, the patient spontaneously provided a total of 24 complaints, the most serious of which he claimed was his "severe memory loss." The patient was given a variety of standardized neuropsychological tests by the examiner's psychological assistant, who reported that the patient tested in the severely impaired range on nearly all of the tests he was administered. The neuro- psychologist, based on these test findings, concluded that the patient had sustained a severe traumatic brain injury as a result of his slip and fall accident approximately two and a half years ago. He also concluded that the patient had been rendered permanently disabled as a result of this accident, based on his severe memory and cognitive difficulties, and was incapable of competitive employment.

Unfortunately, the neuropsychologist did not bother to review the patient's academic, medical, or vocational records prior to rendering his opinion regarding the patient's cognitive functioning and/or brain injury. Had the neuropsychologist done this, he would have realized that the patient had dropped out of school during the 10th grade and a had a pre-existing history of learning difficulties and hyperactivity. These records also indicated that the patient had been involved in three prior personal injury cases for similar injuries, for which he had collected a total of over $500,000 over a 10-year period. These records also noted that the patient had been arrested on five separate occasions in the past for assault and battery, burglary, breaking and entering, embezzlement, and extortion, for which he had served a total of 14 years in prison. These records also indicated that the patient was a heavy drinker and had been arrested twice for driving under the influence. He was also believed to have had drug problems in the past, and had been referred by the courts to a drug diversion program in his early 20s. While the neuropsychologist had not conducted interviews with the patient's co-workers, the attorney for the defendant had deposed three of the patient's co-workers, who described him as a "pathological liar" and as "highly manipulative." They also denied that they had observed any changes in the patient's behavior after he returned to work the day following his slip and fall accident. They described him as the "same old guy, who was always trying to outfox the other guy." Thus, the neuropsychological test data in this particular case can be seen as having low ecological validity.

REFERENCES

Acker, M. B. (1986) Relationships between test scores and everyday life functioning. In B. P. Uzell & Y. Gross (Eds.), *Clinical neuropsychology of intervention* (pp. 85-117). Boston: Martinus Nijhoff.

Bach, P. J. (1993). Demonstrating relationships between natural history, assessment results, and functional loss in civil proceedings. In H. V. Hall & R. J. Sbordone (Eds.), *Disorders of executive functions: Civil and criminal law applications* (pp. 135-159). Delray Beach, FL: St. Lucie Press.

Benson, D. F. (1989). Frontal influence on higher behavioral function. Paper presented at The brain/behavior relationships: An integrated approach" Conference, Rancho Mirage, California.

Bond, M. R. (1975) Assessment of the psychosocial outcome after severe head injury. In CIBA Foundation Symposium 34, *Outcome of severe damage to the central nervous system* (pp. 141-157). Amsterdam: Elsevier/Excerpta Medica.

Bond, M. R., & Brooks, D.N. (1976). Understanding the process of recovery as a basis for the investigation of rehabilitation for the brain-injured. *Scandinavian Journal of Rehabilitation Medicine, 8,* 127-133.

Brown, G. G., Baird, A. P., & Shatz, M. W. (1986). The effects of cerebrovascular disease and its treatment on higher cortical functioning. In I. Grand & K. M. Adams (Eds.). *Neurological assessment of neuropsychiatric disorders* (pp. 384-414). New York: Oxford.

Cummings, J. L. (1985). Clinical neuropsychiatry. New York: Grune and Stratton.

Damasio, A. R. (1993). The frontal lobes. In K. M. Heilman & E. Valenstein (Eds.), *Clinical neuropsychology*, (3rd ed.) pp. 409-460. New York: Oxford Press.

Fisher, D. G., Sweet, J. J., & Pfaelzer-Smith, E.A. (1986). Influence of depression on repeated neuropsychological testing. *The International Journal of Clinical Neuropsychology, 8,* 14-18.

Fromm-Auch, D., & Yeudall, L. T. (1983). Normative data for the Halstead-Reitan Neuropsychological Tests. *Journal of Clinical Neuropsychology, Vol. 5,* (3), *221-238.*

Goldstein, H. (1942). *After effects of brain injuries in man.* New York: Grune and Stratton.

Hart, T., & Hayden, M. D. (1986). The ecological validity of neuropsychological assessment and remediation. In B. P. Uzzell & Y. Gross (Eds.*), Clinical neuropsychology of intervention* (pp. 21-50). Boston: Martinus Nijhoff.

Hathaway, S. R., & McKinnley, J.C. (1951*). The Minnesota Multiphasic Personality Inventory Manual* (rev.). New York: The Psychological Corporation.

Jones, B. P., & Butters, N. (1983). Neuropsychological psychological assessment. In M. Hersen, A. E. Kazdin, & A. S. Bellack (Eds.), *The clinical psychology handbook* (pp. 377-396). New York: Pergamon Press.

Klonoff, H., Low, M. D., & Clark, C. (1977). Head injuries in children: A prospective five year follow up. *Journal of Neurology, Neurosurgery and Psychiatry, 40, 1211-1219.*

Lezak, M. D. (1976). *Neuropsychological assessment.* New York: Oxford.

Luria, A. R. (1966). *Human brain and psychological processes.* New York: Harper and Row.

Luria, A. R. (1969). The neuropsychological study of brain lesions restoration of brain functions. In M. Cole, & I. Maltzman (Eds.), *A handbook of Soviet psychology*
(pp. 277-301). New York: Basic Books.

Luria, A. R, & Tsvetkova, L. S. (1990). *The neuropsychological analysis of problem solving.* Delray Beach, FL: St. Lucie Press.

Matarazzo, J. D. (1990). Psychological assessment versus psychological testing: Validation from Binet to the school, clinic and Courtroom. *American Psychologist, 45 (9),* 999-1017.

Miller, H., & Stern, G. (1965). The long-term progression of severe head injury. *Lancet, 1,* 225-229.

Plato (1952). The dialogues of Plato, translated by B. Jowett. In R. M. Hutchins (Ed.), *Great books of the western world.* (Vol. 7) Chicago: Encyclopedia Britannica.

Reitan, R. M., (1958). Validity of the trail making test as an indicator of organic brain damage. *Perceptual and Motor Skills, 8,* 271-276.

Reitan, R. M., & Wolfson, D. (1993*). Theoretical, methological and validation bases of the Halstead-Reitan neuropsychological test battery.* Tucson: Reitan Neuropsychology Laboratory.

Sbordone, R. J. (1987). A neuropsychological approach to cognitive rehabilitation within a private practice setting. In B. Caplan (Ed.*) Handbook of contemporary rehabilitation psychology.* New York: Charles Thomas, pp. 323-342.

Sbordone, R. J. (1988) Assessment and treatment of cognitive communicative impairments in the closed head injury patient: A neurobehavioral systems approach. *Journal of Head Trauma Rehabilitation, 3,* (2), 55-62.

Sbordone, R. J. (1991). *Neuropsychology for the attorney.* Delray Beach, FL: St. Lucie Press.

Sbordone, R. J., Liter, J., & Pettler-Jennings, P. (1990). Recovery of function following severe traumatic brain injury: A retrospective ten year follow-up. *Brain Injury, Vol. 9, No. 3,* 285-299.

Smith, A. (1968). The symbol digit modalities test: A neuropsychological test for economic screening of learning and other cerebral disorders. *Learning Disorders, 3,* 83-91.

Stuss, D.T. (1989). Contribution of frontal lobe injury to cognitive impairment after closed head injury: Methods of assessment and recent findings. In H. S. Levin, J. Grafman, & H. M. Eisenberg (Eds.), *Neurobehavioral recovery from head injury* (pp. 166-177). New York: Oxford.

Sweet, J. J., & Moberg, P. J. (1990). A survey of practices and beliefs among ABPP and non-ABPP clinical neuropsychologists. *The Clinical Neuropsychologist, 4*(2), 101-120.

Thomsen, V. (1981). Neuropsychological treatment and long-time follow up in an aphasic patient with very severe head trauma. *Journal of Clinical Neuropsychology, 3*(1), 43-51.

Wechsler, D. (1981). *WAIS-R manual.* New York: The Psychological Corporation.

Zangwill, O. L. (1966). Psychological deficits associated with frontal lobe lesions. *International Journal of Neurology, 5,* 395-402.

Ziskin, J, & Faust, D. (1988). *Coping with psychiatric and psychological testimony* (Vols. 1-3, 4th Ed.) Marina Del Rey, CA: Law and Psychology Press.

3

HISTORICAL, PHENOMENOLOGIC, AND OBSERVATIONAL DATA:
A Context for Neuropsychological Test Findings

Andrew W. Siegal, Ph.D.

INTRODUCTION

The acknowledgment of an integral role which is to be played by historical, observational, and symptomatologic data is currently made by proponents of the fixed-battery, actuarially based model (Reitan & Wolfson, 1993), as well as by clinicians utilizing a process-oriented, flexible-battery approach (Christensen, 1975, 1979; Howieson & Lezak, 1992; Kaplan, 1988; Luria, 1966; B.C.Wilson, 1986, 1992). Those theoretical considerations requisite for the construction of comprehensive neurobehavioral anamneses, and for a specification of the rationale for the elicitation of those data points which are to be collected during such anamneses, have yet to be systematically articulated or explicated in the neuropsychologic literature.

Standards for assessing the comprehensiveness of neurobehavioral anamneses require articulation, since, without such agreement among investigators, opportunities for replication of findings across clinicians or investigators is unlikely. The specific goal of this chapter is to specify the range of dimensions which are to be assessed during the neurobehavioral anamnesis, as well as to describe a range of techniques for studying those historical, symptomatologic/phenomenological, and observational databases which constitute the neurobehavioral anamnesis.

It is the author's contention that the levels of theoretical sophistication which have been applied to the study of "higher cortical," or cognitive functions utilizing neuropsychologic tests, now need to be demanded in the study of the process of history-taking in clinical neuropsychology. The anamnestic study of, not only cognitive functions, but the domains of appetitive- homeostatic, drive-states, and affective dysfunction requires refinement. Similarly, the patient's subjective experience of their own symptomatology, their condition, and the patient's assessment of their own functional impairments, and those compensatory strategies which they utilize, are all worthy of study, at levels of sophistication and rigor, which are commensurate with those previously reserved for the psychometric study of losses of cognitive function.

This chapter reviews several theoretical considerations which are necessary for the design of anamneses which provide the basis for a comprehensive system for both clinical and research investigations of the historical antecedents, phenomenologic correlates, and systematic description of those observable alterations of behavior which follow neurologic disease, dysfunction, and injury. The purpose of the model articulated in this chapter is to specify, both the nature and scope of, those historical, phenomenological and observational data which must be collected in order to permit meaningful comparisons of these classes of data with sophisticated psychometric indices of cognitive dysfunction. A further requirement of such a model of the anamnestic parameters of neurobehavioral assessment is that such a model should be able to provide a matrix, of both sufficient breadth and inclusiveness, that psychometric findings which pertain to losses of cognitive function become inherently meaningful in the clinical assessment process once these data are viewed within the context which can be provided by the anamnestically derived matrix.

Neuropsychologists of varying orientations appear to be united in their contention that historical, observational, and symptomatologic data are required in the process of clinical neuropsychologic assessment (Report of the Task Force on Education, Accreditation, and Credentialing of the INS, 1981, pp. 5-6). Differences among subfactions of neuropsychologists appear to involve issues pertaining to whether history-taking should precede (e.g., Christensen, 1975, 1979; 1989; Howieson & Lezak, 1992; Kaplan, 1988; Sbordone, 1987, 1991; Wilson, 1986, 1987, 1992; Wilson & Davidowicz, 1987) or follow (Reitan & Wolfson, 1993; personal communication) the collection of psychometric data. A lack of agreement exists as to whether a questionnaire format alone, interview format alone, or whether a combination of questionnaires, which can then be used to guide follow-up interviews, represent adequate anamnestic technique. Similarly, an issue involving which professional discipline should actively elicit historical, observational, and symptomatologic data exists (i.e., should neuropsychologists collect their own histories, or utilize those which have been collected by other disciplines requires consideration). Lastly, a major issue inherent in consideration of whether psychometric data should be interpreted independently of, and if so, prior to, consideration of anamnestic databases as advocated by Reitan and Wolfson (1993; personal communication, see Appendix I at end of this chapter), or whether psychometric data should be both collected and interpreted based upon the findings of the anamnesis as advocated by various process-approach adherents (Bilder & Kane, 1989; Christensen, 1975, 1979; Howieson & Lezak, 1992; Kaplan 1988; Luria, 1966; Sbordone, 1991, this volume; Wilson, 1986, 1987, 1992).

Rather than further reconsider the aforementioned issues which deal with models of integrating psychometric data with data which are derived from nonpsychometric sources, in this chapter, the author will specifically address the issue of detailing a rationale for specifying which of those historical, observational, and subjective/phenomenologic data require inclusion in the anamnestic phases of the neuropsychological assessment process. A supra-ordinate model is presented in this chapter which specifies a range of neurobehavioral systems subserving both the cognitive and appetitive/homeostatic functions which, in the author's opinion require inclusion in the clinical study of neurobehavioral patients. This model is intended to direct consideration of potential interactions between cognitive and appetitive/homeostatic functions. The model which is presented also directs attention to a wide range of clinical study techniques, which represent a synthesis of various multidisciplinary approaches, which have been applied to the study of both those cognitive and appetitive/homeostatic neurobehavioral systems which may manifest as sequellae of neurologic injury, disease, or maldevelopment.

The model presented, by utilizing a multidisciplinarily based range of study techniques, attempts to generate a database which is capable of accommodating data which describe a sufficiently broad range of phenomena to adequately characterize and describe a wide spectrum of neuropsychopathology. The model also attempts to provide a schematic in which the classification of neuropsychopathologic phenomena can be achieved both in terms of specifying the method by which each phenomenon was apprehended, and also by specifying the neurobehavioral system which was, presumably, studied in order to observe or elicit the neuropsychopathologic phenomenon in question. This model is intended to provide a framework for depicting interactions among neuropsychopathologic phenomena across an expanded range of neurobehavioral systems in comparison to that which would be possible when neuropsychological tests of cognitive functions are used in isolation. Each neurobehavioral system within this model can be studied utilizing a broadly based range of study techniques. The model attempts to provide multiple-complementary objects and methods of study which pertain to each neurobehavioral system; cognitive and appetitive/homeostatic. The consideration of interactions of those various cognitive systems and drive states is hopefully facilitated by the routine description of each patient on both sets of parameters. The use of a comprehensive neurobehavioral anamnesis is advocated as a suitable technique for the collection of a database of sufficient breadth for this task. This model is detailed in Figure 1.

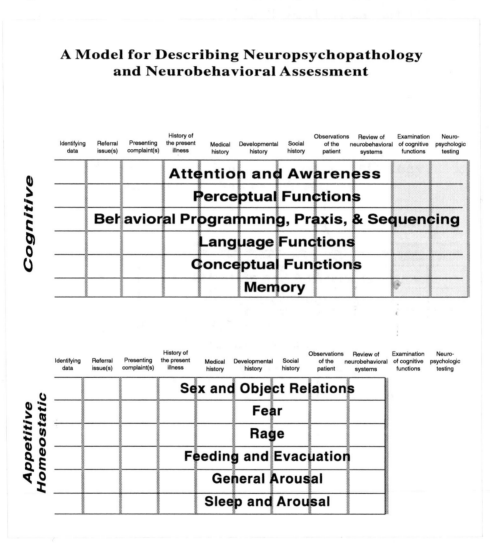

Figure 1. A Model for Describing Neuropsychopathology and Neurobehavioral Assessment: Cognitive Parameters, Appetitive/Homeostatic Parameters, and a Range of Methods for the Study of Each.

Investigators and clinicians are invited to review the current working models of clinical assessment which they utilize in the assessment process in terms of both breadth and intensiveness of coverage of the neurobehavioral systems studied. Also encouraged is review of current working models in terms of the diversity of the assessment strategies they now deploy, and the degree to which those strategies utilize and accommodate a broad spectrum of clinical data. Currently available interview and observational techniques developed for the study of the neurobehavioral systems are indicated by the column headings in Figure 1. Multiple-complementary data collection and analysis techniques are advocated if the validity which is inherent in each study technique are to be profitably utilized in ascending to concurrent validity approaches to clinical data analysis. Increasing the number and types of predictor variables utilized in clinical and forensic neuropsychologic assessments permits the emergence of a process of converging operations. A relatively wide range of techniques for the clinical study of the neurobehavioral disorders is currently available and is depicted in Figure 1. The use of multiple-complementary data analysis techniques provides a variety of internal reliability checks which are requisite to the emergence of ecologic validity of neuropsychologic test data.

The model presented in Figure 1 was designed as an heuristic device for describing the various signs, symptoms, and historical antecedents of neuropsychopathology. This description permits more broadly defined syndromal configurations of neuropsychopathology to emerge which include and extend beyond the syndromal configurations which can be described on the basis of neuropsychologic tests taken in isolation. That same model can be utilized to define the scope of anamnestic approaches to the assessment of the neurobehavioral disorders. One such set of structured interview items, the Neurobehavioral Assessment Format (see Appendix A at the end of the book) also includes a specification of observational data points (Siegal, Schechter, & Diamond, 1983). That system addresses the informational requirements of each cell which is generated by the model for describing neuropsychopathology and neurobehavioral assessment depicted in Figure 1. The general model is presented as an heuristic device intended to foster systematization of the process of collecting historical, observational, and symptomatic/phenomenologic information in studies of neurobehavioral patients. Facilitation of intercommunication among clinicians and investigators who study neurobehavioral disorders may emerge as the result of the author's attempt to provide a supra-ordinate model of the anamnestic aspects of the neurobehavioral database. Clinicians and investigators may then wish to articulate their own models or to adapt and amend the model described in this chapter, while retaining any core, fundamental assumptions they find useful in defining the informational requirements of a neurobehavioral anamnesis.

Several principles are useful in the construction of a model for guiding theoretically based neurobehavioral anamneses which are capable of reflecting current knowledge regarding the diversity of manifestations of the various neurobehavioral disorders. It should be noted that those disorders currently described under the rubric of "functional" psychopathologic disorders can also be described and studied utilizing the model depicted in Figure 1. The requirement that "functional" and "organically" based disorders be equally well described utilizing any given informational system is regarded by the author as a precondition for neurologic aspects of presumably "functional" disorders to emerge, and for the discovery of "functional" parameters in the description of neurobehavioral disorders.

PRINCIPLES RECOMMENDED FOR USE IN THE CONSTRUCTION OF NEUROBEHAVIORAL ANAMNESES

COGNITIVE FUNCTIONS CAN BE STUDIED UTILIZING A VARIETY OF CLINICAL TECHNIQUES IN ADDITION TO NEUROPSYCHOLOGICAL TESTS

The gray stippled area in the upper, right-hand corner of Figure 1 denotes the current emphasis of clinical neuropsychology in its study of losses of cognitive function, whether studied utilizing behavioral-neurologically derived examinations of cognitive functions or whether standardized, psychometric studies of losses of cognitive functions are conducted. The reader's attention is directed to the equal, or greater, breadth of those neurobehavioral systems which are not directly assessed by neuropsychologic testing. Similarly, the broad scope of currently available, multiple-complementary, methods of clinical study of those cognitive systems which can be investigated utilizing historical, observational, and self-report techniques is depicted by the area under all columns in Figure 1 which do not show gray stippling. The breadth of these information sources and types which supplement those derived from neuropsychological tests are depicted, as well, and suggest that the variety of currently available anamnestic techniques are sufficiently diverse that their integration with neuropsychological test data requires consideration.

Those neurobehavioral systems which subserve cognitive functions are typically studied by neuropsychologic tests, but can also be studied using a wider variety of techniques. Neuropsychologic tests emphasize the study of losses of cognitive function (i.e., "negative signs"). These "negative signs" of dysfunction within each neurobehavioral system subserving cognition, can be examined with respect to varying objects of study (e.g., the development of that cognitive system over time [i.e. Developmental History]). The patient's subjective awareness of the integrity, dysfunction, or changes in the experience of their "sense of" that system, may also be studied (i.e., Presenting Complaint; Review of Neurobehavioral Systems). Similarly, the ability of that cognitive system to successfully execute the ecologic demands which have been made upon it developmentally, and/or post-morbidly, constitute additional objects of study (i.e., History of the Present Illness, Developmental History, Social History). The appearance of the patient as they attempt to function utilizing that cognitive system when observed by examiners (i.e., Observations of the Patient) and by significant others (i.e., Referral Issues; Developmental History, Social History) constitute additional study techniques. The conjoint utilization of these multiple-complementary informational sources and methods of study permits both internal reliability checks, and provides data points for corroboration with external, independently obtained data. Both types of reliability checks may foster both the clinical relevance and the ecologic validity of the neurobehavioral assessment process and the data which it generates.

POSITIVE AND COMPLEX-POSITIVE PHENOMENA REQUIRE DIRECT STUDY IN THE ASSESSMENT OF BOTH COGNITIVE AND APPETITIVE/HOMEOSTATIC SYSTEMS

Neuropsychologic testing has emphasized the study of losses of cognitive functions (i.e., negative symptoms/signs) if viewed from within a Jacksonian (1958) model. Both positive and complex positive signs and symptoms may profitably be studied for each neurobehavioral system which subserves cognitive processes (cf., Gastaut & Broughton, 1972; Jackson, 1881/1958; Luria, 1966; Penfield & Jasper, 1954). Phenomenologic inquiry, must be structured to remain sensitive to all three classes of symptomatology. Similarly, observational techniques must also provide a schema which permits the apprehension of augmentations and distortions of function as well as directing the examiner's attention to losses of function.

The top half of Figure 1 depicts a model for describing cognitive neuropsychopathology. Six principal cognitive domains are specified within the proposed model. These cognitive domains include: 1) attention/awareness; 2) perceptual functions including visual, auditory, olfactory, and gustatory modalities as well as somatosensory systems, including haptic perception, proprioception, and kinesthesis; 3) behavioral programming, praxis, sequencing, and executive functions are identified as relevant cognitive domains as are,

4) language functions, 5) conceptual functions, and 6) memory functions. These six domains are routinely included in models of neuropsychologic assessment. The symmetrical inquiry for, and observation of, negative, positive, and complex-positive phenomena within each of these six cognitive domains is advocated as a goal in the construction of a comprehensive neurobehavioral anamnesis.

APPETITIVE/HOMEOSTATIC SYSTEMS REQUIRE DIRECT STUDY TO COMPLEMENT THE STUDY OF COGNITIVE PROCESSES

The degree to which oversimplification permits the aforementioned cognitive processes to be designated, "higher cortical functions;" appetitive/homeostatic functions, and drives can be described, with equal oversimplification, as "subcortical," "limbic," and "brain stem functions." If a neurobehavioral anamnesis is required to maintain sensitivity to disruptions of cortical function, then symmetrical attention to subcortical function and dysfunction should be required of a neurobehavioral anamnesis. Symmetry of higher-cortical functions and subcortical functions coverage is required if the full range of neuropsychopathologic phenomena are to have an opportunity to emerge during the clinical assessment process.

The lower half of Figure 1 depicts six categories of appetitive/homeostatic dimensions of behavior including 1) sex and object relations, 2) feeding and evacuative functions, and 3) sleep and arousal. These homeostatic mechanisms were described as "welfare emotions" by Walter B. Cannon and were distinguished from sympathetically mediated, "emergency emotions," including 4) fear, 5) rage, and 6) general arousal systems (Rado, 1955, 1956, 1958, 1969). These homeostatic drive states are included in the present model as parameters of study which require routine inclusion in neurobehavioral anamneses. Figure 1 depicts the aforementioned appetitive/homeostatic systems and includes them for consideration in models which purport to describe the full range of neuropsychopathology. The resultant model of neuropsychopathology may then guide clinical assessment within the context of a theoretically driven anamnesis.

One particular biologically based, psychoanalytic personality theory, Adaptational Psychodynamics (Rado, 1956, 1962, 1969) emphasized the notion of dynamic balances which are achieved between systems subserving "motivation and control" in describing psychopathology and its neurologic anlage. Luria's (1966) tripartite model of neural organization emphasized ascending and descending pathways for "the maintenance of cortical tone" which were posited as acting to modulate the potentials for both information processing and for volitional action. Both theories of neural integration were built upon Jackson's (1958) notion of vertical integration within the nervous system. The need for inclusion of vertical, and hierarchically organized, model integration in the study of neuropsychopathology and neurobehavioral organization has been emphasized (Monroe, 1970). It has been recommended as a new focus for clinical neuropsychologic research by requiring an integration of those findings derived from the study of the emotions with the knowledge base and study techniques of the cognitive neurosciences (Tucker, 1993).

TECHNIQUES DERIVED FROM ALLIED DISCIPLINES CAN BE INTEGRATED WITH NEUROPSYCHOLOGIC STUDY TECHNIQUES

Neuropsychology's allied disciplines, including psychiatry (cf., Department of Psychiatry Teaching Committee, The Institute of Psychiatry, London, 1973; Detre & Jarecki, 1971; Hall, Gardner, Stickney, LeCann, & Popkin, 1980; Hoch, 1972; Koranyi, 1979; Lishman, 1978), neurology (Bannister, 1992; Cummings, 1985; DeJong, 1979; Mesalaum, 1985), child psychiatry (Goodman & Sours, 1967; MacKeith & Bax, 1963; Rutter, 1983; Schechter, 1970, 1991; Shaffer & Dunn, 1979; Wender, 1987), and pediatric neurology (Levine, Brooks, & Shonkoff, 1980; Paine & Oppe, 1965a, 1965b; Rapin & Wilson, 1978; Schain, 1972; Tupper, 1987) have all made methodological inroads to the systematic study of patient's life history, course of illness, symptomatology, and to the study of observable signs of dysfunction (DeJong, 1979; Luria, 1966; Spillane, 1975) in the various neurobehavioral disorders.

Basic disciplines, such as descriptive and categorical phenomenology (Ellenberger, 1958; Jaspers, 1963; Jennings, 1986), have evolved into sophisticated clinical techniques. These techniques permit detailed study of the experiential sequellae of neurologic dysfunction which can complement the contribution of neuropsychologic testing in the latter's objective description of the effects of brain disease. Each discipline has evolved techniques for study of different aspects of the neurobehavioral disorders. This inherent diversity of objects and methods of study of the neurobehavioral disorders carries the potential for an integration of a variety of unique methodologic contributions to anamnestic technique which can be deployed by neuropsychologists. The columns in Figure 1 depict the types of inquiry which can be identified in surveying the various anamnestic techniques and methodologies derived from approaches which are more heavily utilized in psychiatry (Detre & Jarecki, 1973; Hoch, 1972; Jaspers, 1963) and neurology (Mesalaum, 1985). These clinical methodologies can be reviewed for their heuristic value by neuropsychologists considering the potential utility of a broader, and more methodologically diverse, structure for an expanded neurobehavioral anamnesis. A variety of study techniques are denoted by the column headings in Figure 1. The various anamnestic techniques can be used to study the same cognitive systems which are assessed by neuropsychological tests, but also provide a methodology for the study of appetitive homeostatic drive systems as well.

Each of these study techniques, taken collectively, define the neurobehavioral anamnesis and are introduced briefly and defined below:

Identifying Data. The patient's age, gender, socioeconomic status (i.e., number of years and type of education, ethnicity, and handedness), constitute relevant identifying data points. The patient's native language and subsequent languages learned are specified. The patient's occupation and employment status are specified, as well as a notation of supplementary or disability-related income. Specification of the method of payment for healthcare services is informative. The type and level of examiner training are also specified.

Referral Issues. Systematic elicitation of referral issues involves the exploration and recording of concerns of referring professionals, agencies, and/or family members, and specification of the referral source.

Presenting Complaints. Elicitation of the patient's presenting complaints provides a phenomenologic, and patient-structured, inquiry into those experiential aspects of neuropsychopathology which are within the awareness of the patient. The reporting of complaints is limited to those phenomena the patient is both willing and able to describe to the examiner.

History of the Present Illness. This should consider both the course, and the subsequent elaboration of the patient's symptoms over time, as reported by the patient, observed and reported by significant others, and as recorded in relevant medical records. Consideration of interventions, palliatives, and exacerbating factors, are of special relevance to diagnostic, treatment, and prognostic perspectives.

Medical History. The medical history is elicited from patients, and/or family members, and is supplemented by independent review of medical records. The medical history provides a review of primary CNS insults and systemic illnesses capable of causing secondary CNS insult. Functional psychopathologic disorders, exposure to toxins, seizures, and both clinical and side effects of prior treatments in the patient's personal medical history constitute objects of study in the medical history.

The family medical history's coverage is symmetrical with that of the personal medical history in that each category of illness which is queried for the patient is also queried for occurrence in family members.

Developmental History. In the developmental history, the development of each of the aforementioned parameters of cognitive and appetitive/homeostatic neurobehavioral functions are assessed in terms of each of those functions' development over time. Methods of clinically inferring dysfunction clinically, from developmentally derived data, such as adherence to, or deviation from, predictable, age-stage progressions, have been developed (Erikson, 1950; A. Freud, 1966; S. Freud, 1905, 1915; Piaget, 1973). A variety of research approaches applicable to the analysis of psychometric data in the study of developmental issues (Spreen, Tupper, Rieser, Tiokko, & Edgell, 1984) have been reviewed. Reitan (1966) described four methods for inferring the presence of brain damage or cerebral dysfunction from psychologic test data. These methods included analysis of level of performance, analysis of differential scores/pattern or configurational analyses, analysis of lateralized sensorimotor phenomena, and an analysis of signs which are considered to be "pathognomonic" of cerebral dysfunction. These four inferential systems have been utilized to classify developmental research approaches which utilize psychometric data (Rourke, 1983).

The clinical and research utility of the systems described by Reitan (1966) in identifying the presence of cerebral dysfunction from psychometric data may also hold promise, if applied with equal rigor, to the analysis of anamnestic databases. Data points which are amenable to each of the four types of inference need to be systematically included in the anamnestic inquiry if all four inferential systems are to be utilized. To aspire to such methodologic sophistication, specification of relevant parameters of study, and items required to assess each parameter, and the subsequent development of scoring and coding systems for historical, observational, and subjective-report data, would be required by practitioners within our field. The full utility of the multiple, complementary inferential systems, and the enhancement of diagnostic power and opportunity to utilize inherent systems of reliability checks, may be applied to developmental historical data if the application of this methodologically proven research tactic is afforded consideration when anamneses are constructed.

A variety of performance level indices, as well as development patterns of neurobehavioral systems which subserve various adaptive abilities, may be studied with respect to both form and velocity of development in the developmental history by utilizing patient and/or family as informants. Lateralized dysfunction in various perceptual and motor systems may be noted by these informants, as may the occurrence of pathognomonic signs and failures to achieve variously defined developmental landmarks within each system, both cognitive and appetitive/homestatic.

Social History. In the social history, inquiry is made regarding the patient's interactions with each of the social systems with which the patient interacts (e.g., kinship system, socioeconomic system, educational system). In the social history, neurobehavioral function may be considered as a dependent variable when considering the shaping role which social systems have played in the development of any given behavior and its neural substrate (Bakker, 1984, Richardson, 1964). Similarly, past and current adaptive abilities of the patient may be inferred as an independent variable when considering the adaptive competencies, failures, or anomalous adaptational strategies utilized by the patient in interacting with any of the social systems queried within the context of a social history which is gathered from patient, significant others, and corroborated by relevant records.

Observations of the Patient. Observations of the patient can be made systematically over the 12 basic dimensions of neurobehavioral function depicted in Figure 1's rows. Observations may be made "in vivot" in the form of home visits, visits to the workplace, or, "in vitro" observations can be made of the patient as they approach and participate in the neuropsychologic examination situation. The observation of the presence versus absence, as well as the types of compensatory strategy utilized, and a specification of those situations in which compensatory strategies are, or are not, used provides information both regarding acuteness versus chronicity, as well as in clarifying the nature of the underlying impairment. In addition to the observation of cognitive, affective, and behavioral alterations, a wide range of physical stigmata affecting facies, posture, gait, carriage, and physical appearance have proven useful in identifying and describing the neurobehavioral disorders (DeJong, 1979; Spillane, 1975).

Review of Neurobehavioral Systems. In the review of neurobehavioral systems, structured phenomenologic inquiry may be directed toward each category of the patient's experience of the integrity, function, or dysfunction, of each neurobehavioral system (see Figure 1). The review of neurobehavioral systems can be structured in a form which permits the neuropsychologist to study not only losses of cognitive function (i.e., negative symptoms), but also to study positive and complex-positive phenomena, symmetrically. Interrelations between data derived from subjective reporting of symptoms may then be contrasted with objective data and with the subjective reports of corollary informants.

Appetitive/homeostatic systems can similarly be studied directly utilizing symptomatologic inquiry for the presence of negative, positive, and complex-positive phenomena.

The aforementioned types of historical, observational, and phenomenological techniques provide a broad context into which neuropsychologic test data can be placed. This broader perspective may provide a sufficiently wide context for addressing an expanded range of referral issues regarding interactions of multiple-etiologic factors, description of course of illness, and the assessment of the impact of that illness—upon adaptation. These data would appear to add both diagnostic precision and prognostic power when describing neuropsychopathology in a broader context than would be possible utilizing neuropsychologic test data, if taken in isolation. Thus, phenomenologic study of both cognitive and affective states provides a broader basis for understanding cognitive deficits and their dynamic, adaptational, interactive, and experiential significance to the patient, and to the ecology as perceived by the patient.

PHASIC FLUCTUATIONS IN COGNITIVE AND APPETITIVE/HOMEOSTATIC FUNCTIONS REQUIRE STUDY

Clinical neuropsychology has traditionally emphasized the assessment of cognitive abilities as relatively stable traits. The description of cognitive abilities as traits which were studied under highly controlled conditions was necessary to ensure the reliable measurement of cognitive functions for use in studies demonstrating the sensitivity of neuropsychologic tests to the presence of brain damage, lateralization and localization of lesions, and to the prediction of acuteness, chronicity, and etiology of the underlying neuropathology (cf., Benton, 1967; Reitan, 1966; Reitan & Wolfson, 1993; Smith, 1975; 1981). The requirement of testing patients under optimal performance conditions in the neuropsychologic examination has been critically reconsidered by Sbordone (this volume) as limiting the range of life-performance situations to which generalizations can be made on the basis of neuropsychologic test data when those data are studied in isolation. The anamnesis provides clinicians with an opportunity to extend the number and types of predictor variables which assess past behavior in ecologically relevant, and in extraordinary situations, which have taxed the patient's abilities. The precise situations elicited in the history may be expected to trigger emergency behavior, catastrophic affect, or to typify compensatory maneuvers if these situations are replicated in the future situation to which the clinician is attempting to predict.

Referral issues in current neuropsychologic practice may involve predictions of job performance, the ability to conduct one's self in community versus institutional settings, the ability to provide factual testimony in court, to care for children, manage funds, or to be held responsible for criminal acts. In assessing cognitive functions under optimal performance conditions, it is important to realize that behavioral predictions are being made to situations in which patients are exposed to less than optimal conditions (Sbordone, 1991, this volume, Ch. 2) and represent situations in which suboptimal performance can often be anticipated. Sbordone (this volume, Ch. 2) also emphasized that performance on neuropsychologic tests may not fully reflect the efficacy of well-rehearsed compensatory techniques which the patient may have developed for use in situationally specific environmental demands which are posed by the patient's habitat. Thus, adaptive capability can also be underestimated by predicting on the basis of neuropsychologic test data alone.

The necessity of considering the degree of sophistication, plasticity, efficacy, and organization of cognitive processes at varying activation levels has inhered in biologically oriented personality theories (Freud, 1905; 1915; Rado, 1956). Rado's (1969) Adaptational Psychodynamics provides a neurobehaviorally sophisticated theory of personality which lends itself ideally to clinical neuropsychological theory and assessment. Adaptational Psychodynamics emphasized the concepts of ascending dyscontrol, in which lower brain centers disrupt the functioning of higher cortical functions. Descending dyscontrol was the term utilized in Rado' s theory to describe the triggering of emotional and visceral emergency signaled by environmental cues which bode danger to the organism. Rado (1956a, 1956b, 1958/1962, 1969) described four levels of neurobehavioral integration, each of which was described in terms of the complexity and sophistication of those adaptive responses of which the individual was capable when functioning at each of those four ascending complex levels of neurobehavioral integration. Rado (1958/1962) termed this neurologic schematic *The Psychodynamic cerebral system.* This schematic is presented in Figure 2.

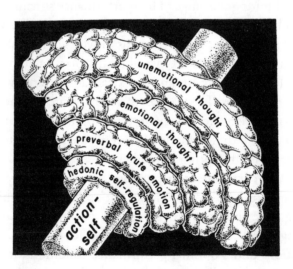

Figure 2. Sandor's Schematic Diagram of Four Levels of Neurobehavioral Integration and Their Heirarchical Organization: "The Integrative Apparatus of the Psychodynamic Cerebral System."

Reprinted with permission from Grune & Stratton, Inc. from *Psychoanalysis of Behavior, Vol. 2,* by Sandor Rado.

Four levels of neurobehavioral integration, including the "hedonic level," the "brute emotional level," and the "emotional thought level" of response were described as levels of emergency functioning. The most sophisticated level of neurobehavioral integration and the most difficult level to attain once, and if, achieved, was described as "the unemotional thought level." The unemotional thought level was described as the last level of neurobehavioral development to be attained in the hierarchy, both phylogenetically and ontogenetically (Rado, 1955/1956a). The notion of ascending levels of complexity along a vertically, and hierarchically organized neuraxis was described as being correlated with progressively more conceptual and less emotionally driven behavior as differentiation along the neuraxis was achieved. Rado's (1955/1956b) schematic for depicting the levels of emergency behavior is presented in Figure 3. Such notions of hierarchically organized levels of neurobehavioral integration have formed bulwarks of neurobehavioral theories beginning with the writings of Jackson (1881/1958) but were developed to the level of formal psychoanalytic personality theory by Rado (1956) and were extended to provide reinterpretations of the psychodynamics of the full spectrum of psychopathology within a neurobehavioral model.

If the sole database pertaining to a neurobehavioral patient consists of psychometric observations which have been obtained under optimal performance conditions, predictions of that patient's behavior when functioning at lower levels of neurobehavioral integration must be viewed with caution since only the "unemotional thought level" will have been sampled to the degree to which optimal performance conditions have been maintained. Thus, the anamnesis provides a database into which conclusions regarding the integrity and asymmetry of cognitive abilities which are based upon psychometric data can be placed for use in predicting behavior in a wider range of performance situations.

It is proposed that the utilization of historical methods in which the patient's past adaptational patterns can be described by the patient, corollary informants, and supporting records, are instructive in contributing to the prediction of the patient's behavior in a variety of "in vivo" situations. Similarly, observation of the patient in the widest range of situations possible to supplement that of the neuropsychologic examination may prove contributory to assessing the degree to which affective control or dyscontrol can be assumed to characterize a given patient's behavior outside of the testing situation. Thus, a model of neurobehavioral anamnesis which is capable of describing phasic fluctuations in the delicate and changing balance between motivational and cognitive-control systems is portrayed in fuller complexity by Figure 4 which includes the author's modification of the model depicted in Figure 1 to include the param-

Emergency Behavior: Basic Mechanisms at the Hedonic, Emotional, and Emotional Thought Levels

Level	Alerting Signal	Emergency Move	Evolutionary Aspects	
			Expanding Range of Anticipation	Improved performance due to more and better equipment
Emotional thought	Angry thought	Combat, defiance	Long-range anticipation of pain from damage	Intellectual exploration of past and future, from near to far: cortical system
	Apprehensive thought	Escape, submission, cry for help		
Emotional	Brute rage	Combat, defiance	Anticipation of pain from impending damage	Sensory exploration of "shell of immediate future surrounding the animal's head": distance receptors
	Brute fear	Escape, submission, cry for help		
Hedonic	Pain	Riddance (prevention of further pain)	Anticipation of further pain	Sampling of pain from damage incurred: contact receptors

Figure 3. Sando Rado's Schematic for Depicting Heirarchical Levels of Neurobehavioral Integration Subserving Emergency Behavior. Reprinted with permission from Grune & Stratton, Inc. From *Psychoanalysis of Behavior*, by Sandor Rado (1956).

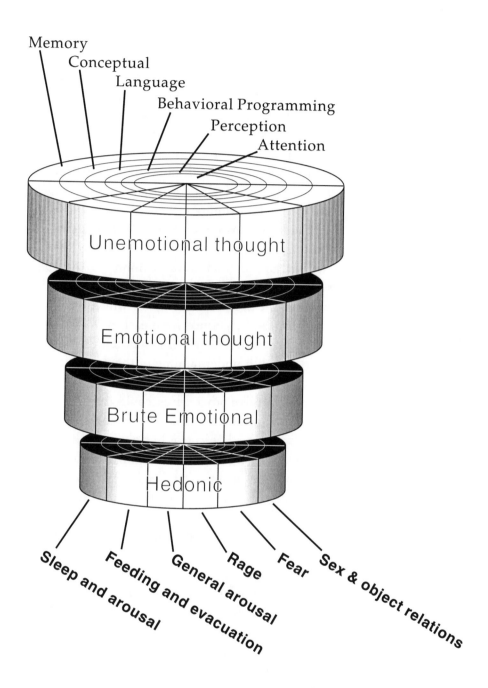

Figure 4. The Model for Describing Neuropsychopathology and Neurobehavioral Assessment, Expanded to Depict Heirarchic Levels of Neurobehavioral Integration.

eter of ascending, hierarchically organized levels of neurobehavioral organization as described in Rado's (1969) Adaptational Psychodynamics.

The need for clinical neuropsychology as a discipline to address the issue of "state theory" has been highlighted (Wilson, 1986). Neuropsychology's allied disciplines, psychiatry and neurology, have demonstrated methodologies which are useful in the study of phasic changes in behavior. Monroe (1970, 1974, 1978a) extended Rado's (1956) theoretical work in his detailed clinical and research studies of epileptic patients with episodic impulse control disorders. Detailed study of hundreds of patients who had been studied clinically, were also studied electrophysiologically with both depth and surface electrodes. These same patients were also studied pharmacologically with medications which either raised or lowered seizure thresholds (Monroe, 1975). Monroe (1970; 1978) studied these patients psychometrically (Monroe, 1970, 1978b) with both tests of cognitive functions and with personality tests (Monroe, 1970, 1978b). Many of these patients were studied psychoanalytically as well (Monroe, 1970, 1982b). These case studies are presented in detailed form and stand as models of meticulously studied neurobehavioral cases (Monroe, 1970) which embody the spectrum of contributions which can be gleaned from each of the disciplines within the neurobehavioral community. The use of the aforementioned convergent operations yielded an in-depth understanding of the dramatic, phasic fluctuations in levels of dyscontrol could be demonstrated in these patients over time. Violence, and the dyscontrol of other drives, could at one time occur with principally volitional control, and at other times the dyscontrol was demonstrated to be ictal or ictally released. Electrophysiologic, self-reported phenomenologic data, and EEG correlates, were all required to differentiate ictally driven behavior from more volitionally controlled behavior which could then be described as being mediated at any of four levels of disintegration. Dyscontrol episodes could be categorized as occurring at the levels of "seizure dyscontrol," "instinct dyscontrol," "impulse dyscontrol," and "acting-out dyscontrol" (Monroe, 1970).

Description on multiple dimensions, simultaneously, was required to define the interplay between personality variables, situational cues and stimuli, and electrophysiologically recorded, neural events which clarified the brain's degree and level of activation on the vertical neuraxis. Such detailed consideration of the multiple determinants of behavior (e.g., response capability, stimulus input levels, personality variables, and level of subjective awareness, specification of activation level were all required to determine the level of disorganization of behavior at any given time for any given patient. Similarly, the degree to which the behavior was described as ego-syntonic vs. ego-dystonic by the patient was required in the phenomenologic differentiation of these four states of dyscontrol. It is significant that the use of these multiple descriptors were essential in generating Monroe's (1970) model of hierarchical levels of episodic dyscontrol, even in patients in whom the exact type and locus of lesion were known and in whom the diagnosis (i.e., epilepsy) had been previously demonstrated. While Monroe (1978b) could identify an individual as being likely to suffer from epileptoid dyscontrol psychometrically using an 18-item self-report psychometric measure, the classification of the epileptoid vs. volitional motivation of any particular disordered behavioral event required multidimensional consideration. The multivariate and interactive nature of the variables necessary to differentiate between seizure dyscontrol, instinct dyscontrol, impulse dyscontrol, and acting-out dyscontrol, are depicted in Figure 5.

Phasic fluctuations in mental activity in states of waking, sleeping, and dreaming have consistently vexed sleep and dream researchers (Grosser & Siegal, 1971; Molinari & Foulkes, 1969; Moruzzi, 1963; Pivik, 1978). Sleep researchers have studied rapid changes in psychophysiologic parameters during various stages of sleep and have attempted with varying success to establish concomitant changes in the degree to which mental activity in sleep occurs is specifically associated with phasic physiologic changes. The degree to which sleep mentation is dreamlike vs. thought-like, imagric vs. linguistic, fantasy-like vs. reflective of day-residue have constituted parameters of study (Grosser & Siegal, 1971). The changes in the quality of mental activity during sleep have all been studied with respect to their phasic changes during waking, sleep, and dreaming in attempts to correlate these with cognitive changes with central nervous system and autonomic nervous system activation levels (Grosser & Siegal, 1971; Pivik, 1978,1991). The inconsistencies among empirical studies of the cognitive correlates of various short-term, phasic changes within sleep may be best reconciled by considering individual differences in excitability and arousal (Pivik, 1991). The complexity of the multiple determinants of these various characteristics of dreams, and other types of sleep mentation, have been addressed in the articulation of the Activation Level, Input Source, and Mode of Processing (AIM) Model (Hobson, 1992). The AIM Model utilizes parameters which are nearly identical to those described by Luria (1966) in his description of the tripartite model of neurobehavioral systems underlying waking cognition. The necessity for specifying activation level of the brain is addressed in the study of waking cognition (Luria, 1966), ictal disorganization of thinking and behavior (Monroe, 1970), and in the study of dreams and sleep mentation (Hobson, 1992). In each of the aforementioned models, the quality of cognitive activity is described as a function of the activation and inhibition which occurs at vertically organized levels of brain organization. The striking similarity of parameters which are currently being studied by researchers in both epilepsy and dreams should remind neuropsychologists that the "via regiae" which were designated by both Jackson (i.e., epilepsy) (1958), and by Freud, (dreams) (1900),

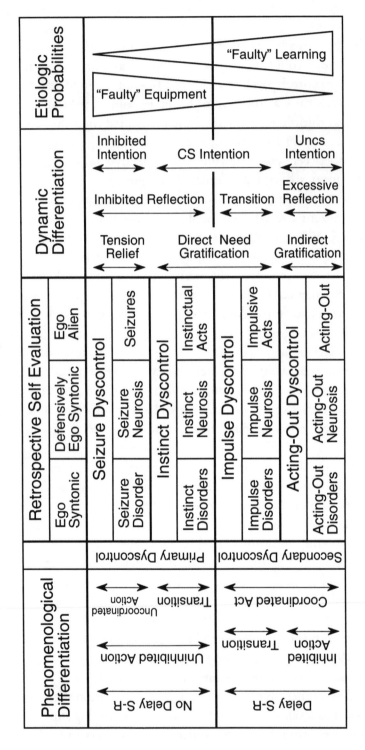

Figure 5. R. R. Monroe's Schematic for Describing Four Heirarchically Organized Levels of Episodic Dyscontrol. Reprinted with permission. From Russell R. Monroe (1970). *Episodic Behavioral Disorders.* Cambridge, MA: Harvard University Press.

are now both pointing in exactly the same direction; a renewed emphasis upon considering cognitive processes as state-dependent phenomena which fluctuate as a function of arousal, appears to be emerging. Research in sleep and epilepsy has paralleled the cognitive neuroscience researcher's (Borod, 1993; Tucker, 1993) recent directive that it is now necessary to explicate state-theory in the study of cognitive processes and to specifically describe cognitive processes under varying conditions of both internal and external arousal. State-dependent phenomena are recommended by the author for routine inclusion in models of neurobehavioral anamnesis to provide a methodology which is capable of reflecting the nature and degree of variability in the organization of cognition, affect, behavior, and experience.

A systematic methodology for follow-up inquiry is detailed in the discussion of a methodology for conducting a Review of Neurobehavioral Systems. In this method, each symptom is queried in a fashion which permits paroxysmal, and more general transient features to be reported, if present. This provides phenomenologic descriptions of state-dependent, or phasic, aspects of experience.

Kurt Goldstein (1942, 1959) paid systematic attention to the deterioration in the level of cognitive organization which occurred in the wake of the "catastrophic anxiety." Catastrophic anxiety was described by Goldstein as being engendered by the patient's realization of the presence of impaired performance. Goldstein (1942, 1959), similarly described the adaptational maneuvers of patients to attempt to simplify, either or both, task and response demands (simplification or stereotypy) in states of "cognitive deficit." The interactive nature of cognitive capability was considered as a function of ecosystem demands in relation to adaptive capability in determining the nature and level of activation (Goldstein, 1963).

The need for neuropsychology to systematically address the vertical organization of the brain and to inter-digitate cognitive neuropsychology with methods of study which have been designed to explicate the "psychology of emotion" has been advocated (Tucker, 1993). The roles of emotion and drive states in its various roles in guiding display behavior (Borod, 1993), in perceiving same (Bowers, Bauer, & Heilman, 1993), and in both driving, organizing, and disorganizing behavior (Heller, 1993) and in mediating qualitative changes in the subjective experience of emotion (Buck, 1993) have been advocated as variables requiring integration with clinical neuropsychology. Consideration of emotional parameters for both lateralization (Borod, 1993) and vertical organization of functions were reviewed recently (Tucker, 1993). The recent recognition of emotional parameters and the need for clinical neuropsychology to devote closer consideration to the study of the emotions was highlighted by the publication of a special edition of the new journal, *Neuropsychology,* (1993) under the editorship of Professor Nelson Butters. This publication constitutes a noteworthy advance in synthesizing consideration of tonic and phasic aspects of both cognitive and appetitive homeostatic systems.

Active consideration of phasic fluctuations in the nature and level of neurobehavioral integration requires systematic inclusion in the construction and conduct of the neurobehavioral anamnesis is paralleled by the recent attention which is being paid to these parameters in basic neuropsychologic research literature.

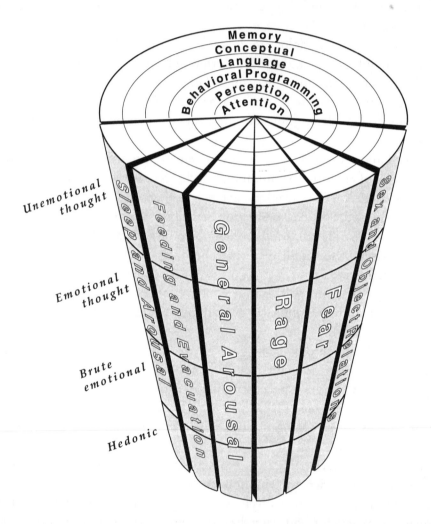

Figure 6. Visually Simplified Schematic for Depicting Interactions of Cognitive and Appetitive/Homeostatic Systems and Phasic Changes in Their Balance and Integration for Use in Constructing Models of Neurobehavioral Anamnesis.

Figure 6 portrays the representation of ascendingly complex levels of neurobehavioral integration which may be considered during the anamnestic study of neurobehavioral patients as the systematic study of the various negative, positive, and complex-positive signs and symptoms of dysfunction are reviewed within each cognitive and appetitive/homeostatic neurobehavioral system.

For purposes of clarity and simplicity, the two-dimensional model which was portrayed in Figure 1 is more profitably used by investigators and permits examiners to note those domains to be assessed during anamnesis literally as the examination proceeds. The third dimension (i.e., the vertical organization of behavior and the recognition of phasic changes in each system), requires a full appreciation of the significance of these factors. Examiners' sensitivities to the report, and elicitation of critical incidents, during the study of each appetitive and cognitive dimension, as it is studied, is requisite if sufficient attention is to be paid to the organizing and disorganizing roles of phasic changes in behavior, and to inferences drawn regarding concomitant neurologic substrata and to the variability in behavior which can be predicted for the given patient over time.

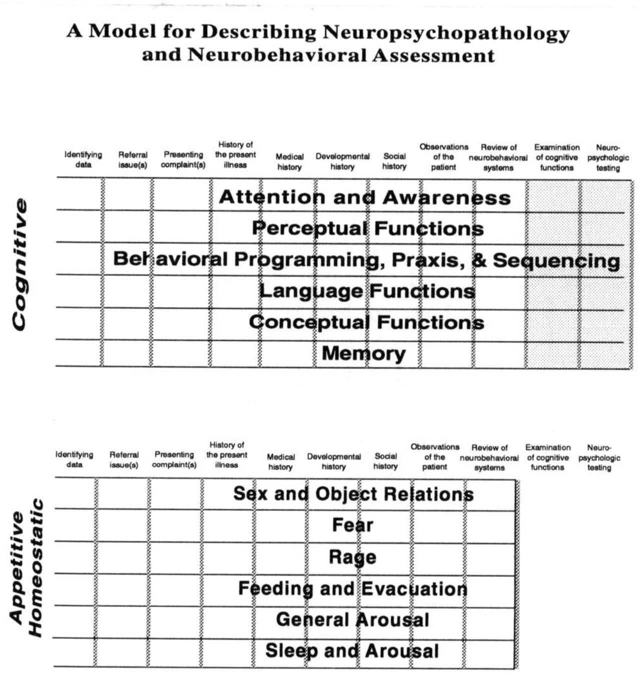

A Model for Describing Neuropsychopathology and Neurobehavioral Assessment

Figure 1. A Model for Describing Neuropsychopathology and Neurobehavioral Assessment: Cognitive Parameters, Appetitive/Homeostatic Parameters, and a Range of Methods for the Study of Each.

CONCLUSION

Expanding both the number and types of neurobehavioral functions which are studied during routine clinical neuropsychological assessment, and by subjecting each neurobehavioral function to multiple-complementary techniques of study, one can generate a sufficiently diverse array of data to permit the emergence of configurations of information which are inherently meaningful in diagnostic, treatment-planning, and prognostic aspects of clinical assessment.

Similarly, the generation of a comprehensive data set lends enhanced confidence in the validity of conclusions reached in forensic situations (Eruenwold, 1991; Matarazzo, 1990, 1991; Sbordone, 1991, Ch. 2, this volume), and should contribute to a more complete understanding of a wide range of basic research issues in the study of brain behavior relations

ACKNOWLEDGMENTS

The permission of Grune and Stratton Publishers to reprint figures from the published work of Sandor Rado is appreciated, as is the permission of Russell R. Monroe to utilize his schematic for depicting levels of episodic dyscontrol.

Ralph M. Reitan is thanked; both his candor and his permission to quote are appreciated.

The editorial assistance of Dr. Lief Crowe in the preparation of The Neurobehavioral Assessment Format is appreciated as are critical readings of this chapter by Drs. J.B. Orange, M. Spica, J.R. Julian, N. Varney, and Ms. M.B. Spina. The chapter is dedicated to the memories Louis J. Gerstman and Emerick Friedman.

REFERENCES

Bakker, D. J. (1984). The brain as a dependent variable. *Journal of Clinical Neuropsychology,* *6*(1), 1-16.

Bannister, R. (1992). *Brain and Bannister's clinical neurology* (7th ed.). New York: Oxford University Press.

Benton, A. (1967). Psychological tests for brain damage. In A. M. Freedman & H. I. Kaplan (Eds.), *Comprehensive textbook of psychiatry* (pp. 530-539). Baltimore, MD: Williams and Wilkins.

Bilder, R. M., & Kane, J. M. (1989). Assessment of organic mental disorders. In S. Wetzler (Ed.), *Measuring mental illness: Psychometric assessment for clinicians,* pp. 183-211, Washington, DC: American Psychiatric Press.

Borod, J. (1993). Emotion and the brain-anatomy: An introduction to the special section. *Neuropsychology,* 7(4), 427-432.

Bowers, D., Bauer, R., & Heilman, K. (1993). The nonverbal affect lexicon: Theoretical perspectives from neuropsychological studies of affect perception. *Neuropsychology, 7*(4), 433-444.

Buck, R. (1993). What is this thing called subjective experience. *Neuropsychology, 7*(4), 490-499.

Christensen, A. L. (1979). A practical application of the Luria methodology. *Journal of Clinical Neuropsychology, 1*(3), 241-247.

Christensen, A. L. (1989). The neuropsychological investigation as a therapeutic and rehabilitative technique. In D. W. Ellis & A. L. Christensen (Eds.), *Neuropsychological treatment after brain injury* (pp. 127-157). Norwell, MA: Kluwer.

Christensen, A. L. (1975). *Luria's neuropsychological investigation.* New York: Spectrum Publications.

Cummings, J. L. (1985). *Clinical neuropsychiatry.* New York: Grune & Stratton.

DeJong, R. N. (1979). *The neurologic examination.* New York: Harper & Row.

Department of Psychiatry Teaching Committee, The Institute of Psychiatry, London. (1973). *Notes on eliciting and recording clinical information.* New York: Oxford University Press.

Detre, T. P., & Jarecki, H. G. (1971). *Modern psychiatric treatment.* Philadelphia, PA: J. P. Lippincott.

Ellenberger, H. F. (1958). A clinical introduction to psychiatric phenomenology and existential analysis. In R. May, E. Angel, & H. F. Ellenberger (Eds.), *Existence: A new dimension in psychiatry and psychology.* New York: Basic Books.

Erikson, E. H. (1950). *Childhood and society* (2nd ed.). New York: W. W. Norton.

Eruenwold, D. (1991). *Comment on psychological assessment versus psychological testing. American Psychologist, 46,* 882.

Freud, A. (1966). *The ego and the mechanics of defense* (rev.). New York: International Universities Press.

Freud, S. (1900). The interpretation of dreams. In J. Strachey (Ed.), *Standard edition: The complete psychological works of Sigmund Freud, Vol. 18* (pp. 1-64). London: The Hogarth Press.

Freud, S. (1905). Three essays on the theory of sexuality. In J. Strachey (Ed.), *Standard edition: The complete psychological works of Sigmund Freud, Vol. 18* (pp. 1-64) London: The Hogarth Press.

Freud, S. (1915). Introductory lectures on psychoanalysis. In: J. Strachey (Ed.), Standard Edition: *The complete psychological works of Sigmund Freud.* Vol. 15, pt. 2 (pp. 83-228).

Gastaut, H., & Broughton, R. (1972). *Epileptic seizures: Clinical features, diagnosis, and treatment.* Springfield, IL: C. C. Thomas.

Goldstein, K. (1942). *After effects of brain injuries in man.* New York: Grune & Stratton.

Goldstein, K. (1959). The organismic approach. In S. Arieti (Ed.), *American handbook of psychiatry, Vol. 2.* New York: Basic Books.

Goldstein, K. (1963). *The organism: A holistic approach to biology derived from pathologic data in man.* Boston: Beacon Press.

Goodman, J. D., & Sours, J. A. (1967). *The child mental status examination.* New York: Basic Books.

Grosser, G. S., & Siegal, A. W. (1971). The emergence of a tonic-phasic model for sleep and dreaming. *Psychological Bulletin, 75,* 60-72.

Hall, R. C. W., Gardner, E. R., Stickney, S. K., LeCann, A. F., & Popkin, M. K. (1980). Physical illness manifesting as psychiatric disease. *Archives of General Psychiatry, 37,* 989-995.

Heller, W. (1993). Neuropsychological mechanisms of individual differences in emotion, personality, and arousal. *Neuropsychology, 7*(4), 476-489.

Hobson, J. A. (1992). A new model of brain-mind state activation level, input source, and mode of processing (A.I.M.). In J. S. Antrobus & M. Bertini, (Eds.), *The neuropsychology of sleep and dreaming.* Hillsdale, NJ: Lawrence Erlbaum Associates.

Hoch, P. M. (1972). *Differential diagnosis in clinical psychiatry: The lectures of Paul M. Hock, M.D.* New York: Science House.

Howieson, D. B., & Lezak, M. D. (1992). The neuropsychological examination. In S. C. Yudofsky & R. E. Hales, *The American Psychiatric Press textbook of neuropsychiatry,* (2nd ed.), 127-150. Washington, DC: American Psychiatric Press.

Jackson, J. H. (1958). Epileptiform convulsions from cerebral disease. In J. Taylor (Ed.), *Selected writings of John Hughlings Jackson,* 330-340. London: Staples Press. (Reprinted from Transactions International Medical Congress, Vol. II, 1881.)

Jaspers, K. (1963) *General psychopathology.* Chicago: University of Chicago Press.

Jennings, J. L. (1986). The forgotten distinction between psychology and phenomenology: Husserl revisited. *American Psychologist, 41*(11), 1231-1240.

Kaplan, E. (1988). A process approach to neuropsychological assessment. In B. T. Bryant, (Ed.), *Clinical neuropsychological and brain function* (pp. 125-167). Washington, DC: American Psychological Association.

Koranyi, E. K. (1979). Morbidity and rate of undiagnosed physical illnesses in a psychiatric clinical population. *Archives of General Psychiatry, 36,* 414-419.

Levine, M. D., Brooks, R., & Shonfoff, S. P. (1980). *A pediatric approach to learning disorders.* New York: Wiley.

Lishman, W. A. (1978). *Organic psychiatry: The consequences of cerebral disorder.* London: Blackwell Scientific Publication.

Luria, A. R. (1966). *Higher cortical functions in man.* New York: Basic Books.

MacKeith, R., & Bax, M. (Eds.). (1963). *Minimal cerebral dysfunction: Clinics in developmental medicine No. 10.* Spastics International Medical Publications, Lavenham Press, Suffolk, U.K.

Matarazzo, J. D. (1990). Psychological assessment versus psychological testing. *American Psychologist, 45*(9), 999-1017.

Matazarro, J. D. (1991). Psychological assessment is reliable and valid: A reply to Ziskin and Faust. *American Psychologist, 46,* 882-884.

Mesalaum, M. M. (1985). *Principles of behavioral neurology.* Philadelphia: F. A. Davis.

Molinari, M. N., & Foulkes, D. (1969). Tonic and phase events during sleep: Psychological, correlates, and implications. *Perceptual and Motor Skills, 29,* 343-368.

Monroe, R. R. (1974). Episodic behavioral disorders: An unclassified syndrome. In S. Arieti & E. B. Brody (Eds.), *American handbook of psychiatry, Volume 3,* 237-254. New York: Basic Books.

Monroe, R. R. (1975). Anti-convulsants in the treatment of aggression. *The Journal of Nervous and Mental Desiase, 160*(2), 119-126.

Monroe, R. R. (1978a). *Brain dysfunction in aggressive criminals.* Lexington, MA: D. C. Heath Co.

Monroe, R. R. (1978b). Criterion of dyscontrol: A self-reporting scale. In R. R. Monroe (Ed.), *Brain dysfunction in aggressive criminals.*

Monroe, R. R. (1970). *Episodic behavioral disorders: A psychodynamic and neurophysiologic analysis.* Cambridge, MA: Harvard University Press.

Monroe, R. R. (1982a). DSM-III style diagnosis of the episodic disorders. *Journal of Nervous and Mental Disease, 170*(11), 664-669.

Monroe, R. R. (1982b). The psychotherapy of the impulsive and acting-out patient. *Journal of the American Academy of Psychoanalysis, 10*, 1-26.

Moruzzi, G. (1963). Active processes in the brain stem during sleep. *Harvey Lecture Series 58*, 233-297.

Paine, R. & Oppe', T. Ed. (Ed.) (1965). *Neurological examination of children: Clinics in developmental medicine*, No. 20. Spastics International Medical Publications, Lavenham Press, Suffolk, U. K.

Paine, R. & Oppe', T.Ed. (Ed.) (1965b). *Neurological examination of children: Clinics in developmental medicine*, No. 21. Spastics International Medical Publications, Lavenham Press, Suffolk, U. K.

Penfield, W., & Jasper, J. (1954). *Epilepsy and the functional anatomy of the brain*. Boston, MA: Little, Brown and Company.

Piaget, J. (1973). *The child and reality: Problems of genetic psychology*. New York: Grossman Publishers.

Pivik, R. T. (1978). Tonic states and phasic events in relation to sleep mentation. In A. M. Arkin, J. S. Antrobus, & S. J. Ellman, (Eds.), *The mind in sleep: Psychology and psychophysiology*, 245-276. Hillsdale, NJ: Lawrence Erlbaum Associates.

Pivik, R. T. (1991). Tonic states and phasic events in relation to sleep mentation. In S. J. Ellman & J. S. Antrobus (Eds.), *The mind in sleep: Psychology and psychophysiology*, 214-276. Hillsdale, NJ: Lawrence Erlbaum Associates.

Rado, S. (1969). *Adaptational psychodynamics: Motivation and control*. J. Jameson, & H. Klein. Science House, New York City, NY.

Rado, S. (1956). Adaptational psychodynamics: A basic science. In S. Rado (Ed.), *Psychoanalysis of behavior*, Vol. I, 332-346. New York: Grune & Stratton.

Rado, S. (1955/1956a). Hedonic control, action-self and the depressive spell. In S. Rado (Ed.), *Psychoanalysis of behavior*, Vol. 1, 286-311. New York: Grune & Stratton.

Rado, S. (1955/1956b). Mind, unconscious mind, and brain. In S. Rado (Ed.), *Psychoanalysis of behavior*, Vol. 1., (pp. 180-186). New York: Grune & Stratton.

Rado, S. (1946/1956). Psychodynamics as a basic science. In S. Rado, *Psychoanalysis of behavior*, Vol 1., 167-173. New York: Grune & Stratton.

Rado, S. (1955/1956) Emergency behavior with an introduction to the dynamics of conscience. In S. Rado (Ed.), *Psychoanalysis of behavior*, Vol. 1, 214-234. New York: Grune & Stratton.

Rado, S. (1958/1962). From the metapsychologic ego to the biocultural action-self. In S. Rado (Ed.), *Psychoanalysis of behavior*, Vol. 2, 42-48. New York: Grune and Stratton.

Rado, S. (1961/1962). Toward the construction of an organized foundation for clinical psychiatry. In S. Rado, (Ed.), *Psychoanalysis of behavior*, Vol. 2, 152-162. New York: Grune and Stratton.

Rapin, I., & Wilson, B. C. (1978). Children with developmental language disability: Neurological aspects and assessment. In M. A. Wyke (Ed.), *Developmental dysphasia*. London: Academic Press.

Reitan, R. M., & Wolfson, D. (1993). *Theoretical, methodological, and validational bases of the Halstead-Reitan Neuropsychologic Test Battery*. Tucson, AZ: Reitan Neuropsychologic Laboratory.

Reitan, R. M. (1966). A research program on the psychological effects of brain lesions in human beings. In N. R. Ellis (Ed.), *International review of research in mental retardation*, Vol. 1. New York: Academic Press.

Reitan, R. M. (1959). *Effects of brain lesions on adaptive abilities in human beings*. Indianapolis, IN: Author.

Report of the Task Force on Education, Accreditation, and Credentialing of the International Neuropsychological Society. (1981). *The International Neuropsychological Society Bulletin*, 5-10.

Richardson, S. A. (1964). The social environment and individual functioning in H. G. Birch (Ed.), *Brain damage in children*. Baltimore, MD: Williams & Wilkins.

Rourke, B. P. (1983). Outstanding issues in research on learning disabilities. In M. Rutter (Ed.), *Developmental neuropsychiatry* (pp. 564-577). New York: Guilford Press.

Rutter, M. (1983). *Developmental neuropsychiatry*. New York: Guilford Press.

Sbordone, R. J. (1987). A neuropsychological approach to cognitive rehabilitation within a private practice setting. In B. Caplan (Ed.), *Rehabilitation psychology desk reference* (pp. 323-343) Rockville, MD: Aspen Publishers.

Sbordone, R. J. (1991). *Neuropsychology for the attorney*. Delray Beach, FL: St. Lucie Press.

Schain, R. J. (1972). *Neurology of childhood learning disorders*. Baltimore, MD: Williams & Wilkins.

Schechter, M. D. (1970). Etiology of mental disorders: Prenatal factors. In B. B. Wolman (Ed.), *Manual of child psychopathology*. New York: McGraw Hill.

Schechter, M. D. (1991). *Clinical assessment of child neurobehavioral cases: Integrating signs, symptoms, historical, and laboratory data with examination and testing results*. Presented at Siegal, A. W., Schechter, M. D., Diamond, Costa, L. D., & Wilson B. C., Integrative Neurobehavioral Assessment Workshop, Ninth Annual Meeting of the International Neuropsychological Society.

Shaffer, D., & Dunn, J. (1979). *The first year of life*. New York: Wiley.

Siegal, A. W., Schechter, M. D., & Diamond, S. P. (1983). *Neurobehavioral assessment format*. Albany, NY: Author.

Smith, A. (1975). Neuropsychological testing in neurological disorders. In W. J. Friedlander (Ed.), *Advances in neurology: Current reviews of nervous system dysfunction, Vol 7*. New York: Raven Press.

Smith, A. (1981). Principles underlying human brain functions in neuropsychological sequellae of different neuropathological processes. In S. B. Filskov & T. J. Boll (Eds.), *Handbook of clinical neuropsychology*. New York: Wiley.

Spillane, J. D. (1975). *An atlas of clinical neurology*. New York: Oxford University Press.

Spreen, O., Tupper, D., Rieser, A., Tuokko, H., Edgell, D. (1984). *Human developmental neuropsychology*. New York: Oxford University Press.

Tucker, D. N. (1993). Emotional experience and the problem of vertical integration: Discussion of special sections on emotion. *Neuropsychology, 7*, 500-510.

Tupper, D. (1987). *Soft neurological signs*. Orlando, FL: Grune & Stratton.

Wender, P. H. (1987). *The hyperactive child, adolescent, and adult: Attention deficit disorder through the lifespan*. New York: Oxford University Press.

Wilson, B. A. (1987). Single-case experimental designs in neuropsychological rehabilitation. *Journal of Clinical and Experimental Neuropsychology, 9*(5), 527-544.

Wilson, B. C. (1986). An approach to the neuropsychologic assessment of the preschool child with developmental defects. In S. B. Filskov & T. J. Boll (Eds.), *Handbook of clinical neuropsychology*, Vol. 2, 121-171. New York: Plenum.

Wilson, B. C. (1987). Neuropsychologic assessment. In V. B. Van Hasset & M. Herson (Eds.), *Psychologic evaluation of the developmentally and physically disabled*. New York: Plenum.

Wilson, B. C., & Davidovicz, H. M. (1987). Neuropsychological assessments of the child with cerebral palsy. *Seminars in Speech and Language, 1*, 1-18.

Wilson, B. C., & Rourke, B. (1980, December). *Neuropsychological assessment of the learning disabled child.* Second Annual Perspectives in Child Clinical Neuropsychology lecture presented at North Shore University Hospital, Manhasset, New York.

Wilson, B. C. (1992). The neuropsychological assessment of the preschool child: A branching model. In I. Rapin & S. J. Segalowitz, (Eds.), *Handbook of neuropsychology,* Vol. 6: 377-394. New York: Elsevier.

APPENDIX I

Methodologic Caveats in the Use of Anamnestic Data in Clinical Neuropsychological Assessment, in the Development and Validation of Neuropsychological Tests, and in Clinical Training in Neuropsychologic Test Interpretation*

A Personal Communication from Ralph M. Reitan

1/12/93

I have had a difficult time making my position clear regarding my use of history information and findings from other relevant disciplines with relation to neuropsychological test results. In your chapter you may be able to clarify the situation.

First, a differentiation should be made between research and clinical procedures. In research, standard protocol requires that independent and dependent variables be identified separately. One must take steps to be sure that the neuropsychological test results are not influenced by neurological findings and vice versa. Nevertheless, the overall aim is to establish consistent and meaningful relationships between the two sources of data. I tried to simulate this procedure in my clinical research efforts to test and validate neuropsychological interpretations by doing the interpretations without having referred to history information and neurological findings (independent variables). In this way I was able to find out how well the neuropsychological test data related along selected clinical dimensions to the independent criterion variables or classification.

At this point I should mention that I have never ignored or de-emphasized the anamnestic technique or findings from other disciplines. Just the opposite is true and it would have to be in order to fulfil the plan outlined above. In fact, my files are full of detailed history information and neurological findings, of research quality and detail, on all of the subjects we examined. Of course, our procedures for collecting and filing this information was separate from our testing and research-oriented interpretations of the test data in order to meet the requirement that no cross-influence occur between independent and dependent variables. As you can see, I was serious about neuropsychology developing competencies that identified it as a separate discipline; other disciplines are equally competent in reaching neurological conclusions, but neuropsychology is the only discipline that is known for its competence in using standardized and objective psychological tests to draw valid inferences regarding both the biological condition of the brain and its behavioral manifestations.

My own clinical work in neuropsychology has always dealt with exactly the same types of variables as is generally true in the field. One thing, however, is quite different, and that is the sequence with which I use the data and information. I review the test results first and record my conclusions. Only then do I turn to the history information and other findings. At this point, I relate the test results to referring questions, patient's complaints, results of other examinations, patient's past history, etc. As you can see, I carry over my belief in the uniqueness, validity, and independence of neuropsychological test findings into the clinical situation, even though separate professional personnel are required to obtain the two sources of data and information.

I think the above is quite clear and straightforward, and I often wonder why my position and practice is so inaccurately represented in the literature. The reason, in part, probably stems from my emphasis on separation of independent and dependent variables not only in formal research studies but also in the process of learning how to do clinical neuropsychological interpretations of the test data. The second point, however, probably concerns that reluctance of clinical neuropsychologists to commit their conclusions to paper, patient by patient, considering the fact the indisputable neurological findings might show up their limitation. In situation that especially call for objectivity in interpretation of test data (e.g., litigation), I routinely write my evaluation based on the test results first, and then write a separate section of the report which considers all additional information (the complete history, opinions of other experts, results of specialized neurological diagnostic procedures, etc.), and only then attempt to reconcile the two sections if necessary. Many neuropsychologists seem to much prefer clinical practices which are not constrained by validity-checks. Thus, they develop a host of reasons for "looking up the answer in the back of the book" (that is, reviewing the history and findings from other disciplines) before interpreting their test results. Another even less rigorous approach is to use a casually-selected test battery that has never been researched as a test battery and for which no standards of interpretation have been developed. Combination of these two latter procedures, in fact, provides many neuropsychologists with the best of all worlds—knowing the answer in advance and almost complete freedom to adapt the test results to explain (or explain away) the clinical problems and circumstances.

> Ralph M. Reitan
> Personal Communication
> 1/12/93

* Title for this appendix was provided by this writer (A.W.S.).

4

FUNCTIONAL CONSIDERATIONS IN NEUROPSYCHOLOGY

Gerald Goldstein, Ph.D., A.B.P.P.

This chapter pursues the problem of relating neuropsychological data to behavior in natural environments. The chapter begins with a critique of current practices in this research area, and then makes some suggestions for future work. The basic premise of this critique is that neuropsychologists have attempted to work in the area of ecological validity without adequate training, experience, or access to technologies that are necessary for such work. These inadequacies lie in three disciplines; ecological psychology, behavior theory, and rehabilitation technology and methodology. It is asserted that these lacks of expertise typically limit neuropsychologists' capacities to conceptualize and study the environment, systematically observe the behavior of individuals in environments, and understand the distinction between behaviors measured by tests and functions performed in natural settings.

ECOLOGICAL PSYCHOLOGY

Ecological psychology is the study of behavior in natural settings. The discipline had its origins in the field theory of Lewin (1951), but its founders and major contributors were Roger Barker and Herbert Wright. These psychologists made at least two major contributions to our understanding of the relationship of behavior to the environment. First, they developed precise and detailed methods for observing, recording, and analyzing the behavior of individuals in natural settings (Wright, 1967). Second, they made a profound contribution to conceptualization of the human environment. Using such key concepts as the behavior setting, they were able to describe relationships between behavior and the environment in which it occurred in precise detail. A behavior setting has been defined by Barker (1968) as consisting of "one or more standing patterns of behavior-and-milieu, with the milieu circumjacent and synomorphic to the behavior" (p. 19). By circumjacent and synomorphic Barker means surrounding the behavior spatially or temporally, and similar in structure. Barker and Wright (1951, 1955) eschewed the use of tests, and did their work by systematically observing individuals, mainly children, in natural settings. This work is documented particularly well in *Midwest and Its Children* and *One Boy's Day*. Illustrative of the detail and complexity of this area is that *One Boy's Day* consists entirely of the behavioral description and analysis of a single child over the course of a single day.

Some degree of mastery of the theory and technologies of ecological psychology should provide the neuropsychologist with two skills that would appear to be crucial for establishing the ecological validity of tests. First, there is the matter of accurately observing, recording, and analyzing behavior in natural settings with sophisticated and established technologies. Second, there is the capacity to characterize environments, and to relate behavior to being in different environments or behavior settings. It is difficult to understand how one can develop ecological validity criteria without the capacity to systematically observe and record behavior in natural settings, or to characterize the environments in which behaviors occur.

BEHAVIOR THEORY

There is a long-standing debate in theoretical psychology concerning the appropriate unit of behavior for scientific study. The distinction between "molar" and "molecular" approaches to the analysis of behavior was made many years ago (Brunswik, 1955). The ecological psychologists have a strong preference for molar behavior. Their unit of study is meaningful interactions with the environment, which might be characterized as episodes or events. At the extreme, advocates of the study of behavior at a molecular level use such response measures as reaction times, single reflexes, or simple motor responses as units of observation. Advocates of molecular theory believe that more complex behaviors are built up out of these simpler elements. Advocates of molar theories do not accept that view, believing that molar behaviors have emergent properties. This debate has been characterized as the reductionist argument.

Does neuropsychology do better with a molecular or molar approach to behavior? The author proposes that neuropsychology probably should not view this matter as a debate, since it may benefit from working at both levels. As assessors and, to a large extent, as researchers, we tend to be molecular. We divide behavior into abilities such as language, memory, abstraction, and spatial skills. Implicitly, we assume that differing levels of performance among these abilities will be determinants of behavior in the environment. However, behavior in the environment rarely, if ever, involves use of any single ability in isolation from other abilities. We probably use most of our abilities, to a greater or lesser extent, most of the time. Indeed, the neuropsychological analysis of individual tasks is quite complex.

For example, if we looked at the molecular structure of reading a newspaper we would have to involve, at a minimum, numerous linguistic skills, visual perception, working memory, visual-motor function, and higher cognitive functions. As neuropsychologists, we know that such molecular analyses are helpful in relating complex behavioral processes to brain function, and in delineating specific difficulties a patient may have in performing a complex behavior. However, it is not particularly helpful in describing and analyzing behavior as an event in daily life. The ecology of reading a newspaper involves an episode in what Barker (1963) characterizes as "the stream of behavior" within a behavior setting. Typically, people read newspapers at home or in libraries rather than in church or while performing surgery.

An alternative method of evaluating behavior in natural settings comes from the field of behavioral assessment. Behavioral assessment tends to be more molecular than the methods of Barker and Wright. Hartmann and Wood (1990) describe and discuss a number of observational methods used in behavioral assessment, and like the ecological psychologists, incorporate the environment in what they characterize as observation settings. Their methods, such as time sampling or interval recording tend to be more appropriate for molecular, repeated behaviors than are the ecological methods, that focus on full episodes. Thus, behavioral assessment may evaluate such behaviors as eye contact, or activity level as measured with a pedometer. While there are numerous substantive and theoretical differences between ecological psychology and behavioristically oriented behavioral assessment, both theories and their theorists would agree that the environment plays a critical role in the determination of behavior.

FUNCTIONAL ASSESSMENT

SOME DEFINITIONS

The language associated with the description of cognitive and physical capacities and disorders contains a number of words that are often not clearly defined, or distinguished from one another. The most important of the capacity words, for our present purposes, are ability and function. In neuropsychology, we unfortunately often use these words synonymously, as when we speak of language abilities or functions. From a rehabilitative standpoint, however, they are not the same thing. An ability is a skill or talent within the individual, and may be assessed with instruments of the neuropsychological test type. A function is the exercise of an ability in an environmental context. Thus, speech is an ability; requesting information is a function. Motor skill is an ability, riding a bicycle is a function. Spatial skill is an ability; dressing is a function. This distinction is why occupational and physical therapists perform their assessments either by asking about or observing patients perform practical tasks. They are primarily interested in functions rather than ability. This distinction is reflected in speech/language pathology through development of standard aphasia tests, to assess ability, and tests of functional language, notably the Sarno Functional Communication Profile (FCP) (Sarno, 1969) and the Holland Communicative Abilities in Daily Living (CADL) test (Holland, 1980) to evaluate function.

Under conditions of disorder, when an ability becomes disrupted, we say that the person has acquired an *impairment.* That impairment may produce a functional deficit, which is generally called a *disability.* A disability may prevent a person from performing certain functions in society, in which case we say that the person has a *handicap.* Thus, a sprained ankle (impairment), may produce a problem with walking (disability), thus preventing the individual from playing basketball (handicap). An aphasia (impairment) may prevent an individual from conversing on the telephone (disability) leading to not being able to work as a telephone operator (handicap).

IMPLICATIONS OF THE DEFINITIONS

From the standpoint of the ecological validity of neuropsychological tests, these definitions might suggest that ecological validity has to do with the relationship between abilities and functions in general. In the case of disorder, it has to do with the relationship of impairment to disability or handicap. In essence, that is what investigators have done in the research already accomplished. As Acker (1990) pointed out, the functional criterion measures have traditionally been statistical relationships (correlations) between test scores and outcome measures, comparisons between test scores and anecdotal evidence of functioning (testimony), or classification tables containing hit rates of tests and functional categories (e.g., employed/unemployed). Depending upon test characteristics and subject variables, such as stage of recovery, some tests are relatively good predictors and some are relatively poor predictors of outcome.

PROBLEMS OF PREDICTION AND OUTCOME

PREDICTION

We now return to the matter of the extent to which neuropsychological tests relate to behavior in the environment. As alluded to above, and described in detail in Acker's (1990) review, investigators have found moderate correlations between test results and various forms of functional assessment. Franzen (this volume) describes the strength of this relationship as the veridicality of the test. Apparently, this term applies to empirical validity based upon studies of correlation between test scores and measures of relevant behaviors. He also characterizes tests in terms of verisimilitude, or the extent to which the test in question is similar to the naturally occurring behavior of interest. Based on considerations offered here, we would suggest that the attainment of verisimilitude is a virtual impossibility. Even if the test used completely duplicated the naturally occurring behavior, it would not be duplicated in a setting in which that behavior typically occurs. The test would of necessity be given in the behavior setting of a laboratory or clinic, rather than that of the street or a supermarket. The contributions of the environment would be substantially different. One naturally behaves differently in front of a doctor than in front of a checkout clerk. Thus, there seems little point in making up tests that on the surface look like real life, because they probably will not be like real life for the patient at all.

There appears to be substantially more hope for veridicality. Regardless of the surface appearance of the test, empirical validity studies can and have documented relatively robust relationships between test scores and functional outcome measures (e.g., Acker & Davis, 1989; McCue, Rogers, & Goldstein, 1990). Unfortunately, however, the literature suggests that the correlations obtained appear to have an upper limit of about 40% explained variance. Thus, while psychometrically satisfactory validity coefficients may be obtained, our present capacity to make individual predictions is quite limited.

A potentially productive approach to designing ecologically relevant neuropsychological tests is that of functional analysis, in which we divide functions, which are generally complex, into the simpler, individual abilities required to perform them. Here, we are aided by theoretical conceptualizations proposed some time ago by Werner (1937) and Scheerer (1946), and represented at present in the process approach to neuropsychology (Kaplan, 1988). However, in this case, the purpose of the functional analysis, or "performance analysis" as Scheerer called it, is not that of inferring brain localization but rather that of inferring from a test or series of tests what the individual may be able to do or not do in a natural setting. Thus, we ask questions like what skills and abilities would an individual need to use a telephone or write a check? In our research, we correlate test or test profile results against appropriate activities of daily living. Here, multiple regression and related techniques are quite helpful (e.g., McCue, et al., 1990).

The major caveat we would offer here is that these functional analyses are "armchair activities," and must be followed by empirical observation or experimentation to prove whether or not the analyses are correct or not. It is generally necessary to do a study in which the test or test combination results are correlated with the individual's capacity to perform the function. In view of considerations raised above, the examination of capacity to perform the function should ideally not be done in the clinic or laboratory, unless those are natural settings for the subject. Rather, they should be done at home or wherever the individual customarily performs the function. Even more ideally, the function should be observed in several places, so that generalization across settings can be evaluated.

As a general hint provided by the available literature, complex tests appear to be better predictors of activities of daily living than simple tests. For example, the Halstead Category Test (Halstead, 1947), a complex problem-solving task, has been shown to have high predictive power in a number of studies. Correspondingly, tests of elementary perceptual and motor skills have less power. In a study by Acker and Davis (1989), for example, the correlation between the Wechsler Memory Scale MQ and a global measure of functional outcome was -.48 ($p<.001$); the correlation for the color recognition component of the Stroop test was -.16 ($p>.05$). The notion that one can predict performance levels of complex functions from an analysis of what are assumed to be component individual skills has proven to be largely illusory. Thus, tests that may have high relevance as components of the neurological evaluation may have little capacity to predict functional outcome.

The advantage of a process or performance analysis approach in development of ecologically relevant tests is that it is not necessarily the test score itself that is most predictive of functional outcome. While the data are certainly not in regarding this matter, one may wonder about whether or not the manner in which an individual proceeds through a complex cognitive task may be more reflective of the way that individual performs at work than would be the fact that the task is successfully completed or not. Watching a patient struggling with the Tactual Performance Test, trying to force blocks into holes that they don't fit, or preseverating through the Category test, regardless of the informative feedback provided by the buzzer and chime, may be quite revealing of the way in which an individual would perform a job or manage a household. On the more positive side, watching a severely aphasic patient "breeze through" Block Design might suggest capabilities far beyond what is immediately suggested by the severely limited, halting speech. The effort to formulate objective scoring systems for process analysis, as in the case of the WAIS-R-NI (WAIS-R for Neuropsychological Interpretation) (Kaplan, Fein, Morris, & Delis, 1991), is quite likely to significantly aid the study of ecological validity.

OUTCOME

Often, abnormal neuropsychological test results do not bespeak life-threatening illness or clearly treatable conditions. That situation has raised, in a somewhat trivialized form, the "So-what?" question. Now that you know that the patient has these impairments what do you do? Where do you go from there? Underlying this question may be the question of what meaning these deficits have for the patient's life. Physician's typically describe some of their positive findings with phraseology like "not disabling" or "not clinically significant." Thus, symptomatology of this type is not felt to be consequential for the patient's health or longevity. The author's impression is that neuropsychologists are less likely to do this, and are more inclined to view most, if not all abnormal findings as serious. They may not be viewed as serious in terms of morbidity and mortality, but they may be understood as having implications for the patient's functioning in the "real world."

We often seem to assume implicitly that the office or clinic in which we give our tests is not part of the "real world." The tests themselves may not be "real." The "real world" is somewhere else, and is not a place where people take tests. In view of the remarks above, we would view the clinic or office as behavior settings that produce forces influencing individuals to behave in certain ways; doctors behave "doctor," and patients behave "patient." Taking tests is behavior occurring in that setting. Perhaps one of the most cogent ways of describing that behavior is found in Rapaport's (1946) distinction between intelligence-concept formation and personality tests.

In the former, the subject is required to live up to a standard, and his type of deviation from it becomes a basis of his diagnosis; in the latter, it is the characteristic course of his own spontaneous thought processes—his own reactions to, understanding and organization of, and selective choice from, different more or less complex situations—which is the basis of diagnosis. (p. 4)

Elsewhere, Rapaport has informally described testing as a situation in which one induces anxiety to determine how the patient copes with it. Whether or not one agrees with these formulations, they make clear that the testing situation is a kind of behavior setting that has particular characteristics.

The question to be asked then becomes "Does behavior in the testing behavior setting generalize to related behaviors in other settings?" This question is really another way of putting the various definitions of ecological validity provided by Franzen (this volume) (e.g., generalization from controlled assessment situations to naturally occurring phenomena). This author only disagrees in one respect. A testing clinic is as natural as is any other place in the world; it is simply a different behavior setting. As Rapaport (1946) has indicated, when cognitive testing is being done, it is a place where one is required to live up to standards. Other characteristics are doubtlessly present, and it would be of great benefit to our studies of generalization if someone did a full characterization of a testing clinic as a behavior setting.

OUTCOME EVALUATION METHODS

This chapter indicated that the major methods used to evaluate outcome are testimony, classification into functional categories, and quantitative outcome measures. These three methods are discussed in terms of their value as criterion measures in studies of ecological validity, concentrating on quantitative outcome measures of function.

TESTIMONY AND CLASSIFICATION

Anecdotal testimony is rarely used seriously as an outcome measure in research because of obvious validity and reliability problems. However, testimony has some heuristic value, which the author would like to illustrate in the following anecdote:

A stroke patient received a neuropsychological evaluation, partially in response to a referral question concerning his ability to return to driving. The report indicated that because of the patient's cognitive deficits, he would not be capable of driving a car. Nevertheless, the patient applied for restoration of his license, passed the examination, and was reported to be driving safely.

This kind of anecdotal material is useful because it illustrates the presence or absence of ecological validity of tests, or of inferences made from tests, in a rather clear-cut fashion. In this case, it also might constitute a cautionary tale for the neuropsychologist, who might wish to become more circumspect about making predictions from test results. Ecological psychology makes extensive use of anecdotal data, but they are collected in a highly rigorous and detailed way. In this case, the data are referred to as specimen records (Barker & Wright, 1955; Wright, 1967), and consist of the notes of trained observers concerning the individual and the setting.

The outcome classification most commonly used appears to be employment status. In this case, test results are compared with whether or not subjects are or are not working. This matter was reviewed some time ago by Heaton, Chelune, and Lehman (1978) and by Heaton and Pendleton (1981). One important conclusion was that neuropsychological tests and indices, particularly the Average Impairment Rating from the Halstead-Reitan battery (Russell, Neuringer, & Goldstein, 1970), are reasonably good predictors of employment status. In studies of patients with more severe disorders, classification was based on independent living categories such as ability to eat, dress, and walk (Winograd, 1984).

Utilizing discrete categories as criteria for ecological validity studies has obvious practical value, and there are essentially no difficulties with the reliability of the criterion measure. However, these measures are not at all refined, and one might wish to know more about functioning after giving a lengthy battery of neuropsychological tests. We would only note that the available literature suggests that neuropsychological tests are reasonably good predictors of employability in the case of brain-damaged patients.

QUANTITATIVE MEASURES

The use of quantitative measures of function is based largely on an alliance between neuropsychology and the rehabilitation specialties; notably occupational and physical therapy. Linn and Linn (1983) categorized the assessment instruments designed by rehabilitation specialists into Activities of Daily Living (ADL) scales, and Instrumental Activities of Daily Living (IADL) scales. ADL refers to the most basic activities; eating, toileting, walking, dressing, and bathing, while IADL refers to more complex activities such as shopping, cooking, using transportation, using devices such as telephones, and managing money. Brief descriptions of many of these instruments may be found in Crook, Ferris, and Bartus (1983). They may be divided into three types; self-report interview or questionnaire reports by patients, interview or questionnaire reports by informants, and performance tests. The most well-known and comprehensive instruments incorporating several of these assessment types are the OARS Multidimensional Functional Assessment (Duke University Center for the Study on Aging,

1978) and the Comprehensive Assessment and Referral Evaluation (CARE) (Gurland et al., 1977).

In recent years, efforts have been made to develop ADL scales that place a relatively heavy emphasis on instrumental and cognitive activities. One such instrument, the Performance Activities of Daily Living (PADL) (Kuriansky & Gurland, 1976), contains items that ask the patient to make a phone call, tell time, and sign his or her name. More recently, the Performance Assessment of Self-Care Skills (PASS) (Rogers, 1987) was developed. It contains a considerably larger number of items with heavy emphasis on cognitive content. As indicated above, specific performance tests in the area of language were developed by Sarno (1969) and Holland (1980).

Vocational and rehabilitation counselors have developed a number of instruments that can be useful to neuropsychologists when patients are seeking employment or are already working. These include the Functional Assessment Profile, the Functional Assessment Inventory, the Personal Capacities Questionnaire, the Preliminary Diagnostic Questionnaire, the Scale of Employability, the Vocational Behavior Checklist, and the Vocational Diagnosis and Assessment of Residual Employability. Some of these instruments are self-rating scales or questionnaires, while others are completed by informants. Basically, these instruments assess vocationally relevant strengths and weaknesses of clients receiving vocational rehabilitation services. While they were not intended to be used as criteria for neuropsychological ecological validity studies, they have potential to be used for that purpose because they provide functional assessments in the sense we have defined the term. Actually, these instruments are probably more pertinent for young patients who are potentially employable than are the ADL and IADL scales, which are probably more appropriate for elderly and more severely disabled patients who are not employable. For example, the Functional Assessment Inventory specifically evaluates memory, learning ability, and speech.

An effort to make a functional assessment instrument that is specifically relevant to neuropsychology is represented in the Patient Assessment of Own Functioning Inventory (PAF) (Chelune, Heaton, & Lehman, 1986). Originally designed as a patient self-rating, unpublished versions for relatives and other informants have been constructed. The items are exactly the same for each form, except for change in person (You or He/She). The inventory is divided into sections covering memory, language and communication, use of hands, and higher level cognitive and intellectual functions. The items, such as "How often do you have difficulties understanding what is said to you?" are answered on a 6-point scale ranging from "almost always" to "almost never." Sunderland, Harris, and Gleave (1984) developed a similar instrument specialized for memory failures. A sample item is "Completely forgetting to do things you said you would do, and things you planned to do." Responses range from "Not at all in the last three months" to "More than once a day."

RESULTS OF STUDIES UTILIZING OUTCOME EVALUATION METHODS

Detailed reviews of ecological validity studies are found in Acker (1990), Chelune and Moehle (1986), and Heaton and Pendleton (1981). The major conclusions of those reviews are that there are reasonable correlations between test results and outcome methods. However, although Acker reports correlations as high as .85, the explained variance rarely exceeds 40%. An important proviso, however, is that brain-damaged patients are poor informants concerning their actual capacity levels. This phenomenon is of interest in and of itself (Chelune, et al., 1986), but for purposes of this discussion, it is unwise to use patient self-ratings as accurate criterion measures for ecological validity studies. In a recent study, Goldstein and McCue (1992) reconfirmed the finding that patients were, in general, poorer judges of their own capacities than were informants. However, there were some abilities, notably basic perceptual and motor skills, in which the correlations between ratings and neuropsychological test scores were statistically significant and equally high for patients and informants. That finding, however, should not detract from the more general one that patients are poor judges of their own ability levels.

There does not appear to be any particular test or test battery that is superior to other procedures with regard to ecological validity. Except for the general finding that complex tests tend to be better predictors than simple tests, the superiority of one predictor over another will vary greatly with different patient populations. Acker (1990) points out that tests are more or less valid predictors depending upon the recovery stage at which the tests are administered. Goldstein, McCue, Rogers, and Nussbaum (1992) showed that in elderly patients, accurate neuropsychological predictors of outcome were vastly different for patients with dementia and depressed patients.

SUGGESTIONS FOR FUTURE WORK

Tests or predictors and outcome measures or criteria are both surrogates for actual abilities and behaviors. A test assesses an ability, but is not the ability itself. Likewise, outcome rating scales or performance tests represent behaviors of interest, but are not themselves such behaviors. In neuropsychological terms, the interest then becomes a matter of determining how deficits associated with brain dysfunction impact on behaviors in specified behavior settings of interest.

How can we go about making more ecologically valid neuropsychological tests? First, most neuropsychological tests were not meant to be ecologically valid. They are typically evaluated against indicators of brain function and structure, such as neurosurgical or radiological data. Rather than remain in hope that these same tests will also have ecological validity, it would appear to be more productive to design tests with ecological validity in mind. Perhaps the Rivermead Behavioral Memory Test (RBMT) (Wilson, Cockburn, & Baddeley, 1985) is the best current example of this effort. The RBMT may well be ecologically valid not because of the practical nature of some of the items, but because from the beginning, the development of the test was oriented toward prediction of behavior in the environment. Indeed, it was derived from a checklist of patients' and informants' reports about various memory problems (Sunderland, et al., 1984).

The first task then becomes one of developing tests that are neuropsychological in nature, but are also ecologically relevant. The task is a difficult one because most of the current tests were not designed to be ecologically relevant although, by good fortune, they may turn out to have that characteristic. The RBMT was used as the example because it was designed to be ecologically relevant. However, it is also a plausible memory test that may be quite useful in conventional neuropsychological assessment. As a general principle, it might be a good idea during test development to validate new procedures not only against standard medical criteria but also against ecological criteria. This practice is not uncommon in the fields of educational and industrial testing, where outcome studies are often done to see if tests are predictive of academic or vocational success. For example, extensive work of this type has been done with the General Aptitude Test Battery (GATB) (Hartigan & Wigdor, 1989). We may look forward to the day in which outcome studies are tightly woven into the fabric of neuropsychological research.

As indicated above, tests based on a process or performance analysis approach to assessment may be particularly helpful. For example, the practice of allowing a client to complete a task after the time limit has expired can provide useful information concerning possibly relevant work-related considerations with regard to whether or not a particular function can be performed at all. If slowness is the major problem, then several possibilities arise, such as accommodation in the workplace, or specific retraining to increase speed.

THE NEED FOR BETTER OUTCOME MEASURES

Efforts to predict outcome may come to nothing if adequate measures of outcome are not available. As in other areas of validation research, the criterion is a crucial matter. In this review of quantitative measures it was indicated that most of these measures consisted of questionnaires, rating scales, interviews, and performance tests. All but the performance tests may be accomplished by the patients themselves or by informants. These instruments were developed mainly within the frameworks of the rehabilitation specialties and vocational rehabilitation counseling, and are primarily functional assessment procedures. The author offers the view that none of the available instruments or techniques provide sufficiently adequate criterion measures for establishing the ecological validity of neuropsychological tests. Like the tests themselves, with the exception of the PAF, none of these instruments were developed with neuropsychology in mind. Rather, they were called into service by neuropsychologists as the best available outcome measures.

A criticism often heard about assessments developed within the framework of the rehabilitation specialties is that while the instruments used may do an excellent job of evaluating physical capacities and personal self-care skills, relatively less emphasis is placed on tasks with heavy information processing loads. Efforts to alter this situation have included the development of the PADL and PASS as general functional assessments, the Sunderland, Harris, and Gleave (1984) functional assessment of memory, the Functional Communication Profile and CADL, as functional assessments of language, and the PAF as a functional assessment instrument specifically designed to be neuropsychologically relevant. Nevertheless, more needs to be done in this area, particularly with regard to vocationally relevant outcome measures.

The matter of self-rating vs. informant interview vs. performance test requires some discussion. It now seems clear that self-ratings of function made by brain-damaged patients do not typically reflect the objective situation. Interviews or questionnaires given to knowledgeable informants have been shown to be better, but problems with possible bias remain. Reliability studies accomplished with multiple informants observing the same subject appear to be needed. The performance test, in which individuals are asked to actually accomplish ADL tasks, preferably at their residences, appears to be ideal. Nevertheless, these instruments also require inter-rater reliability studies, as accomplished in the case of the PASS (Rogers, 1987). A potential problem with performance tests is that they could become too "test like," a situation that would compromise their value as validation criteria. For example, the actual performance requirements may be quite similar for dialing a phone number from instructions and repeating a set of digits on an intelligence test. Particular care must be taken to assure that items on ADL performance tests are closer to behaviors in the subject's everyday environment than they are to test behaviors.

THE NEED FOR ANALYSIS OF THE ENVIRONMENT

Common sense dictates that the best way to determine whether or not an individual performs some task well or poorly is to directly observe the individual attempting to perform that task. Since tasks are typically performed in environments, we would extend this consideration to indicate that the observation is best made in an appropriate behavior setting or across a number of such settings. Unfortunately, within neuropsychology, we have essentially no experience with or technologies for making such observations. This chapter suggested that the methods of ecological psychology could be productively applied here, but there has been no *One Boy's Day* (Barker & Wright, 1951) written for a brain-damaged patient.

The practical problem is that when we make predictions about outcome based upon test data, we typically have little knowledge of the structure of the environment in which the patient exists. We don't know, for example, the number of behavior settings with which the patient interacts, nor do we know about the constraints and supports those settings impose. The use of functional assessment outcome measures are of limited value here, since such measures may often be obtained in settings similar to the ones in which the neuropsychological test findings were obtained. In any event, even if these measures are obtained in a "natural environment," the structure of that environment is generally not evaluated. We do not look at its synomorphs or its standard patterns of behavior. We typically do not look at generalization of behavior across behavior settings. This lack of data has unfortunately led to a tendency toward "guess-work" with some authorities suggesting that test settings are more benign than home or work settings because of the availability of hints and cues, while others have claimed the opposite because of the availability of a familiar support network at home or work. Either of these uninformed beliefs could potentially lead to inaccurate prognostic formulations.

We should look forward to the day when, based upon knowledge of the environment to which our patients return, and scientific analyses of those environments, we will be able to make data-based, accurate predictions of the probable nature of the interactions between the patient and the various behavior settings in which the patient lives. Until that occurs, the establishment of ecological validity becomes highly problematic, simply put, because of lack of information concerning the specifics of the ecologies in which our patients exist.

Indebtedness is expressed to the Department of Veterans Affairs for support of this work. The author wishes to acknowledge Dr. Michael McCue for the information and materials he provided for the Outcome Evaluation Methods section of the chapter.

REFERENCES

Acker, M. B. (1990). A review of the ecological validity of neuropsychological tests. In D. E. Tupper & K. D. Cicerone (Eds.), *The neuropsychology of everyday life: Assessment and basic competencies* (pp. 19-55). Boston: Kluwer Academic Press.

Acker, M. B., & Davis, J. R. (1989). Psychology test scores as predictors of late outcome in brain injury. *Neuropsychology, 3*, 101-111.

Barker, R. G. (Ed.). (1963). *The stream of behavior.* New York: Appleton-Century-Crofts.

Barker, R. G. (1968). *Ecological psychology.* Stanford, CA: Stanford University Press.

Barker, R. G., & Wright, H. F. (1951). *One boy's day.* New York: Harper & Row.

Barker, R. G., & Wright, H. F. (1955). *Midwest and its children.* New York: Harper & Row.

Brunswik, E. (1955). The conceptual framework of psychology. *International encyclopedia of unified science. Vol 1., Part 2* (pp. 656-750). Chicago: University of Chicago Press.

Chelune, G. J., Heaton, R. K., & Lehman, R. A. W. (1986). Neuropsychological and personality correlates of patients' complaints of disability. In G. Goldstein & R. E. Tarter (Eds.), *Advances in clinical neuropsychology, Volume 3* (pp. 95-126). New York: Plenum Press

Chelune, G. J., & Moehle, K. A. (1986). Neuropsychological assessment and everyday functioning. In D. Wedding, A. M. Horton, Jr., & J. Webster (Eds.), *The neuropsychology handbook* (pp. 489-525). New York: Springer Publishing Company.

Crook, T., Ferris, S., & Bartus, R. (Eds.). (1983). *Assessment in geriatric psychopharmacology.* New Canaan, CT: Mark Powley Associates, Inc.

Duke University Center for the Study on Aging. (1978). *Multidimensional functional assessment: The OARS methodology* (2nd ed.). Durham, NC: Duke University Press.

Goldstein, G., & McCue, M. (1995). Differences between patient and informant functional outcome ratings in head-injured individuals. *International Journal of Rehabilitation and Health, 1,* 25-35.

Goldstein, G., McCue, M., Rogers, J., & Nussbaum, P. D. (1992). Diagnostic differences in memory test based predictions of functional capacity in the elderly. *Neuropsychological Rehabilitation, 2,* 307-317.

Gurland, B., Kuriansky, J., Sharpe, L., Simon, R., Stiller, P., & Birkett, P. (1977). The Comprehensive Assessment and Referral Evaluation (CARE) - rationale, development, and reliability. *The International Journal of Aging and Human Development, 8,* 9-42.

Halstead, W. C. (1947). *Brain and intelligence: A quantitative study of the frontal lobes.* Chicago: University of Chicago Press.

Hartigan, J. A., & Wigdor, A. K. (Eds.). (1989*). Fairness in employment testing: Validity generalization, minority issues, and the General Aptitude Test Battery.* Washington, DC: National Academy Press.

Hartmann, D.P., & Wood, D. D. (1990). Observational methods. In A. S. Bellack, M. Hersen, & A. E. Kazdin (Eds.), *International handbook of behavior modification and therapy* (2nd ed.) (pp. 107-138). New York: Plenum Press.

Heaton, R. K., Chelune, G. J., & Lehman, R. A. W. (1978). Using neuropsychological tests to assess the likelihood of patient employment. *Journal of Nervous and Mental Disease, 166,* 408-416.

Heaton, R. K., & Pendleton, M. G. (1981). Use of neuropsychological tests to predict adult patients' everyday functioning. *Journal of Consulting and Clinical Psychology, 49,* 807-821.

Holland, A. L. (1980). *CADL Communicative abilities in daily living: A test of functional communication for aphasic adults.* Baltimore: University Park Press.

Kaplan, E. (1988). A process approach to neuropsychological assessment. In T. Boll & B. K. Bryant (Eds.), *Clinical neuropsychology and brain function: Research, measurement, and practice.* Washington, DC: American Psychological Association.

Kaplan, E., Fein, D., Morris, R., & Delis, D. C. (1991). *WAIS-R-NI manual.* San Antonio: Psychological Corporation, Harcourt Brace Jovanovich, Inc.

Kuriansky, J., & Gurland, B. (1976). The performance test of activities of daily living. *The International Journal of Aging and Human Development, 7,* 343-352.

Lewin, K. (1951). *Field theory in social science.* New York: Harper & Row.

Linn, M. W., & Linn, B. S. (1983). Assessing activities of daily living in institutional settings. In T. Crook, S. Ferris, & R. Bartus, (Eds.) *Assessment in geriatric neuropsychology* (pp. 97-104). New Canaan, CT: Mark Powley Associates, Inc.

McCue, M., Rogers, J. C., & Goldstein, G. (1990). Relationships between neuropsychological and functional assessment in elderly neuropsychiatric patients. *Rehabilitation Psychology, 35,* 91-99.

Rapaport, D. (1946). *Diagnostic psychological testing, Vol. 2.* Chicago: The Year Book Publishers, Inc.

Russell, E. W., Neuringer, C., & Goldstein, G. (1970). *Assessment of brain damage: A neuropsychological key approach.* New York: Wiley-Interscience.

Rogers, J. C. (1987). *Performance Assessment of Self-Care Skills (PASS).* Unpublished performance test.

Sarno, M. T. (1969). *The Functional Communication Profile: Manual of directions.* New York: Institute of Rehabilitation Medicine, New York University Medical Center.

Scheerer, M. (1946). Problems of performance analysis in the study of personality. *Annals of the New York Academy of Science, 46,* 653-678.

Sunderland, A., Harris, J. E., & Gleave, J. (1984). Memory failures in everyday life following severe head injury. *Journal of Clinical Neuropsychology, 6,* 127-142.

Werner, H. (1937). Process and achievement, a basic problem of developmental and educational psychology. *Harvard Educational Review, 7,* 355-368.

Wilson, B., Cockburn, J., & Baddeley, A. (1985). *The Rivermead Behavioral memory test manual.* Reading, England: Thames Valley Test Company.

Winograd, C. H. (1984). Mental status tests and the capacity for self-care. *Journal of the American Geriatrics Society, 32,* 49-61.

Wright. H. F. (1967). *Recording and analyzing child behavior.* New York: Harper & Row.

5

CONCEPTUAL FOUNDATIONS OF ECOLOGICAL VALIDITY IN NEUROPSYCHOLOGICAL ASSESSMENT

Michael D. Franzen, Ph.D.
Karen L. Wilhelm, Ph.D.

INTRODUCTION

Ecological validity is a term which is being used increasingly in discussions of the evaluations of neuropsychological tests and assessment techniques. Equal to its currency of usage is its lack of definitional specificity. The term "ecological validity" has been used primarily to describe aspects of the assessment task and the perceived relation of that task to everyday tasks, that is, tasks which are found in the open environment. For example, Crook, Youngjohn, and Larrabee (1990) devised a set of procedures they describe as being more ecologically relevant and valid than previously devised techniques for the assessment of memory. Although their test, the Misplaced Objects Test, is a standardized procedure that is administered in the assessment clinic, the behaviors involved have a topographical similarity to behaviors in "real life." Implicit in the current usage of the term "ecological validity" is the idea that somehow the assessment procedure is similar to some aspect of free behavior in the open environment and that the results of the assessment procedures can somehow predict free behavior in the open environment.

In general, the validity of an assessment instrument is related to its ability to achieve the objectives of the assessment process. Therefore, ecological validity may not be an important consideration in all assessment techniques. When the main objective of assessment is the localization of a lesion, there are not specific ecological concerns. When the main objective of the assessment is to provide diagnostic information, ecological concerns are implicit if prognosis and statements regarding need for treatment or supervision are made. However, when the objective of assessment is the prediction of behavior in the open environment or the prediction of functional capacity, the relation of the assessment data to the environmental or ecological variables becomes pertinent.

DEFINITIONS OF ECOLOGICAL VALIDITY

Brinberg and McGrath (1985) define ecological validity research as the process by which we reduce the uncertainty regarding the correspondence between research results or other empirical measurements and some actual aspect of the phenomenon under study. They state, "Ecological validity is the extent to which a researcher can specify the scope and limits of a set of empirical findings with respect to the elements and relations selected from the substantive domain" (p. 138). Therefore, we can see that ecological validity refers to those inferences drawn when we make statements about behaviors or situations other than those behaviors and that situation involved in the assessment procedure.

Behavioral assessment is one of the areas where the concept of ecological validity is also frequently mentioned but infrequently defined. An exception is Barrios (1988) who gives a definition of ecological validity that appears to be related to the stability of obtained scores. He states that, "If scores on one instrument in one setting correlate highly with scores on the same instrument but in a different setting, then the instrument is said to be of high ecological validity" (p. 30). Ecological validity is also infrequently defined in the neuropsychological literature. An exception is Hart and Hayden (1986) who give a rudimentary definition of ecological validity, dividing it into assessment and treatment. They utilize Brunswick's (1955) definition of ecological validity for assessment, namely the ability to generalize from the results of controlled assessment situations to naturally occurring phenomena in the open environment. In defining ecological validity for treatment, the authors state that it refers to "the success of an intervention in enhancing the everyday functioning of the patient" (p. 22). Thus, ecological validity may be applied to both assessment and treatment procedures in clinical neuropsychology; however, consideration of treatment issues would unnecessarily broaden the scope of this chapter. The writer confines his comments to a consideration of the ecological validity of assessment procedures with full knowledge that this is only an incomplete discussion of the concept of ecological validity and that treatment issues are no less important than assessment issues.

DEFINITION OF NEUROPSYCHOLOGICAL ECOLOGICAL VALIDITY

There are two general aspects of ecological validity. The first is verisimilitude, or the similarity of the data collection method to tasks and skills required in the free and open environment. The second is veridicality, or the extent to which test results reflect or can predict phenomena in the open environment or "real world." Verisimilitude may be more important in the design of neuropsychological assessment instruments. In designing the procedures of the instrument, one needs to carefully consider the intended use of the information. For example, in designing an instrument to evaluate the ability of a patient to remember instructions at work, one needs to assess verbal memory, memory for narrative, and memory for conceptually linked discrete behaviors because all of those memory types are likely to be involved in the relevant task. Additionally, Smith (1985) argues that at least in the case of communication skills, the assessment instrument should be graded in terms of familiarity and difficulty to more accurately predict performance in the natural environment. Once the instrument is designed, aspects of veridicality become more important. What is needed at that point is evidence that the results of the assessment predict performance on the relevant task in the work situation. The types of information necessary and the levels of analysis for each of these aspects are discussed later in the chapter.

The current usual consideration of ecological validity in neuropsychological assessment involves a description of deficits in specific cognitive skills. The presence of a deficit is then related to the capacity of the subject to perform a certain behavior. For example, an assessment may uncover a deficit in verbal memory for short narratives. On that basis, the clinician may make some statement about the capacity of the subject to remember verbal instructions in a work setting. However, as Chelune (1982) points out, a more complete conceptualization of ecological validity involves the correlation of a neuropsychological assessment technique with a behavior and not just a correlation with a deficit. This consideration is an expansion of the aims of neuropsychological assessment beyond the traditional aim of uncovering a deficit, which is the legacy of behavioral neurology. The consideration of behavior and not just deficit increases the relevant population of interest from impaired subjects to normal subjects; do the scores derived from the test correlate with performance on the criterion behavior in a sample of nonimpaired individuals?

One study examining this question found that neuropsychological test scores could be related to scores on the Sickness Impact Profile and the Katz Adjustment Scale, Relatives' Version for a sample of 303 patients with chronic obstructive pulmonary disease but not for a sample of 99 normal control subjects matched for demographic variables (McSweeney, Grant, Heaton, Prigatano, & Adams, 1985). These results indicate that deficient performance on traditional neuropsychological measures may represent limiting factors on everyday functioning. That is to say, performing in the impaired range on a neuropsychological test may mean that the subject is unlikely to be able to perform a certain environmental behavior. However, in this particular instance, the lack of correlation in the normal control sample may have been due to a restriction of range imposed by the ceiling effects of assessment instruments that do not measure reliably in the unimpaired or superior ranges of performance.

Behavior prediction can be evaluated in either the universe of specific, although complex behaviors, such as driving skills as well as in the prediction of molar outcomes, such as success in rehabilitation or return to work. In the first case, a single test may be useful in predicting the criterion, as in the example noted above of the use of a verbal memory test to predict capacity to remember work instructions. In the second case, because molar outcome is dependent upon a combination of behavioral skills, a group of tests may be necessary for accurate predictions. Additionally, the capacity of the subject to link together molecular skills may need to be assessed. Acker (1990) published a review of investigations of ecological validity, and interestingly, most of the criteria were global measures of gross outcome, such as quality of life, community participation, informal reports of performance at work, or the Glasgow Outcome Scale (Jennett & Bond, 1975). A few studies investigated the relation of neuropsychological functioning to classes of independent activities such as money management and laundry activities. In one of those studies, relations between scores on the Halstead-Reitan and questionnaires completed by significant others were significant but not specific enough to allow discrete predictions (Searight, Dunn, Grisso, Margolis, & Gibbons, 1989).

RELATION TO SOCIAL VALIDITY

Another consideration in the examination of ecological validity is the extent to which the target behavior is important to the functional capacity of the subject. This is a term that has been called "social validity" by some behaviorists (Hawkins, 1988). The issue is the extent to which the chosen unit of observation, or target behavior, is related to an issue of concern to the subject or to others in the social environment. For example, an assessment instrument used in the clinic may be found to be a good predictor of memory for shopping lists, but the task of remembering shopping lists may be irrelevant to a certain subject's life. The information relevant to this decision would involve self-report by the subject, the report of others in the subject's environment such as family members or caregivers, or expert opinion derived from neuropsychologists, nursing staff, or occupational therapists.

An implication of including social relevance in the evaluation of ecological validity is that the cultural and personal values of the information source become an important part of the evaluation process. The question cannot be simply answered by examining whether a subject can perform a behavior; we must additionally ask, is the behavior important, and if so, to whom is it important? There might be instances in which there are differences of opinion as to whether the target behavior or the assessment index is important. For example, an elderly resident of a nursing facility may not feel it is important for her to be able to remember the names of staff or connect the names with the correct faces because the staff will provide care regardless of how she addresses them. In comparison, the care facility staff may feel that learning and using the staff's names will help the staff behave positively toward the subject, and the clinical neuropsychologist may possess the opinion that it is always better to improve a subject's functional memory. Another example might involve a severely head injured patient's opinion that it is important to be able to plan and execute a cooked meal when the professional staff feel that his or her severe motor deficits significantly reduce the likelihood of such a behavior occurring.

The inclusion of values in the consideration of ecological validity is not meant to cloud the issues, but instead is meant to make explicit processes which already occur in the clinical setting. Clinical work does not exist in a social vacuum. Instead, all clinical activity occurs in the context of social contingencies partly under the control of the funding agent whether it is the government, the insurance company, a family member, or the patient. Additionally, the social contingencies are under partial control of spouse and family members, care provider staff members, and other members of the clinical assessment team. By including social considerations, we allow ourselves a chance to examine the relevance, fairness, and utility of the values underlying some of our clinical decisions.

Including the issue of social validity complicates the evaluation of assessment instruments. One problem is that the demands of each person's open environment are different. The tasks and skills required in one job setting or in one cultural setting may not be applicable to another setting. The problem of individual environments does not obviate the need for basic assessment instruments. For one thing, basic assessment instruments, or instruments that have been designed to answer questions of organic integrity, localization, or diagnosis maintain an important place in the overall assessment process. Most of these

instruments are nomothetic with available comparisons to normative information. The normative comparisons can help provide information related to the
level of skill demonstrated by the individual subject. The diagnostic information presented by the instruments can help in indicating treatments that may
be helpful. Or alternately, the diagnostic information may help particularize
the treatment approach most likely to be successful.

For example, a memory assessment instrument may indicate that Alzheimer's
disease is a probable diagnosis, indicating that serial assessments may be necessary or that arrangements for family members to help take responsibility should
be made. Alternately, a memory assessment instrument may indicate that the
manifest memory failure is due to difficulty in encoding, pointing to treatments which facilitate encoding. Although the problem of individual environments may seem to discourage the assessment of social validity, this challenge
actually underlines the need for developing a more full armamentarium of assessment techniques. In that way, the clinician can obtain a more full view of
the functioning of the subject.

METHODS OF ASSESSMENT OF ECOLOGICAL VALIDITY

The assessment of ecological validity has different forms and utilizes different methods. Aspects of appropriate criterion measures in the evaluation of
ecological validity are given a more thorough discussion in Chapter 4. However, some aspects of experimental design are discussed in this section. Experimental design considerations involved in the investigation of ecological validity can be seen to be relatively independent of which component of ecological
validity is being evaluated and relatively independent of what criterion measures have been chosen. A complete assessment of the ecological validity of a
neuropsychological instrument involves investigations of both verisimilitude
and veridicality.

VERISIMILITUDE

The investigation of verisimilitude includes an examination of the instrument with reference to theoretical considerations. The instrument is examined
regarding the theoretical relation between the task demands of test procedures
and the situational demands of the behavior supposedly predicted by the test
results. For example with a test of visual-spatial skills, such as the Line Orientation Test, it is important to consider the extent to which line orientation discriminations are required in the visual-spatial tasks of driving an automobile.

Part of this investigation asks the question: does the task have a topographical similarity to the behavioral domain of interest? Furthermore, one would need to evaluate the extent to which the assessment task sufficiently taps the behavioral domain.

A second part of the evaluation of verisimilitude includes an examination of the instrument with reference to situation descriptions. Does the manner in which the skills are tapped in the task required of the subject in the assessment paradigm match the requirements of the relevant situations in the open environment? Here, the evaluation moves beyond a consideration of the task and into a consideration of variables such as the rate of information processing necessary to complete the behavioral task, the degree of interference or distraction in the situation, and the extent to which compensatory mechanism are available and utilized. For example, a test of memory that does not allow rehearsal may not accurately predict memory behaviors in the open environment where rehearsal is applicable.

VERIDICALITY

The evaluation of veridicality partly involves an examination of relations between scores from the neuropsychological instrument and scores from other instruments found to have predictive relations with behavior in the free environment. As an example of this type of investigation, Klesges (1983) reported that scores on the Halstead-Reitan Neuropsychological Battery for Children correlated with scores on the Children's Assessment of Cerebral Dysfunction, a behavioral checklist. As another example, if a standardized behavioral assessment instrument is known to predict performance on self-care tasks, the relation between the two sets of test data (behavioral assessment and neuropsychological test) might be used to provide information about the ecological validity of the neuropsychological instrument of interest. However, this should be seen as weak information because of the possibility that the two instruments are related for reasons other than variance shared with the target behavior. Correlations between the two instruments might help identify possible predictors which would then need to be further evaluated in terms of their ecological validity. For example, The Loewenstein Direct Assessment of Functional Status (Loewenstein et al., 1989) is a standardized behavioral assessment technique that contains a subtest that evaluates recognition of common traffic signs. If an analog test of general visual-spatial matching, for example the Benton Visual Discrimination test (Benton, Hamsher, Varney, & Spreen, 1983) correlates with the naturalistic traffic sign subtest of the Loewenstein, we can then examine the relation of the Visual Discrimination test to actual driving skill.

This type of investigation is not limited to skills assessment, but may also include conative variables such as emotion and affective state which have a known relation to the behavior of interest. For example, the Paced Serial Addition Test, or PASAT (Gronwall, 1977) can be used to evaluate the integrity of attentional processes. If performance on a measure of depression has been found to correlate with performance on the PASAT, and the PASAT has been found to predict performance on tasks requiring attention, then the measure of depression may have a relation to performance on those tasks. This information would allow us to make predictions regarding the performance of a depressed person.

The stronger type of evidence involves an examination of relations between the instrument and behavior in the open environment. The methods of assessing behavior in the open environment include self-report, report by others, formal behavioral observation, and questionnaires. The methods do not include naturalistic methods such as laboratory observations in simulated environments which would be classified under standardized behavioral assessment techniques.

EXPERIMENTAL DESIGN

There are two basic classes of experimental design that can be utilized in evaluations of the ecological validity of neuropsychological assessment instruments. These design classes are the concurrent and the longitudinal designs. In the concurrent designs, the results of neuropsychological assessment instruments are evaluated in terms of their ability to statistically predict performance on everyday tasks. For example, the relation between score on a test of sequencing skills and the ability to follow a recipe in cooking may be investigated.

The longitudinal design involves prediction not only in the statistical sense, but also in the temporal sense. For example, scores on a test of abstract problem solving may be examined in terms of their ability to predict success in rehabilitation or return to work. Application of the longitudinal design would also allow the neuropsychologist to investigate whether relevant predictors change over time. The scores on memory tests may be reasonable predictors of return to work when the memory assessment is conducted in an acute setting, but scores on a test of executive functioning may have greater predictive power in a re-entry setting. Dodrill and Clemmons (1984) report the results of a longitudinal design to investigate the ability of neuropsychological evaluations to predict adjustment in young adult epileptic patients between three and 11 years after the evaluations were conducted. The authors reported that the neuropsychological variables, especially the language variables, were more effective in prediction than were the emotional variables (MMPI scale scores).

Regardless of whether a longitudinal design or a concurrent design is used, the statistical design may be either correlational or factorial. In the correlational design, the goal is to identify tests which have shared variance with behavioral tasks. In the factorial designs, the goal can include attempts to identify interactions among variables when subjects are classified according to some characteristic. For example, independent variables may include diagnosis, the ability of a subject to live independently versus live under supervision, and the presence of impaired versus intact skill.

LIMITS ON THE DETERMINATION OF THE ECOLOGICAL VALIDITY OF NEUROPSYCHOLOGICAL ASSESSMENT

There are at least three reasons why prediction of behavior in the open environment is not an easy presently task. First, there is little information regarding relations between test results and actual behavior. Second, the evaluation of relations between test results and behavior in the open environment will itself be difficult. The set of relations between these two sets of phenomena is likely to be complex and moderated by other variables. These moderating variables may include the speed of information processing and the degree of distractibility. Third, the controlled aspect of the assessment situation may rule out the use of learned compensatory mechanisms that have proven to be successful for the subject. In the second case, test results may overpredict behavioral performance; in the third case, test results may underpredict performance.

Clinical neuropsychology has developed from the perspective of identifying behavioral patterns associated with lesion locations or etiological variables. As a result, certain tests, such as the Halstead Category test, while useful in the determination of organic dysfunction have little in the way of topographical similarities to real-world activities. The component skills of the Category test may have real-world referents. For example, the Category test requires visual recognition skills, aspects of memory, nonverbal abstraction skills, and systematic problem-solving skills. However, it would be difficult to find an environmental situation in which a person was asked to perform the actual task involved in the Category test. Additionally, for some neuropsychological constructs, there may be limited practical implications. As an example of this situation, Hart and Hayden (1986) discuss the lack of real-world examples of ideomotor apraxia.

THE IMPACT OF INTERACTIVE VARIABLES

The test situation traditionally involves procedures designed to isolate capacity to perform tasks requiring discrete skills. An example of this sort of procedure would be the Benton Judgment of Line Orientation test (Benton et al., 1983) where the subject is assessed simply for the capacity to recognize and match angular relations among line segments. In comparison, some assessment procedures require that subjects perform somewhat more complex tasks so that comparison of performance on two tasks, which differ only slightly, can result in isolation of the impaired molecular skill. An example of this sort of procedure can be found in the Luria-Nebraska Neuropsychological Battery where verbal memory items are administered with either verbal or visual interference to determine which type of interference is more disruptive. In these instances the ability of the subject to perform the task in a controlled setting, such as the assessment laboratory, may be an overestimate of the capacity of the subject to perform the same behaviors in the open environment where multiple distractors may impede accurate performance. Future research may identify variables, additional to attentional capacity and speed of information processing, that moderate relations between test performance and behavior in the open environment. Clinical neuropsychologists already use information regarding motivational and affective status in interpreting cognitive test results, but systematic research investigating the precise nature of interactions among cognitive and conative variables is needed.

Heaton, Chelune, and Lehman (1976) investigated the relation of cognitive variables (scores from the Halstead-Reitan Battery, Wechsler Adult Intelligence Scale, and achievement measures) and conative variables (scores from the MMPI) to employment status in a sample of subjects referred for neuropsychological evaluation. Unfortunately, the number of subjects in the derivation sample for the discriminant function analysis (n = 148) in ratio to the number of predictors (31) was not sufficient to assume stability of the solution. However, the discriminant function solution was then applied to a cross-validation sample of 147 subjects with similar results allowing us some confidence in the results. The discriminant function was able to correctly classify subjects as either full-time employed or unemployed 83.7% of the time, averaged across both samples. Interestingly, six of the predictor variables were neuropsychological in nature and 11 of the predictor variables were conative in nature. Using the neuropsychological variables alone, the correct classification rate was 74.2%, and using the MMPI variables alone, the correct classification rate was 78.6%, indicating that the MMPI variables may have been more influential in statistically predicting concurrent employment status. Of course, we can not determine whether the MMPI variables were causative in the determination of employment status.

Typically, the neuropsychological evaluation involves particularization of performance. As noted above, the assessment situation may result in overestimates of actual capacity in the open environment due to laboratory control over interfering or moderating variables such as attentional capacity. It may also occur that the assessment situation may result in underestimates of actual capacity. The subject may have found or developed methods of compensating for any neurocognitive impairments. For example, an individual with frontal lobe dysfunction may have developed a self-cueing strategy to guide her- or himself through behavior chains. In the assessment situation, the examiner may deprive the subject of this compensation resulting in a poor performance and underestimates of the capacity of the subject to successfully perform the behavior in the open environment. For example, Aten, Caligiuri, and Holland (1982) report that intensive language therapy resulted in improvement on a more functionally based and ecologically relevant evaluation instrument (Communication Abilities in Daily Living) than on a more linguistically based evaluation instrument (Porch Index of Communicative Ability).

Further examples of moderated relations between test results and real-life behaviors are found in the occupational therapy literature. Williams (1967) examined the relation between constructional apraxia and dressing difficulties in right and left hemisphere stroke patients. All of the examined patients were hemiplegic, but the patients who demonstrated constructional apraxia on a drawing task were much more likely to demonstrate dressing difficulty both at the time of testing and at the time of discharge following training in self-dressing skills. The results were interpreted as indicating that the relation between results of motor skills testing and self-dressing skills were moderated by skill at a two-dimensional construction task. Unfortunately, no other cognitive skills were assessed allowing the possibility that other impairments may account for the dressing difficulty. A later investigation (Warren, 1981) indicated that both constructional apraxia and body schema accuracy were related to dressing ability in stroke patients even after other apraxias, agraphia, and aphasia were ruled out as possible influences. However, in this study, body schema accuracy and design copy performance correlated .54 with each other, indicating the need for a statistical analysis model that calculates partial correlation coefficients in order to examine unique variance shared with the criterion. As further evidence for this statistical model, Baum and Hall (1981) reported that in a sample of head-injured patients, dressing skill was correlated approximately equally with two-dimensional constructions (r =.59), three-dimensional constructions (r =.59), and drawing skill (r =.60).

STATISTICAL MODELS OF INTERACTIVE PREDICTOR VARIABLES

Contemporary neuropsychological theoretical models are multivariate, and the above evidence indicates that ecological validity models will, of necessity, be multivariate as well. The multivariate nature of neuropsychology should be no surprise to any student of psychology. Although the inferences drawn from the end product of assigning numbers to neuropsychological assessment procedures may frequently relate to physiological processes and structures, it is important to remember that neuropsychology predominantly involves the study of behavior. As such, the same issues attending the study of behavior in general (i.e., psychological investigations), will impact upon the study of neuropsychological phenomena, albeit with the further complication of issues of physiology and anatomy. In explicating his notion of ecological validity, Brunswick (1955) stated his view that behavior is multiply determined and probabilistic in nature. If this position is true for the study of behavior in general psychology, it can be no less true for the study of behavior in neuropsychology.

HEURISTIC MODELS OF INTERACTIVE PREDICTOR VARIABLES

The relations between brain and behavior are complex, and adequate representations will need to reflect the intercorrelations among the predictors. These representations are currently applied in the form of clinical judgment. The individual clinician attempts to combine information derived from the assessment and match that information to what is known about the demands of the subject's environment. Clinical judgment is fraught with potential error (Wedding & Faust, 1989), and objective decision techniques would help improve the accuracy of these predictions. Research to develop the decision techniques might first examine the logical steps followed by clinicians who are accurate predictors. Mathematical models of these steps could then be examined and compared for degree of accuracy and utility. Alternately, test results thought to be relevant to the predictors could be entered into multiple regression models in order to determine the best weighted combination of those test results.

LEVELS OF ANALYSIS

In evaluating the ecological validity of neuropsychological tests, there are multiple levels of analyzing the data obtained, but not all of these levels will be relevant to evaluating the twin aspects of verisimilitude and veridicality. Verisimilitude will require an analysis of information at a theoretical level. The questions asked will include whether the test demands can be theoretically related to the behavioral tasks or criterion. That is, one would want to know if there is a theory which can use information about discrete skills in order to make statements about environmental behaviors. For example, one theory of memory consolidation posits that memory consolidation is partly a function of rehearsal whether active or passive. A test that allows a comparison between memory accuracy when active rehearsal is allowed versus when passive rehearsal is allowed (that is, in the absence of interference) may theoretically be related to performance on environmental tasks where passive rehearsal is precluded. Yet another level of analysis for verisimilitude is conceptual where the relevant question involves the conceptual similarity between the test task and the environmental behavior. For example, solving abstract problems on the Halstead Category test may be conceptually similar to solving "diagnosing" problems in a malfunctioning automobile engine. Finally, the level of analysis for verisimilitude may be rational. The relevant question here may be whether a logical argument can be made regarding the relation of a discrete skill to a molecular behavior, or is line orientation a component of visual placement in space of environmental objects.

Veridicality will involve two levels of analysis; theoretical and empirical. The first level of analysis attempts to answer the question of whether there is theoretical justification for considering the relation between test results and criterion behavior. A negative answer on the theoretical level should not preclude the examination of relations in all cases. Current theory may be inadequate to the understanding of relations among the classes of variables. However, a positive answer to this question should indicate the probable utility of an examination of the relations. The second level of analysis is empirical where systematic controlled observations are examined to determine the qualitative and quantitative boundaries of the relations.

CRITERIA OF ECOLOGICAL VALIDITY

Once investigations of ecological validity have been conducted, one would need some criteria by which to judge the results of the investigations. One criterion is the extent of objectification achieved in the endeavor. To what extent can the results of the activity be specified, either quantitatively or qualitatively? It is not necessary that the results be assigned a number, only that they be assigned a quality that elicits agreement from other observers. Given the results of a neuropsychological evaluation, is another clinical neuropsychologist likely to make the same predictions regarding return to work? A second criterion is the sufficiency of the information obtained. Will the information allow us to draw reasonable conclusions about real-life phenomena, or will we require additional information in the form of conative variables or other test data? Yet another criterion is the relation of the results to other data (e.g., inferences drawn by professionals in other disciplines regarding the same issues). If the neurosurgeon and the neuropsychologist disagree about the ability of a patient to perform activities of daily living, what is required to resolve the dispute?

RELATION TO OTHER FORMS OF VALIDITY

Perhaps the best way to conceptualize ecological validity is to consider it in the context of general aspects of the validity of assessment techniques. Validity is best conceptualized not as a characteristic of tests, but rather as a characteristic of inferences (Franzen, 1989, p. 32). That is to say, we do not evaluate the validity of a test, but instead we evaluate the validity of an inference in using a test with a certain population. The different forms of validity become different methods of evaluating the utility and accuracy of the inferences drawn from the test results. The different forms of validity may be seen to overlap. For example, factorial validity may overlap with construct validity in an instrument that purports to evaluate both visual and verbal memory.

In the same way, ecological validity is not an entirely independent concept. Aspects of ecological validity, for example, the degree of verisimilitude, may be seen to overlap with aspects of face validity. The relevant question here would be whether a test that is said to measure memory contains tasks that resemble everyday tasks that require memory processes. In the same way, aspects of ecological validity related to empirical relations may overlap with predictive validity. The relevant question here would be whether an instrument said to measure memory can predict memory performance in the open environment.

Just as there can be no general answer to the question: which is more important, discriminant validity or concurrent validity; there can be no general answer to the question: which is more important, ecological validity or traditional validity. The related issues revolve around questions of understanding versus questions of application. Brooks and Baumeister (1977) have considered these issues in the context of research investigating mental retardation, but the points made are relevant here as well. Two themes become apparent. The first theme is the development of a theory of brain-behavior relations and the second theme is an understanding of the condition of brain impairment. The first theme, which relates to traditional validity, requires the researcher to consider issues of internal and external validity. The second theme, which relates to ecological validity, further requires the researcher to consider what Brooks and Baumeister (1977) term "metatheoretical constraints," namely the implications of motivation, the nature of the underlying condition, and the idiosyncratic manifestation of cause and effect in a specific real-life situation.

In comparison, House (1977) points out the importance of traditional validity and research concerns because true causes may not be discernible from direct natural observation. The natural environment contains such a mix of interacting and potentially confounding influences that inferences regarding causation are tenuous at best. The author earlier stated that comparisons between traditional validity and ecological validity involve questions of understanding versus questions of application. The author now adds that the laboratory or "bench" researcher need only consider questions of understanding whereas the clinical researcher must consider both sets of questions.

Similar to the questions regarding comparisons between traditional and ecological validity, we may consider whether verisimilitude is more essential to ecological validity than is veridicality. This question is also specious for both aspects need to be investigated in order for any definitive statements to be made regarding the ecological validity of clinical neuropsychological activity. The two aspects can be seen as complementary. As an example, consider the clinical interview, which is perhaps the most ecologically valid in terms of verisimilitude. It is here that the clinical neuropsychologist collects the information that has the highest degree of ecological relevance. Unfortunately, the clinical interview also has the lowest degree of certainty regarding the accuracy of the data and the least amount of information relating the data to other sources of data, (e.g., correlations with standardized test data, relation to clinical decision making). Therefore, knowledge about the ecological validity of the interview may be said to be incomplete.

RELATION OF CLINICAL ASSESSMENT TO FUNCTIONAL ASSESSMENT

As defined above, one of the considerations of ecological validity is the extent to which the neuropsychological instrument obtains ecologically relevant information (verisimilitude). One way to obtain ecologically relevant information is to design test procedures that elicit behaviors that are topographically related to the target behaviors. Another way to obtain ecologially relevant information is to evaluate the capacity of the subject to perform the behaviors in the environment. For reasons of economy, direct behavioral observations are rarely conducted. Instead, subjects may be given standard stimuli and asked to perform environmental behaviors. An example of this sort of functional assessment is the Loewenstein Direct Assessment of Functional Status (Loewenstein et al., 1989). Here, among other tasks, the subject is given a short list of grocery items and is then taken into a room where multiple grocery items are placed on a table. The task is to select correctly the items on the list. Another task on the assessment involves writing a check and balancing a checkbook.

Alternately, other functional assessment instruments attempt to obtain ecologically relevant material in one of two other methods, either through questionnaires administered to collateral sources or through ratings obtained from professionals. Sometimes, ecologically relevant information is derived from the subject as in the case of the Cognitive Failures Questionnaire (Broadbent, Cooper, Fitzgerald, & Parkes, 1982). However, relying on the neuropsychologically impaired subject to provide information regarding level of skill or deficit is problematic because the subject may be unaware of the deficit or may report inaccurate data (Godfrey, Partridge, Knight, & Bishara, 1993; McGlynn & Schacter, 1989).

Examples of the use of collateral report or professional rating of functioning can be found in Williams (1987) and in Crockett, Tuokko, Koch, and Parks (1989). Williams (1987) presents a questionnaire (the Cognitive Behavior Rating Scale or CBRS) in which a family member rates subjects on behaviors related to dementia. The reported validity study involved the ability of the scales (Language Deficit, Apraxia, Disorientation, etc.) of the CBRS to discriminate between a group of 30 demented patients and a group of 30 pair-matched normal subjects. Unfortunately, there have not as yet been attempts to evaluate the veridicality of the instrument in terms of its ability to accurately identify level of performance on the different scales. Crockett et al. (1989) described the Functional Rating Scale which is completed by a multidisciplinary team. Here the subject is rated on a five-point scale in eight areas (memory, personal care, etc.). The information is derived from interviews with the patient and primary care giver, from the referral source, from laboratory findings, and from clinical evaluations. Crockett et al. (1989) also describe the Present Functioning Questionnaire which includes 60 items across five problem areas and which is administered to a collateral source in a structured interview.

In some cases, the functional assessment instrument has been evaluated against behavioral observations. For example, Skurla, Rogers, and Sunderland (1988) report an investigation of the Clinical Dementia Rating Scale which correlated results of the assessment with performance on four laboratory tasks (e.g., making a cup of coffee, telephoning the pharmacy). Performance on the laboratory tasks was objectively scored on the basis of whether visual, verbal, or physical prompting or some combination was required to complete the task. The authors reported higher correlations of the laboratory task with the Clinical Dementia Rating Scale than with the Short Portable Mental Status Exam and interpreted the results as indicating greater specificity of the rating scale, but the results could also be seen as indicating greater ecological validity for the rating scale in the population of elderly demented subjects.

The clinical neuropsychological assessment and the functional assessment can be seen to be complementary with each contributing unique information. The degree of overlap between the two classes of assessment information may depend upon the characteristics of each. For example, McCue, Rogers, and Goldstein (1990) reported that the degree of correlational overlap between the Luria-Nebraska Neuropsychological Battery and the Performance Assessment of Self-Care (PASS) was small for personal self-care, mobility, and physical activities, but was higher for more cognitive-oriented self-care variables such as use of a telephone, cooking, and shopping. In comparison, Haut, Franzen, Keefover, and Rankin (1991) report that functional assessment results were more highly related to neuropsychological measures of confrontation naming, verbal fluency, constructional ability, and new learning than to neuropsychological measures of memory span, delayed recall, or general cognitive efficiency.

Typically, functional assessments are more likely to have been conducted by an occupational therapist than by a psychologist. As such, the functional assessment methods may differ from the methods utilized in more conventional psychological assessment. Therefore, the functional assessment instruments have not received the same psychometric investigations that are frequently given to psychological assessment instruments.

In reviewing functional assessment instruments, several criticisms become apparent. Many of these instruments are subjectively scored. While subjectivity is not in itself necessarily a drawback, the presence of subjectivity indicates the need for investigations of interrater agreement in order to assess the adequacy of the scoring instructions. Subjective judgments that are replicable across observers can serve the purposes of the assessment. A second related criticism is that the scoring systems are frequently insufficient to allow easy judgments. The judgments required are frequently involved in the ability to perform groups of behaviors under widely varying conditions, for example, the ability to maintain personal hygiene which can include body cleanliness, oral hygiene, dressing, and hair grooming. Scoring systems with specific behavioral anchors would help increase the agreement across raters. Decomposing the judgments into smaller units would also help increase reliability. Sometimes the assessment instrument will have a mix of items ranging from behaviorally specific to conceptually vague. For example, the Functional Dementia Scale (Moore, Bobula, Short, & Mischel, 1983), which is completed by nursing staff, has a behaviorally specific item "Shouts or yells" as well as a somewhat more subjective item "Is unaware of the limitations imposed by illness." Subjectivity also enters in the scoring system where the four-point scale includes the categories "Good part of the time" and "Most or all of the time" without defining the difference between "good part of the time" and "most of the time."

A third problem with many of the functional assessment instruments is that the scale properties of the scores are largely unknown. Functional assessments require that different types of information be combined into summary scores. Because psychometric investigations have not been conducted, we do not have knowledge regarding the specifics of the reliability of the instruments. Because the summary scores are hybrid forms of information we can not make reasonable assumptions about the possible scalar properties.

A final problem is the issue of criteria. Even if the subject can perform the behaviors in an assessment situation, it remains to be seen if the subject can perform the behaviors without supervision in a free environment. Or to use another example from a functional assessment, even if a person can move in bed, can that person know what time to go to bed or make a decision as to how many bedcovers to use? A final criticism of functional assessment methods involves the lack of validational studies relating these instruments to actual behavior.

The problem here is that even though the functional assessment instruments may appear to possess ecological validity on the basis of verisimilitude, the veridicality has yet to be evaluated. This problem is especially evident for functional assessments that rely upon reports rather than upon direct observation; however, the problem can be seen to exist for observation instruments as well. The issue is one of reactivity of the subject to the situation as well as an issue of similarity of the naturalistic situation to the natural environment. By examining a patient in a clinical setting we may be removing the contextual cues and familiarity that may make independent functioning possible for that patient.

While some ADL instruments attempt to avoid this problem by observing the patient in his or her home, we are in effect turning the home into a laboratory which then invites potential reactivity (Kapust & Weintraub, 1988). A visit from an examiner may prompt a subject to make an extra effort to do well. On the other hand, the subject may view the visit as intrusive and may not cooperate fully with the evaluation. In either case, the presence of reactivity is an empirical question.

CONCLUSIONS

Ecological validity is a complex concept that can be conceptualized as involving both verisimilitude, or extent of similarity to relevant environmental behaviors, and veridicality, or degree of accuracy in predicting some environmental behavior or molar outcome. Because of the history of clinical neuropsychology, few clinical neuropsychological assessment instruments have been evaluated in terms of their ecological validity. However, this topic will acquire increased importance as clinical neuropsychologists become more active in applied treatment activities.

Ecological validity can be considered in terms of the intent of the assessment. Ecological concerns become important when the purpose of the evaluation is to predict some aspect of extra-test behavior. These concerns are not so important when the purpose of the evaluation is diagnostic. Ecological validity can also be considered in the context of other forms of validity where validity refers to the inferences drawn from the test results and not from the test itself.

There are multiple problems involved in the determination of ecological validity. Some of these concerns are related to issues of criterion choice, whether it be global outcome measures or discrete environmental behaviors. Some of these issues are related to reactivity of the assessment procedure. However, despite these problems, ecological validity should be evaluated in neuropsychological assessment instruments.

IMPLICATIONS FOR FUTURE RESEARCH

The most obvious direction for future research is to conduct studies that will help elucidate the relations between traditional neuropsychological assessment results and behaviors in the open environment. This would require the development of methods to evaluate the degree of success in performing the behaviors. Relevant sources of information include direct behavioral observation, self-report, and report by significant others. An example of self-report instruments is the Cognitive Failures Questionnaire (Broadbent et al., 1982). An example of report by significant others is the Cognitive Behaviors Rating Scale (Williams, 1987).

An ancillary area would be to identify those variables which are most likely to operate as moderating variables in the relation between test data and free behavior. Some of these variables, such as speed of information processing, degree of executive control required, and extent of distractions, have already been discussed. Other variables include level of motivation, extent of anxiety, and affective status.

The development of assessment techniques may follow two potentially fruitful avenues. First, examination of the task requirements of free behaviors may indicate the direction for future assessment instrument development. An example of this can be found in the everyday memory instrument developed by Crook, Youngjohn, and Larrabee (1990), the memory instrument developed by Wilson, Cockburn, and Baddeley (1991) or the communication skills instrument developed by Holland (1982). Another direction for instrument development may be similar to the Loewenstein Direct Assessment of Functional Status (Loewenstein et al., 1989) where behavioral assessment techniques are used to evaluate the capacity of an individual to complete simple behaviors related to everyday functioning.

REFERENCES

Acker, M. B. (1990). A review of the ecological validity of neuropsychological tests. In D. E. Tupper & K. D Cicerone (Eds.) *The neuropsychology of everyday life: Assessment and basic competencies.* Boston: Kluwer Academic Publishers.

Aten, J. L., Caligiuri, M. P., & Holland, A. L. (1982). The efficacy of functional communication therapy for chronic aphasic patients. *Journal of Speech and Hearing Disorders, 47,* 93-96.

Barrios, B. A. (1988). On the changing nature of behavioral assessment. In A. S. Bellack & M. Hersen (Eds.), *Behavioral assessment: A practical handbook,* pp. 3-41. New York: Pergamon.

Baum, B., & Hall, K.M. (1981). Relationship between constructional praxis and dressing in the head-injured adult. *The American Journal of Occupational Therapy, 35,* 438-442.

Benton, A. L., Hamsher, K. deS., Varney, N. R., & Spreen, O. (1983). *Contributions to neuropsychological assessment.* New York: Oxford University Press.

Brinberg, D., & McGrath, J. E. (1985). *Validity and the research process.* Beverly Hills, CA: Sage Publications.

Broadbent, D. E., Cooper, P. F., Fitzgerald, P., & Parkes, K. R. (1982). The cognitive failures questionnaire (CFQ) and its correlates. *British Journal of Clinical Psychology, 21,* 1-16.

Brooks, P. H., & Baumeister, A. A. (1977). A plea for consideration of ecological validity in the experimental psychology of mental retardation: A guest editorial. *American Journal of Mental Deficiency, 81,* 407-416.

Brunswick, E. (1955). Representative design and probabilistic theory in functional psychology. *Psychological Review, 62,* 193-217.

Chelune, G. J. (1982). Toward a neuropsychological model of everyday functioning. *Psychotherapy in Private Practice, 3,* 39-44.

Crockett, D., Tuokko, H., Koch, W., & Parks, R. (1989). The assessment of everyday functioning using the Present Functioning Questionnaire and the Functional Rating Scale in elderly samples. *The Clinical Gerontologist, 8,* 3-25.

Crook, T. H., Youngjohn, J. R., & Larrabee, G. J. (1990). The Misplaced Objects test: A measure of everyday visual memory. *Journal of Clinical and Experimental Neuropsychology, 12,* 819-833.

Dodrill, C. B., & Clemmons, D. (1984). Use of neuropsychological tests to identify high school students with epilepsy who later demonstrate inadequate performances in life. *Journal of Consulting and Clinical Psychology, 52,* 520-527.

Franzen, M. D. (1989). *Reliability and validity in neuropsychological assessment.* New York: Plenum.

Godfrey. H. P. D., Partridge, F. M., Knight, R. G., & Bishara, S. (1993). Course of insight disorder and emotional dysfunction following closed head injury: A controlled cross-sectional follow-up study. *Journal of Clinical and Experimental Neuropsychology, 15,* 503-515.

Gronwall, D. (1977). Paced auditory serial addition task: A measure of recovery from concussion. *Perceptual and Motor Skills, 44,* 367-373.

Hart, T., & Hayden, M. E. (1986). The ecological validity of neuropsychological assessment and remediation. In B. P. Uzzell & Y. Gross (Eds.) *The clinical neuropsychology of intervention,* Boston: Martinus Nijoff Publishing.

Haut, M. W., Franzen, M. D., Keefover, R., & Rankin, E. (1991). *Relationship between functional status and cognitive functions in dementia.* Paper presented at International Neuropsychological Society Meeting, San Antonio, Texas.

Hawkins, R. P. (1988). Selection of target behaviors. In R. O. Nelson and S. C. Hayes (Eds.) *Conceptual foundations of behavioral assessment,* (pp. 331-385). New York: The Guilford Press.

Heaton, R. K., Chelune, G. J., & Lehman, R. A. W. (1976). Using neuropsychological and personality tests to assess the likelihood of patient employment. *The Journal of Nervous and Mental Disease, 166,* 408-416.

Holland, A. L. (1982). Observing functional communication of aphasic adults. *Journal of Speech and Hearing Disorders, 47,* 50-56.

House, B. J. (1977). Scientific explanation and ecological validity: A reply to Brooks and Baumeister. *American Journal of Mental Deficiency, 81,* 534-542.

Jennett, B., & Bond, M. (1975). Assessment of outcome after severe brain damage. *The Lancet,* March 1, pp. 480-484.

Kapust, L. R., & Weintraub, S. (1988). The home visit: Field assessment of mental status impairment in the elderly. *The Gerontologist, 28,* 112-115.

Klesges, R. C. (1983). The relationship between neuropsychological, cognitive, and behavioral assessments of brain functioning in children. *Clinical Neuropsychology, 5,* 28-32.

Loewenstein, D. A., Amigo, E., Duara, R., Guterman, A., Hurwitz, D., Berkowitz, N., Wilkie, F., Weinberg, G., Black, B., Gittelman, B., & Eisdorfer, C. (1989). A new scale for the assessment of functional status in Alzheimer's disease and related disorders. *Journal of Gerontology: Psychological Sciences, 44,* 114-121.

McCue, M., Rogers, J. C., & Goldstien, G. (1990). Relationships between neuropsychological and functional assessment in elderly neuropsychiatric patients. *Rehabilitation Psychology, 35,* 91-99.

McGlynn, S. M., & Schacter, D. L. (1989). Unawareness of deficits in neuropsychological syndromes. *Journal of Clinical and Experimental Neuropsychology, 11,* 143-205.

McSweeney, A. J., Grant, I., Heaton, R. K., Prigatano, G. P., & Adams, K. M. (1985). Relationship of neuropsychological status to everyday functioning in healthy and chronically ill persons. *Journal of Clinical and Experimental Neuropsychology, 7,* 281-291.

Moore, J. T., Bobula, J. A., Short, T. B., & Mischel, M. (1983). A functional dementia scale. *The Journal of Family Practice, 16,* 499-503.

Searight, H. R., Dunn, E. J., Grisso, T., Margolis, R. B., & Gibons, J. L. (1989). The relation of the Halstead-Reitan Neuropsychological Battery to ratings of everyday functioning in a geriatric sample. *Neuropsychology, 3,* 135-145.

Skurla, A., Rogers, J. C., & Sunderland, T. (1988). Direct assessment of activities of daily living in Alzheimer's disease. *Journal of the American Geriatrics Society, 36,* 97-103

Smith, L. (1985). Communicative activities of dysphasic adults: A survey. *British Journal of Disorders of Communication, 20,* 31-44.

Warren, M. (1981). Relationship of constructional apraxia and body scheme disorders to dressing performance in adult CVA. *The American Journal of Occupational Therapy, 35,* 431-437.

Wedding, D., & Faust, D. (1989). Clinical judgment and decision making in neuropsychology. *Archives of Clinical Neuropsychology, 4,* 233-265.

Williams, J.M. (1987). *Cognitive behavior rating scales manual.* Odessa, FL: Psychological Assessment Resources, Inc.

Williams, N. (1967). Correlation between copying ability and dressing activities in hemiplegia. *American Journal of Physical Medicine, 46,* 1332-1340.

Wilson, B. Cockburn J., & Baddeley, A. (1991). *The Rivermead Behavioural Memory test: Manual* (2nd edition). Bury St. Edmunds: Thames Valley Test Company.

6

ECOLOGICAL VALIDITY AND THE EVOLUTION OF CLINICAL NEUROPSYCHOLOGY

David E. Hartman, Ph.D., A.B.P.N.

ECOLOGICAL VALIDITY AND NEUROPSYCHOLOGY

More than most areas of psychology, clinical neuropsychology has always been constrained by ecological validity. No clinical variation of neuropsychology dares stray too far from direct patient observation and the attempt to link those observations to models of functional neuroanatomy. Nevertheless, being tied to brain-behavior relationships has not been proved restrictive to methodological diversity. In fact, the most novice practitioners of neuropsychology become immediately aware of pronounced differences in procedures and philosophy among groups of neuropsychological practitioners.

Very little has been written to account for these methodological preferences and prejudices of clinical neuropsychologists; possibly all assume that having found the "correct" clinical philosophy, there is no point considering the choices of their "less enlightened" colleagues.

It is the hypothesis of this author that variations in approach are explainable by differences in ecological validity; that is, the variations in neuropsychological methodology were determined by a combination of particular neurological or psychological theories in vogue at the time, and the resulting clinical extensions of those philosophies. Boring (1963) noted that psychological theories may be influenced by their historical context; i.e., "the state of the times works both before and after the discovery...prepar[ing] the way for the discovery and...develop[ing] it into further research and discovery after it is made" (pp. 64-65). For neuropsychology, the "state of the times" generated particular diagnostic paradigms that, in turn, required specialized neuropsychological methods. Understanding the various theories of neuropsychology as products of their historical and clinical context also seems more conflict-free and less inherently polemical than attempting to determine who has the ultimately superior approach to current practice of neuropsychology.

The literature identifies a number of important methodologies in clinical neuropsychology, "fixed" batteries, "flexible" batteries, the more individualistic, "process" approach, "performance testing," and "organicity." Each is a product of scientific constructs and resulting clinical aims. A brief overview of each is particularly important to understanding how ecological validity has been an inherent construct underlying each method.

AMERICAN PSYCHOMETRIC/FIXED BATTERY APPROACHES

In the United States, the ecological context of fixed battery development was the need to investigate and categorize individual differences among large groups; a paradigm whose practical extension became known as the "mental testing movement. Clinical applications of the mental testing movement began with systematic investigation of individual differences with the aim of educating, rehabilitating, or placing school children of differing "native" abilities (e.g., Binet & Simon, 1914). Galton played a major role in the development of mental testing, and while his main interest was human inheritance, some of the individual differences he investigated were in areas now considered "neuropsychological" in nature. As early as 1882, Galton had established a laboratory in London where, for 3 pennies, individuals could be tested for physical and psychophysical measurements, including sensory acuity and reaction time. By 1889, Galton had published *Inquiries Into Human Faculty* detailing individual differences in mental imagery, visual memory, and what we now would term "meta-memory." Evaluation of individual differences were put to very practical use by the application of mental testing to more than a million recruits for the U.S. Army (Franz, 1919). The mental testing movement presaged the development of more clearly neuropsychological methods by developing the basic statistical methods necessary to analyze significant differences among patients and controls, and also in its development of a creative array of testing equipment. Many of these eventually wound up in neuropsychological laboratories. For example, by 1924, available tests included a Stoelting dynamometer, tapping, motor steadiness, color vision, vibration sensitivity, tachistoscopic attentional tasks, the Seguin-Godard Formboard, and cancellation tests that measured "maximal attention...so that reduction of attention is reflected directly in the speed or accuracy of the work" (Whipple, 1924, p. 306). Other tests in use at that time included digit-symbol substitution and rote memory exams for words, objects, and digits. Many of those had norms for normals, "defectives" (retardates), and the brain-damaged (usually epileptics).

The clinical aim of mental testing was to elucidate the multifactorial nature of functional mental abilities. Freeman (1926), for example, concluded that:

> [t]he results of mental tests have shown that no particular single mental process can be identified as the essence of intelligence. All these and more are involved to some degree in those activities which are characteristic of intelligent behavior. We *require memory, discrimination, association, judgment, concept formation, and the others* ...(italics author's). (p. 486).

Even though psychologists of the time were unable to make neuroanatomical inferences from their data, their evaluation of functional strengths and weaknesses was performed very similarly to present-day neuropsychological inference. Referring to the abilities required for a certain test, Bronner, Healy, Lowe, and Shimberg, (1938) noted that it may be solvable:

> ...by some individuals through visualizations or mental representations....But another individual may solve the test without the use of visual imagery and altogether by reasoning....While no one test is probably a reliable measure of any one ability...by utilizing a group of tests involving an identical mental ability, a fair estimate of that ability may be made." (Bronner et al., 1938, p. 23).

Finally, mental testing practitioners had a very modern "neuropsychological" acceptance of the multiple influences upon mental function, as well as a sense of their craft's limitations. Bronner (1938) stated:

> ...[S]pecific abilities and disabilities exist in each human being, whether or not these are due entirely or in part to environmental conditions, earlier experiences, or to original endowment. Though from any mental performance we may not yet be able to decipher primary inherent capacities of various sorts, we are not barred from measuring present capabilities. (p. 11).

During the early twentieth century, the "ecological context" of psychometric testing began to change as the aims of behavioral neurology were gradually melded into psychometric test development. Psychologists stopped simply measuring mental "function"; and gradually began to view themselves as contributing to the accuracy of neurological diagnosis. Trettien's (1917) address before the Toledo Academy of Medicine concluded that psychology was making diagnostic, didactic, and rehabilitative contributions to psychiatric and neurological practice. Trettien stated:

> The second role which psychology is playing today is that of *a diagnostic function in certain neural disturbances* .... Modern psychology is a biological science...in the matter of tracing causes...psychology is rendering important service.... With the aid of the psychiatrist... [psychologists] are teaching the nature and causes of mental arrests as well as the processes of deterioration as they occur in the various forms of psychopathology and neuropathology" (p. 247, italics author's).... "Psychology can also suggest a course of training that may conserve and develop every power of the patient to the fullest and best of which it is capable.... Psychology is just beginning to apply itself to the re-establishment of function through the process of re-education. (pp. 248, 249).

Similarly, Richmond (1924) claimed that "It is possible with the means now at command, to distinguish between original mental defect or feeble mindedness and the deteriorated state resulting from mental disease" (p. 309).

Halstead must be credited as the first to apply the paradigm of mental testing on a large scale toward this new clinical aim. His validation of a fixed battery upon a vast selection of neurologically impaired patients at the University of Chicago Hospital, was probably the first large-scale attempt to systematically determine the psychometric correlates of neurological individual differences.

Initially attempting to provide evidence for abstract reasoning impairment in these individuals, Halstead and his graduate student, Ralph Reitan later extended their scope of investigation to include a wide variety of brain impairments. They accomplished this aim through extensive validation of a fixed series of tests that became known as the Halstead-Reitan Neuropsychological Battery. Credit is theirs for mid-twentieth century neuropsychology's emphasis on higher cortical localization, lateralization, and lesion detection. Matarazzo

(1972), for example, indicated that these factors were increasingly important foci of Halstead's interest and work:

> Apparently so sure was Halstead that the psychological assessment techniques he and others were developing could help in effectively differentiating the brain-damaged individual from the patient who was not brain-damaged that he soon began to concentrate his research efforts, instead, on attempting to localize more precisely such lesions within the brain. (p. 384).

Parson's (1986) reminiscence of Halstead's 1951 talk at Worcester State Hospital corroborates Matarazzo:

> The results of his research, [Halstead] averred, enabled him to predict lesions in the brain with great accuracy. Afterwards, most of us shook our heads and said that it was too good to be true, that brain functions were not as localizable as he was portraying them.(p. 156).

Reitan was similarly predisposed toward empirical validation of HRB performance and cortical function localization. The result was a life-long series of investigations that provided standardized psychometric correlates of brain damage and clinically useful norms. Initial studies which discriminated the presence or absence of brain damage (Reitan, 1955), were soon followed by investigations into the "lateralization, localization, nature, and type of lesion" (Parsons, 1970, p. 6). When Parsons visited Reitan in 1957, he found Reitan "busily concerned with identification of the lesion, lateralization, localization, and ultimately the prediction of the type of lesion." (p. 157).

Halstead and Reitan's large-scale empirical validation of the HRB allowed longitudinal tracking of impairments, and the collection of a normative sample that allowed powerful clinical inferences to be made about the scores of newly presenting patients.

What was the ecological influence that determined Halstead and Reitan's approach? Their initial battery development attempted to validate Halstead's belief in an abstraction factor as the primary cortical function affected by brain damage. A second influence may have been the wish to standardize the skill of the expert neurologist, and in doing so, open up neurology to psychometric research. While the former goal has not met the test of history, there is no doubt that the latter goal initiated a rich field of research and clinical application.

CLINICAL PROCESS/APHASIOLOGY APPROACHES

The so-called "process" or "Boston Process" approach to neuropsychology differs significantly from the fixed battery methodology, and yet also may be understood as a sensible extension of historical roots and clinical aims. The process approach derives from the paradigm of the clinical expert, consistent with European behavioral neurology roots that emphasized qualitative understanding of the patient's behavior as assessed by the expert clinician.

The clinical aim here was a conceptual rather than purely descriptive analysis of brain injury. Early behavioral neurologists attempted to classify deficits by their underlying causes or processes rather than their surface symptoms. One of the first modern descriptions of this type of reasoning was written by Bouillaud in 1825. He proposed that:

> ...the nervous system which directs the formation of signs is not identical with that which produces the movements of the organs of speech, for it is not uncommon to observe suspension of speech sometimes because the tongue and its congenerous organs refuse the pronunciation of words and sometimes because the memory of these words escape us.... It is important to distinguish clearly between these two causes which can lead to loss of speech, each in its own way; one by destroying the organ of memory of words, the other by an impairment in the nervous principle which directs the movement of speech. (in Benton, 1964).

Thus, process methodology seeks to go beyond the score or pattern of scores and test hypotheses underlying the cause of the behavioral disorder.

The work of Werner, in particular, is thought to be especially seminal to process methodology development. Werner attacked the use of achievement scores in isolation and attempted to understand the "process" of how achievement test scores were derived. When this approach was applied to the analysis of brain-damaged behavior, the result was an individually focused, in-depth examination of brain-behavior relationships.

The process approach requires creative application of testing technique, spontaneous hypothesis testing, and flexible analysis of whatever "leads and interests" are suggested during the course of the examination (Gilandas, Touyz, Beumont, & Greenberg, 1984, p. 12). The process expert must be capable of "testing the limits," and the particular set of core tests given to the patient is heavily dependent upon "the examiner's knowledge of available tests of cognitive function and his ingenuity in creating new measures for particular deficit areas."

Luria (e.g., 1973) is probably the most well-known proponent of this form of qualitative neuropsychological analysis. His bedside experience with patients from two World Wars emphasized the importance of the process behind any given impairments. Luria did not adhere to a normative psychometric approach, but developed a set of theories from his observations that allowed for individual hypothesis testing of brain-injured patients.

In the United States, Boston University Medical Center and its associated Veteran's Hospital, apparently played a key role in disseminating process methodology, by supporting presentations of many prominent European neuroscientists and aphasiologists. Kaplan, Goodglass, and other well-known neuropsychologists have been associated with the Boston University Medical Center and have contributed a life's work to the development of this methodology (Milberg, Hebben, & Kaplan, 1986).

Why did the process approach evolve? Differences between the battery approach and process methods are rather pronounced, and occasionally difficult to reconcile within the same field. Again, the construct of ecological validity may provide the missing link. Like the fixed battery approach, process methodology was shaped by the ecological context of its clinical aims (e.g., the investigation of apraxias, aphasias, and other clinical correlates of brain injury). European war victims were available in great numbers to neurologists of the time, and their highly complex, diversely presenting phenomena required detailed exploratory neuropsychological investigation prior to accurate categorization. An in-depth analysis of individual variations in behavior and their relationship to lesion localization became the primary task of early process approach developers. It was this methodology that developed into a more generalized paradigm of neuropsychological investigation.

FLEXIBLE BATTERY APPROACHES

Flexible battery proponents employ both empirical and process philosophies. Batteries are constructed from psychometric tests that have been validated for sensitivity to brain injury. Flexible battery approaches are often used as "screening" measures (e.g., Benton, 1985; Wysocki & Sweet, 1985) where a few preliminary measures determine the need for more extensive clinical investigation. More extensive clinical investigation is equally amenable to the flexible battery approach, with equal emphasis on each neuropsychological domain, or a battery tailored to investigate a single area of observed impairment.

Like the empirically based fixed battery approach, flexible battery proponents rely upon standardized and validated psychometric tests. Flexible batteries also approach the flexibility and hypothesis-testing power of the process approach, as batteries can be changed or expanded during the testing session to investigate areas of increased interest.

Flexible battery approaches have developed from many sources, and probably owe their main influence to the experimental and clinical laboratory, where tests were developed for individual aspect of cognitive functioning. Physicians and psychologists both contributed to the development of flexible batteries. German neurologists of the later nineteenth and early twentieth centuries applied laboratory experimental psychology to the understanding of brain-behavioral relationships. For example, Isserlin, (1923) used Ebbinghaus's list-learning paradigm tests of visual imagery to assess impairment in closed-head injury patients. During the 1800s, Wurzberg neuropsychiatrist Konrad Reiger, developed one of the earliest systematic clinical batteries; a group of about 40 tests to measure various linguistic and neuropsychological skills in patients with nervous or mental disease (Benton, 1985, p. 67).

Psychologists also developed individual psychometric tools to describe neurological and psychiatric abnormalities. General and specific mental disabilities were tested and compared to one another and to control groups. Gatewood (1909) used a battery of 11 tests to compare eight "dementia praecox" against four normals. Cotton (1912), compared normals with dementia praecox or alcoholic psychosis and found that the two experimental groups were similar, with somewhat less impairment in the dementia praecox group. Yerkes, Bridges and Hardwick (1915), used standardized, norm-based mental function tests to assess patients with chorea, epilepsy, syphilis, dementia praecox, hysteria, hypopituitarism, and other disorders (p. 116). They noted the need for a comprehensive assessment of mental abilities and they attempted to fulfill that imprimatur by concatenating tests of cognitive function developed of the time into a battery.

> It seems plain that, to be satisfactory, an examination program must give as little opportunity as possible for interpreting a specialized defect or ability as general. That is, it is important to test all the principle mental functions for each individual and not to infer the development (or lack of development) of some from tests of others. (p. 116)

Developing and refining techniques from the laboratories of Wundt, Ebbinghaus, and Cattell, psychologists investigated abnormal cognition using both natural and artificially induced states of impairment. For example, cognitive functions were assessed under various states of artificially induced neurological or neurotoxicological impairment; subjects under the influence of alcohol, paraldehyde, trional, bromide of sodium, and caffeine were examined. Physical activity, fasting and other general health factors were also assessed for their influence on cognitive performance (Hoch, 1904).

Memory assessment across clinical and normal subjects was another popular area of investigation. For example, Ranschberg compared memory in 12 year old boys, hospital attendants, educated adults, "neurasthenics," and "general paralytics" (syphilitics) (Hoch, 1904). Ranschberg as stated to have found age, education, and occupational effects on memory performance, as well as specific memory disabilities in the 'paralytics,' including "diminution of extent...of total memory...total or almost total destruction of the word memory, name memory of the memory for localization of squares, while that for colors and persons was relatively well preserved."

NEUROPSYCHOLOGICAL "PERFORMANCE" TESTING

The measurement of human *aptitudes and skills*, has lately become integrated with clinical neuropsychology. Considered to be an offshoot of mental testing-style classification of individual differences, the ecological context of test development was the workplace. The resulting "clinical" aim was the creation of tests to quantify work performance, and allow accurate ability estimates for job placement. The *MacQuarrie Test of Mechanical Ability*, originally published in 1925, was one of the first widely distributed tests of this sort. It contained paper-and-pencil measures of motor speed, eye-hand coordination, and visuoperceptual skills; in the service of categorizing the skills of employees.

Thus, rather than categorizing the performance of brain-injured patients and correlating it with a static lesion location, industrial testing developers used mental tests to categorize the performance of *healthy* workers, and correlating test performance with *work efficiency*. In turn, this required tests of active, on-going work behaviors *over time* and investigation of factors that affect work efficiency.

The different aims of performance testing allowed new types of problems to be addressed. The number of butter pats wrapped per hour, the accuracy of aircraft maneuvers under oxygen deprivation or heat stress, and the effects of various drugs on efficient performance are examples of problems capable of being investigated by this paradigm. The United States Government has produced several computerized performance batteries for the latter sort of investigation. *The Unified Tri-service Cognitive Performance Assessment Battery* (UTC-PAB), for example, was designed "to produce a standardized metric that is responsive to required military-mission abilities and skills and will be a sensitive instrument for detecting performance decrements due to the use of biomedical treatment drugs" (Eglund et al., 1987). Several other batteries of similar purpose are currently in use or under development by the Office of Military Performance Assessment Technology (OMPAT).

When integrated within clinical neuropsychology, performance evaluation lends itself to neuropsychological problems not easily addressed with other systems of assessment. In particular, the effects of medications, neurotoxicants, or reversible stresses upon an otherwise healthy nervous system are particularly amenable to performance investigation.

THE ECOLOGICAL VALIDITY OF "ORGANICITY"

The ecological context of organicity testing was different from approaches to neuropsychology that generated previously described approaches. Specifically, organicity testing appears to have unfolded from (1) equipotentialist rather than localizationist theories of brain-behavior relationships, (2) rudimentary diagnostic nosology (e.g., dementia praecox), (3) the anti-localization stance taken by intelligence researchers, and (4) the need to classify the brain-damaged in a separate class from so-called "functional" patients.

In the first, *equipotentiality*, as defined by Flourens and carried on by Lashley and Goldstein, has a long tradition in neurology, and had extended itself into neuropsychology. Much has been written about the naive and reductionistic battle between mental function localizationists and anti-localizationists, which Walsh (1978) has aptly termed the battle of the "skull palpators versus the bird brain ablators" (p. 15), and need not be elaborated upon here. Similarly, Lashley and Goldstein were not naive equipotentialist advocates, but rather counseled a far more complex and integrative form of neural processing. (Goldstein, 1990; Hebb, 1963).

Insofar as equipotentiality theorists like Lashley were (and continue to be) widely misinterpreted as advocating nonlocalizable mental functions, it is not surprising that early clinical applications based on this philosophy attempted to find either a single test of "organicity," or to diminish the importance of localization in higher cortical function analysis.

Intelligence researchers adhered to this latter goal. While Wechsler (1958) admitted that sensory, motor, and perceptual areas had their own circumscribed cortical locations, he believed that more complex cognitive or intellectual functions were not so delimited. Wechsler devalued Halstead's attempt to localize "biologic intelligence" to the frontal lobes; his dismissal of both Halstead's work and higher cortical localization was clear:

> Not only does the bulk of contemporaneous experimental and clinical evidence dispose of the role of the frontal lobes as unique centers of intelligence, it also counter-indicates the possibility of its exclusive localization in any other part of the brain....In brief, neither electroencephalographic nor neurological evidence substantiates the existence of loci in the cerebral hemispheres that serves as centers for...any specifically defined mental processes.....Intelligence has no locus. (p. 20).

The fourth influence on neuropsychological "organicity" testing may have been what Davison (1974) called the "psychodiagnostic testing mission," whose "major use in the United States for many years was answering the question of whether psychiatric patients were suffering from "organic" or "functional" (emotional) disorders" (Golden, 1983, p. 163).

The emphasis may have been a function of the assessment needs of the psychiatric milieu, since "behavioral pathology fell outside the theoretical scope of the treatment orientation....[i]t was important only to identify the brain-damaged as patients of poor therapeutic prognosis, not to learn anything about the scope of brain damage on behavior as a subject of intrinsic interest... " (Davison, 1974, p. 16).

There has been dispute about the value or utility of organicity to modern neuropsychology (e.g., Leonberger, 1989; Mapou, 1988), however, there is little doubt that the term, if not also the clinical techniques, remain in active use. A search of PsyScan through February 1990, identified 239 articles employing the term, with 37 of those also mentioning neuropsychology. The referral for "organicity" testing remains a common request for psychologists performing inpatient evaluations in the psychiatric milieu. Since organicity testing, too, is a product of its ecological context (i.e., the needs of the psychiatric milieu) it may be valid within that context, regardless of its power to uncover complex brain-behavior relationships.

THE FUTURE OF CLINICAL NEUROPSYCHOLOGY

An inevitable conclusion from the preceding review is that clinical neuropsychology is a mutable discipline, with clinical aims that are ecologically valid within the surround of history, medical science, and resulting clinical referrals raised in these contexts. The present decade brings neuropsychology on the uncomfortable cusp of another change in ecological validity. Increasingly sophisticated neuroscientific methods have begun to reveal relationships among neurochemistry, cerebral blood flow, brain metabolism, neuroendocrine function, drug effects and organ system integrity upon brain-behavior relationships (e.g., Buchsbaum, et al., 1991; Sbordone, 1991; Schwankhaus et al., 1989; Swedo, et al., 1991; Tarter, Edwards, & Van Thiel, 1988).

Other aspects of the brain itself are coming under increasing scrutiny in neuropsychology. Investigation of cerebellar disorder, subcortical abnormality, and neurosensory phenomena will also become increasingly important to future neuropsychology. Questions about these systems will require behavioral answers, resulting in new measures and adaptations of older methodologies. This is already occurring for referrals related to neurotoxic exposure, since neuropsychology has begun to adapt *neurosensory* measures to its armamentarium in response to referrals related to neurotoxicant exposure. Recent research has shown a link between early effects of neurotoxic exposure and neurosensory dysfunction. For example, visual impairments are seen in carbon monoxide intoxication. COHb saturation up to 12-13% has no effect on finger tapping or perceptual speed, but appears to affect critical flicker fusion, which decreases as a linear function of single percentage point increases in COHb (Seppanen, Hakkinen, & Tenkku, 1977). Critical flicker fusion has also been found useful in identifying effects of neurotoxic exposure (Winneke, 1981). "Dyschromatopsia," a subtle impairment in color vision, is thought to be produced by neurotoxic insult to the optic pathway, and can be tested by neuropsychological measures. It has been seen to accompany, and even predate conventional neuropsychological impairments in alcohol abusers, solvent workers, printshop employees, and others, (e.g., Braun, Daigneault, Gilbert, Bornstein, & Chelune, 1989; Mergler, Belanger, de Grosbois, & Vachon, 1988; Mergler, Blain, & Lagace, 1987). Testing for dyschromatopsia involves arrangement of desaturated color chips along a chromatic continuum while viewed under a standard light source—a simple neurobehavioral test. Neurosensory evaluation of *auditory* processing has been proposed by Varney (1990) as a potentially sensitive measure for detection of white matter damage from exposure to certain solvents.

In summary, neuropsychology is inevitably changing to fit the new context of its time, much as Boring would have predicted. Benton (1988) predicted that "We are in an era which promises to generate an incomparably deeper and more comprehensive knowledge than we now possess of how the brain functions to mediate cognitive and affective behavior (p. 22)."
It is clear than neuropsychology will continue to change with this new ecological context to become similarly more incisive and comprehensive; its clinical aims will continue to reflect a intrinsic link to ecological validity.

REFERENCES

Benton, A. (1964). Contributions to aphasia before broca. *Cortex, 1.*

Benton, A. J. (1985). Some problems associated with neuropsychological assessment. *Bulletin of Clinical Neurosciences, 50,* 11-15.

Benton, A. (1988). Neuropsychology: Past, present and future. In F. Boller and J. Grafman (Eds.), *Handbook of neuropsychology,* Vol. 1 (pp. 3-27). Elsevier Science Publishers, B.V.

Binet, A., & Simon T. (1914). *Mentally defective children .* New York: Longmans, Green & Co.

Boring, E. G. (1963). *History, psychology, and science.* Selected papers. New York: John Wiley and Sons, Inc.

Braun C. M. J., Daigneault, S., Gilbert, B., Bornstein, R. A., & Chelune, G. J. (1989). Color discrimination testing reveals early solvent neurotoxicity better than a neuropsychological test battery. *Archives of Clinical Neuropsychology, 4,* 1-14.

Bronner, A. F., Healy, W., Lowe, M E., & Shimberg, M. E. (1938*). A manual of individual mental tests and testing.* Boston: Little, Brown and Company.

Buchsbaum, M. S., Kesslak, J. P. Lynch, G., Chui, H., Wu, J., Sicotti, N, Hazlett, E., Teng, E., & Cotman, C. W. (1991). Temporal and hippocampal metabolic rate during an olfactory memory task assessed by positron emission tomography in patients with dementia of the Alzheimer type and controls. *Archives of General Psychiatry, 48,* 840-847.

Cotton, H. A. (1912). Comparative psychological studies of the mental capacity in cases of dementia praecox and alcoholic insanity. *Nervous and Mental Disease Monographs, Series 9,* 123-154.

Davison, L. A. (1974). Introduction. In R. Reitan & L. A. Davidson (Eds.), *Clinical neuropsychology: Current status and applications* (pp. 1-18). New York: John Wiley & Sons.

Eglund, C. E., Reeves, D. L., Shingledecker, C. A., Thorne, D. R., Wilson, K. P., & Hegge, F. W. (1987). *Unified Tri-Service Cognitive Performance Assessment Battery (UTC-PAB) 1. Design and Specification of the Battery* Report No 87-10. Naval Health Research Center, P. O. Box 85122, San Diego, CA 92139.

Franz, S. I. (1919). *Handbook of mental examination methods* (2nd ed.). New York: The MacMillan Company.

Freeman, F. N. (1926). *Mental tests.* Cambridge: The Riverside Press.

Gatewood, L. C. (1909). An experimental study of dementia praecox. *Psychological Monographs, 11,* No. 45.

Gilandas, A., Touyz, S. Beumont, P., & Greenberg. H. (1984). *Handbook of neuropsychological assessment.* New York: Grune & Stratton.

Golden, C. J. (1983). The neuropsychologist in neurological and psychiatric populations. In C. J. Golden & P. J. Vicente (Eds.), *Foundations of clinical neuropsychology*. New York: Plenum Press.

Goldstein, G. (1990). Contributions of Kurt Goldstein to neuropsychology. *The Clinical Neuropsychologist, 4*, 3-17.

Hebb, D. O. (1963). Introduction to Dover edition. In K. S. Lashley, *Brain mechanisms and intelligence* (pp. v-xiii). New York: Dover Publications, Inc.

Hoch, A. (1904). A review of some psychological and physiological experiments done in connection with the study of mental diseases. *The Psychological Bulletin, 1*, 241-257.

Isserlin, M. (1923). Ueber storungen des gedachtnisses bei hirngeschadigten. *Zeitschrift fur die gesammte Neurologie und Psychiatrie, 85*, 84.

Leonberger, F. T. (1989). The question of organicity: Is it still functional? *Professional Psychology: Research and Practice, 6*, 411-414.

Luria, A. R. (1973). *The working brain.* New York: Basic Books.

MacQuarrie, T. W. (1953). *MacQuarrie Test for Mechanical Ability.* Monterey, CA: CTB/MacGraw-Hill.

Mapou, R. L. (1988). Testing to detect brain damage: An alternative to what may no longer be useful. *Journal of Clinical and Experimental Neuropsychology, 10*, 271-278.

Matarazzo, J. D. (1972), *Wechsler's measurement and appraisal of adult intelligence.* Baltimore: Williams & Wilkins.

Mergler, D., Blain, L., & Lagace, J. P. (1987). Solvent-related colour vision loss: An indicator of neural damage? *International Archives of Occupational and Environmental Health, 59*, 313-321.

Mergler, D., Belanger, S., de Grosbois, S., & Vachon, N. (1988). Chromal focus of acquired chromatic discrimination loss and solvent exposure among printshop workers. *Journal of Toxicology, 49*, 341-348.

Milberg, W. P., Hebben, N., & Kaplan, E. (1986). The Boston Process Approach to neuropsychological assessment. In I. Grant & K. Adams (Eds.), *Neuropsychological Assessment of Neuropsychiatric Disorders* (pp. 65-86.) New York: Oxford Press.

Parsons, O. (1986). Overview of the Halsted[sic]-Reitan Battery. In T. Incagnoli, G. Goldstein, & C. J. Golden (Eds.), *Clinical application of neuropsychological test batteries* (pp. 155-192). New York: Plenum Press.

Parsons, O. (1970). Clinical neuropsychology. In *Current Topics in Clinical and Community Psychology, 2*, 1-60.

Reitan, R. E. (1955). An investigation of the validity of Halstead's measures of biological intelligence. *Archives of Neurology and Psychiatry, 73*, 28-35.

Richmond, W. (1924). The psychologist in the psychopathic hospital. *Journal of Abnormal and Social Psychology, 18*, 299-310.

Sbordone, R. J. (August 18, 1991). The side effects of neuropharmacological medications on neuropsychological test performance in the traumatically brain injured patient. Presented at the 1991 Annual Meeting of the American Psychological Association, San Francisco, CA.

Schwankhaus, J. D., Currie, J., Jaffe, M. J., Rose, S. R., & Sherins, R. J. (1989). Neurologic findings in men with isolated hypogonadotropic hypogonadism. *Neurology, 39*, 223-226.

Seppanen, V., Hakkinen, & Tenkku, M. (1977). Effect of gradually increasing carboxyhaemoglobin saturation on visual perception and psychomotor performance of smoking and nonsmoking subjects. *Annals of clinical research, 9*, 314-319.

Swedo, S. E., Rapoport, J. L., Leonard, H. L., Schapiro, M. B., Rapoport, S. I., & Grady, C. L. (1991). Regional cerebral glucose metabolism of women with trichotillomania. *Archives of General Psychiatry, 48*, 828-833.

Tarter, R. E., Edwards, K. L., & Van Thiel D. H. (1988). Perspective and rationale for neuropsychological assessment of medical disease. In R. E. Tarter, D. H. Van Thiel, & K. L. Edwards (Eds.), *Medical neuropsychology: The impact of disease on behavior* (pp. 1-10). New York: Plenum Press.

Trettien, A. W. (1917). Practical applications of psychology in the treatment of certain psychopathics (and other neuropathologies). *Journal of Applied Psychology, 1*, 244-252.

Varney, N. (1990). Neuropsychological sequelae of long-term exposure to organic solvents. Presented at the 11th Annual Meeting of the Midwestern Neuropsychology Group, Madison Wisconsin, May 17, 1990.

Walsh, K. (1978). *Neuropsychology: A clinical approach* . New York: Churchill Livingstone.

Wechsler, D. A. (1958). *The measurement and appraisal of adult intelligence* . Baltimore: The Williams & Wilkins Company.

Whipple, G. M. (1924). *A manual of mental and physical tests.* Baltimore: Warwick & York, Inc.

Winneke, G. (1981). The neurotoxicity of dichloromethane. *Neurobehavioral Toxicology and Teratology, 3*, 391-395.

Wysocki, J. J., & Sweet, J. J. (1985). Identification of brain damage, schizophrenic, and normal medical patients using a brief neuropsychological screening battery. *International Journal of Clinical Neuropsychology, 7*, 40-44.

Yerkes, R. M., Bridges, J. W., & Hardwick, R. S. (1915*). A point scale for measuring mental ability.* Baltimore: Warwick & York, Inc.

* Portions of this chapter appeared in another form as Hartman, D. (1991). Reply to Reitan: Unexamined premises and the evolution of clinical neuropsychology. *Archives of Clinical Neuropsychology, 6* 147-166.

7

A PRACTICAL MODEL OF EVERYDAY ASSESSMENT

J. Michael Williams, Ph.D.

INTRODUCTION

The everyday skill movement has recently influenced virtually every area of cognitive psychology. A formal appreciation of everyday skill assessment has also influenced clinical neuropsychology and has found its way into the clinical reasoning of neuropsychologists, primarily in the rehabilitation and forensic assessment areas. Although these influences have recently been highlighted, certainly the practical assessment problems embodied in the everyday skill area have existed since tests were originally invented. Many were actually developed in response to everyday assessment problems that were not explicitly posed as such. In recent years, models of everyday skills have emerged and represent a formal, pragmatic influence on theories of cognition and clinical practices that utilize cognitive assessment instruments.

The notions of everyday cognition and ecological validity emerged from three major sources in psychology. These were the study of practical intelligence in cognitive psychology (e.g., Neisser, 1979; Sternberg, 1977; Sternberg & Wagner, 1986) the study of everyday cognition in gerontology (Acker, 1986; Poon, 1986; West, 1985) and the prediction of everyday functioning in neuropsychological rehabilitation settings (Chelune & Moehle, 1986; Hart & Hayden, 1986). Movements in all of these areas were at least partially motivated by a reaction to psychometrically based, trait-oriented theories of intelligence and the arcane style of intellectual tests which dominate clinical psychology practice. The following is a brief summary of three major factors which influenced the inclusion of everyday skills in conventional clinical assessment, a general model of everyday cognition, and a description of strategies to incorporate this model into a practical system of clinical assessment. This chapter is a substantial update of Williams (1988).

THE CONSTRUCTION OF CLINICAL INTELLIGENCE TESTS

As a point of historical convenience, applied intelligence testing began in 1902 with the Binet-Simon test battery, developed to evaluate children for school placement. Other investigators had previously invented tests which had practical applications, but the Binet-Simon tests were the first to have an applied focus from the inception of the test battery. Binet developed a set of tasks and a format for presenting them which laid the groundwork for virtually all intellectual test batteries that were to follow. The basic design strategy was to choose a group of tasks for the foundation of the battery which were already developed and had some support among clinicians and investigators. New tasks invented by the developers were then added to this foundation group. Finally, the battery was administered to clinical groups and further modifications were made based upon pilot studies. Although Binet and Simon had fewer previously developed tests for possible inclusion in their battery, by the time of Wechsler's intelligence scales (see Wechsler, 1958), many tests were available and this style of test development was widely accepted without qualification among test developers and clinicians. It still remains the dominant style of test battery development.

The notion of building new batteries from the tests currently available probably represents an adequate, common sense approach to test development. It also enhances the use of the test among clinicians because the subtests are usually known to the potential users. However, this approach stands in contrast to procedures used in developing methods to scientifically examine intellectual constructs, such as memory, language, and problem-solving. Here, the investigator begins with a theory of the construct and then develops methods to test hypotheses based upon the theory. The assessment methodology is logically derived from a theory of the intellectual construct. In contrast, clinical test batteries were developed from virtually no theoretical foundation. Probably as a result of this clinically expedient method of building test batteries, test developers have been, and still are, allowed to invent intellectual and neuropsychological tests without first explaining the constructs the tests were designed to measure.

From the very beginning, intellectual batteries designed for clinical use have had only cursory face validity and fit into models of cognition that were very global and nonspecific. For example, in the words of Binet and Simon (1916), intelligence is, ". . . judgment, otherwise called good sense, practical sense, initiative, the faculty of adapting one's self to circumstances. To judge well, to comprehend well, to reason well, these are the essential activities of intelligence." Wechsler's (1958) definition presented 39 years later was similarly vague: "The aggregate or global capacity of the individual to act purposefully, to think rationally and to deal effectively with the environment."

It is unfortunate that these definitions of intelligence which suggest ecological validity notions, such as environmental adaptation and practical knowledge, led to test batteries which were so abstract and arcane. One must wonder at the ability of some of the Wechsler Adult Intelligence Scale subtests, such as Digit Span, or Digit Symbol, to measure one's ability "to act purposefully, to think rationally and to deal effectively with the environment." Although Wechsler and others certainly recognized the practical aspects of intellectual skills, the test batteries themselves were not developed from a theoretical basis of practical intelligence. The batteries were simply constructed by gathering together tasks already known to clinicians and roughly validating them with clinical populations.

If test developers do not explain the theoretical foundation of the tests and manner in which items or tasks were constructed, then tests will not improve by incorporating any positive innovation, including everyday cognition. These theoretical explanations must also include a clear description of the clinical applications of the test and how they are to be accomplished. If a test is supposed to predict everyday abilities, then this relationship should be explained at a theoretical level as well as established through empirical investigations whenever possible. These investigations should be deemed as important as the standardization and normative studies. In order to invent new tests and conduct such investigations, test developers must first turn to the emerging theoretical basis of practical intelligence.

PRACTICAL COGNITION

One prominent movement in the development of cognitive psychology was the emergence of a variety of theories that stressed information processing as a general model of cognition. The information processing movement gave rise to some extremely reductionistic, abstract models of memory, language, and other cognitive abilities. These in combination with tests of "academic intelligence" were criticized as impractical and conceptually distant from explanations of cognition in everyday life (Neisser, 1979). The emerging reaction to this strict information processing point of view has been loosely described as the study of everyday cognition. This approach always examines some practical ability, usually within the context of traditional cognitive theories. One clear example is the study of eyewitness testimony (Buckout, 1974; Loftus & Palmer, 1974). Here, an everyday domain was chosen for analysis using theories of memory function largely developed in the laboratory.

The everyday cognition movement also represents a departure from traditional methods used in cognitive psychology. In the practical cognition framework, methods reflect the complexity and uncertainty of everyday cognition. In contrast, experimental methods invented in the laboratory usually isolate and control for numerous influences which are extraneous to the specific constructs under study. Experimental methods were not intended to be comprehensive or to have an applied utility. In contrast, everyday measures cover a wide variety of constructs and variability may be accounted for by a number of factors, many of which are unknown to the investigator. For example, memory for eyewitness testimony is influenced by such complex social factors as the degree of empathy perceived by the witness for people in the scene the witness observes (Buckout, 1974). Likewise, the complex role of confabulations and reconstructions in eyewitness recall represent a further manifestation of the complexity and uncertainty present in the study of everyday memory skills. Such complex interactions and multiple factors are usually partialed out of experimental studies so that simple relationships between them are clarified.

Although Sternberg (1985), Neisser (1979), and others proposed that the practical cognition movement began as a reaction to "academic" intelligence, which is presumably that embodied in most intelligence tests, and the testing movement's impoverished theoretical development, it also probably represents the simple infusion of pragmatism into cognitive psychology. Many investigators in the practical cognition movement do not necessarily view their efforts as the study of "intelligence." Many are involved in simply examining an applied skill or some everyday domain without referring to a general model of intelligence and all such a term implies. The testing movement itself represents one applied area of cognitive psychology. Unfortunately, the testing movement developed and gained momentum before there were sophisticated theories of cognition. If the current level of sophistication in theories of cognition were available to Binet or Wechsler, intelligence tests would probably be much more sophisticated.

EVERYDAY COGNITION AND AGING

The practical cognition movement in cognitive psychology has greatly influenced the study of cognition and aging. Many gerontologists are psychologists trained in academic psychology departments in the areas of developmental and cognitive psychology. For some, interests in gerontology emerged from the study of development across the life span (Baltes, 1973).

There has now emerged a gerontology movement that includes every branch of the social sciences. There is a strong clinical and professional group emerging among gerontologists who are establishing geriatric clinical services in hospitals, community mental health centers, nursing homes, and rehabilitation facilities. This movement will expand as our population ages and more emphasis is placed on enhancing the quality of life for older people.

The gerontology movement has prompted numerous studies of cognitive abilities and aging. Early investigations of these relationships revealed pronounced cognitive declines over the life span. These early declines were substantially qualified by later studies (Poon, 1986; Salthouse, 1985; Schaie, 1983). In addition to these qualifications of functional levels, many of these investigators observed that many conventional measures of cognitive abilities were arcane and unrelated to the subject's apparent high level of everyday adjustment. Although the older subjects performed worse on conventional tests, they were not correspondingly unsuccessful in the cognitive demands of everyday life. All these concerns led to a strong ecological validity emphasis in gerontology.

COGNITIVE REHABILITATION

The final relevant setting in which everyday cognition has become prominent is rehabilitation. Here there is strong interest in the ability of intellectual tests to predict functioning in everyday life. This interest has emerged over a time of greatly expanding rehabilitation services for brain-injured patients. As these services have moved from the acute hospital to outpatient and community transitional programs, it has become increasingly apparent that conventional tests are limited in assessing brain-injured patients for rehabilitation purposes.

The basic assessment task of the rehabilitation setting is to predict the patient's post-injury functional levels in occupational, school, and home environments (Williams, 1987b). This task is daunting, given the assessment tools available and lack of prediction studies. The neuropsychological batteries may be adequate in predicting everyday abilities but there is not sufficient knowledge gained through scientific studies which would allow the clinicians any valid basis for such predictions.

All of these factors and interests have worked to produce a high degree of discontent among rehabilitation psychologists and a strong need for a practical assessment technology. In partial response to this need, a variety of rehabilitation-oriented rating scales, inventories, and short neuropsychological batteries were developed (e.g., Prigatano et al., 1984). However, these measures are still tentative and in their early developmental stages.

The rehabilitation, gerontology, and practical cognition movements have all worked to strongly influence the development of new assessment tools. Each has contributed a host of criticisms of current intellectual and neuropsychological tests (see Erickson & Scott, 1977; Poon, 1986). Consistent with the practical cognition movement, these criticisms often focus on the predictive utility of the tests. There are large gaps in knowledge concerning the relationship between conventional intellectual tests and adjustment to occupational, school, and home environments. Although the clinician may know that a patient's IQ is reliably near 85, this knowledge may not reduce the uncertainty in predicting whether this patient can work at a certain occupation, or function independently at home.

THE NATURE OF EVERYDAY SKILLS

Everyday cognition is a term which refers to the great variety of skills, knowledge structures, and reasoning strategies which apply to a particular class of environmental settings. Each setting in which we function has cognitive demands, such as memory for required facts and performance skills, which specifically apply to the setting and may not apply to another. For example, the venerable profession of bartending requires a knowledge of drink ingredients, the skills to combine the ingredients quickly and efficiently, fluent social skills in starting and maintaining conversations, basic academic skills, and a variety of other cognitive skills which an expert bartender could enumerate (see Table 1). Of course, many of these skills are required for successful functioning only in the barroom setting. Skill in mixing drinks is usually not required for successful functioning at home. However, many other abilities, such as social skills and basic academic skills, are part of successful adjustment to many home and work environments.

There is an important distinction between everyday skills that are generic and those which are very specific to certain environmental settings (see Table 1). Generic everyday skills are usually simple, basic skills, often referred to as

Activities of Daily Living Skills (ADLS) (Hart & Hayden, 1986). These are skills required of everyone, such as dressing, maintaining personal hygiene, and feeding oneself. They are generic because they are fundamental to successful functioning in virtually all environments. They are also foundation skills for all others. Geriatric and rehabilitation settings, especially inpatient settings, often refer only to these generic abilities when describing everyday abilities.

The other major type of everyday skills are those specific to individual environments, typically work settings. These represent very specific task demands which an individual masters to successfully adjust to the setting. As a rule of thumb, specific skills are usually more complex and difficult to learn and teach than are generic skills.

This generic-specific distinction is an important conceptual structure for the entire everyday cognition domain. For example, most inpatient brain-injury rehabilitation programs spend their resources training the patients in generic everyday skills, such as ambulation, dressing, cooking, and the like. Outpatient rehabilitation programs typically train generic and specific skills. The transitional nature of outpatient programs compels rehabilitation efforts to include specific environments and consequently, specific skills training, such as job-related skills.

TABLE 1
SOME EVERYDAY SKILLS REQUIRED OF BARTENDERS

Generic:	Specific:
Clean, dress, and care for self	Drink mixing
Driving a car or engaging public transport	Conversational skills
Basic communication skills	Maintaining an inventory
Basic arithmetic	Discriminating sobriety from drunkenness

Generic skills are much easier to predict from test results or other measures because they represent much lower levels of ability and the neuropsychologist is presumably very familiar with performing them. For example, it is much easier to predict whether a patient will be able to dress independently rather than predict whether a patient can keep payroll accounts. Keeping payroll accounts requires skills which are far too specific to have direct referents among neuropsychological test batteries. Also, the neuropsychologist has personal experience with dressing and can perform an informal, qualitative appraisal of the required skills. This subjective context is missing for any setting that is personally unfamiliar to the neuropsychologist making predictions.

There is some precedent for the prediction of such specific job skills. Our colleagues in vocational rehabilitation and general vocational counseling often grapple with this problem. At present, the gains in this area are subsumed within evaluation systems like the General Aptitude Test Battery (GATB) (U. S. Department of Labor, 1970). The GATB includes a variety of tests of generic vocational skills, such as basic clerical and arithmetic skills. Specific occupational skills are assessed using a job task analysis, which includes a combination of informal observations of people in the job setting and formal specifications of tasks which compose the job activities (Anchor, Sieveking, Peacock, & Presley, 1979). Unfortunately, these task analyses are most often applied to simpler, physical occupations that do not have complex cognitive components. There are essentially no task analyses performed for such complex occupations as accountants or managers. However, the general model of job task analysis is one which could be developed to address one aspect of the everyday prediction problem in rehabilitation. The job task analyses could be related to neuropsychological tests and the clinician would have a much more substantial, empirical basis for the prediction of everyday vocational skills.

CONSTRUCT-SPECIFIC EVERYDAY SKILLS

The comprehensive, generalized application of skills in ever-changing environments constitutes the nature of everyday skills. Specific intellectual constructs, such as memory or language, are often indiscernible when such skills are applied. Everyday environments often tax a variety of intellectual abilities in combination and the separate contribution of each skill to the overall performance is difficult or impossible to decipher. However, within this general characterization, there are also construct-based models of everyday skills. There is some integrity to the concepts of everyday language, or everyday memory, which are genuinely distinct and can be distinguished from the variety of skills which are applied to particular everyday problems. The most distinctive of these are language, memory, and visual-spatial skills. Many everyday activities will predominantly express one of these skill domains and a discussion of their unique contribution will highlight many of the points made previously regarding everyday skill environments.

Everyday language skills are expressed predominantly in conversation, giving instructions and following the directions of others, reading road signs, magazines, newspapers, and books, writing letters, filling out forms, and a host of other activities (see Table 2). Memory skills may be refined to include memory for daily activities, memory for instructions, remembering names and faces, and the like. Spatial skills are not as apparent in everyday life as language and memory skills. They may be quite impaired before a disability is noticed. Such skills allow for finding new locations, giving someone else directions to a place, and drawing figures or maps. Everyday motor and sensory coordination includes using tools or cooking utensils and the motor and sensory parts of driving the car.

TABLE 2
CONSTRUCT-SPECIFIC EVERYDAY SKILLS

Everyday Environment	Language	Memory	Spatial Processing	Motor & Sensory Coordination
Living	Conversation, Following instructions, General reading & writing	Remembering the daily schedule of activities, Remembering new names and faces	Finding a new place while driving in the car, drawing a map for someone else	Driving the car, Using tools to fix something
Working	Reading or hearing instructions, Giving instructions, Making notes or reports of work activities, Comprehension of instructions for using a computer	Remembering instructions, Remembering names and faces of customers or clients, Remembering the daily work schedule of activities	Finding the location of objects in a warehouse, or the location of files for record-keeping, Finding new locations to make deliveries	Operating machinery, Driving a forklift or tractor, Using tools to construct products
Learning	Reading Textbooks, Writing school papers and reports, Comprehending lectures or complex presentations, Note-taking skills	Remembering reading material, memorizing facts	Drawing diagrams or other schematics for courses which require them, visualizing the placement or arrangement of objects in schematics (e.g., plumbing diagrams)	Simple writing skills, operating machinery and tool use for technical courses

The interaction of skills is also implied in some of the examples cited here. For example, the process of actually following instructions includes the language comprehension of the instructions and memory for the instructions. Without the application of both abilities, the instructions will not be executed. Failure in environmental adaptation can therefore result from deficits in individual skills that are part of composite everyday activities. Also notice in Table 2 that "Following instructions" appears as a necessary skill for successful functioning at home and at work. This is another representation of a generic skill. The sample skill "Driving a forklift" is a good example of a specific skill.

NEUROPSYCHOLOGICAL STUDIES OF EVERYDAY SKILLS

ACTIVITIES OF DAILY LIVING

There have been a variety of studies examining the utility of neuropsychological tests in predicting basic activities of daily living. Almost all of these studies examined head trauma or stroke patients originally treated in inpatient rehabilitation settings. ADLS were measured at some follow-up time after discharge and neuropsychological assessments performed while the subjects were inpatients were used to predict the ADLS. In general, conventional neuropsychological and intellectual tests predict simple activities of daily living at a low to moderate level (Chelune & Moehle, 1986; Hart & Hayden, 1986; Heaton & Pendleton, 1981). Apparently patients who perform at low levels on neuropsychological tests likewise have difficulty executing simple everyday living skills.

The predictive utility of neuropsychological tests are constrained in this setting for two major reasons. First, many ADLS involve basic sensory and motor skills which are not adequately measured by neuropsychological batteries. Such skills as walking, dressing, or bathing among brain-injured populations probably contain a strong component of sensorimotor coordination and strength in the extremities, which are not carefully assessed by cognitively oriented neuropsychological tests.

Second, ADLS measures are not scaled in the above average to superior range, whereas many neuropsychological tests are scaled across the average to superior range. Many severely impaired patients have great difficulty responding to many neuropsychological tests but will demonstrate a range of function on ADLS scales. For example, patients who cannot dress themselves may be completely untestable on the Tactual Performance Test, a conventional part of the Halstead-Reitan Battery. As a consequence, this neuropsychological test will not appear predictive of these skills due to this contrast in scaling.

EMPLOYMENT STATUS

The neuropsychologist in the outpatient setting is often faced with the straight-forward question of whether a patient can return to former employment. If that is determined to be impossible, then the neuropsychologist is often asked to specify which occupations are now reasonable expectations for the patient. Although this prediction task has become extremely important in outpatient and rehabilitation-oriented neuropsychology, very few studies have examined the prediction of actual employment skills using neuropsychological tests. Most studies in this area have simply predicted employment status rather than specific occupational skills.

A number of these studies have, in fact, validated the use of neuropsychological tests in the prediction of simple employment status (Dikman & Morgan, 1980; Heaton, Chelune, & Lehman, 1978; Newnan, Heaton, & Lehman, 1978). The strength of this relationship is apparently low to moderate. This characterization is tentative, however, because most of the studies performed thus far have used only mean comparisons to establish this relationship and virtually no study used regression techniques to make predictions of employment status. Typically, employed and unemployed patients are compared on neuropsychological tests. Unemployed patients have been observed to have significantly lower neuropsychological test scores. Although such comparisons indicate that some relationship between these variables exist, the strength of such relationships cannot be established with such simple designs.

A very few studies have examined the relationship of neuropsychological tests to actual job-related skills. These have also found a low to moderate relationship between the test findings and the job skills (Chelune & Moehle, 1986). It is apparent from these studies that job skills are extremely specific and make up skill clusters which neuropsychological tests may predict only in very general terms. For patients who have borderline impairment, this situation results in great uncertainty for the clinician's prediction of job success. Our pilot research on this "reasoning under uncertainty" (Kahneman, Slovic, & Tversky, 1982) suggests that neuropsychologists develop idiosyncratic rules of thumb and systematic biases in their reasoning concerning relationships of the tests to job skills (Williams, 1987a). In general, neuropsychologists believe their tests are more reliable and the predictive relationships between tests and job skills are more robust than research would suggest. For example, many neuropsychologists had strong beliefs about the ability of the Tapping test to predict motor skills in job areas, such as assembly line work. However, there has never been a study of this relationship.

MISCELLANEOUS SKILLS

The final domain of interest involves the prediction of general everyday skills which are more sophisticated than ADLS and not specific to occupational environments. This includes a few studies which used intellectual and neuropsychological batteries to predict driving skills, everyday memory skills (e.g., remembering phone numbers), and the like. Among these studies, there has been an almost exclusive focus on two everyday skill domains: driving skills and everyday memory skills. The driving studies are usually performed in brain-injury rehabilitation settings, the everyday memory studies are performed by gerontologists who typically examine normal elderly volunteers.

Driving is a generic skill which is important for successful functioning in most occupational, educational, and home environments. The few prediction studies using neuropsychological tests strongly suggest that the tests are predictive of the cognitive aspects of driving (Golper, Rau, & Marshall, 1980; Gouvier, Webster, & Blanton, 1986). Certainly the basic motor and sensory aspects of driving are best predicted by physical strength and dexterity assessment devices and driving simulators. Neuropsychological tests appear especially useful in predicting the visuospatial components of driving (Gouvier & Warner, 1987).

In the memory assessment arena, numerous gerontologists have criticized conventional memory tests because they are not "ecologically valid." This criticism arises from the simple observation that elderly adults who are functioning competently in the home environment can score poorly on memory and intellectual tests. There is an apparent discrepancy between their tested vs. everyday ability. This basic discrepancy has led to studies examining everyday competencies among the elderly, prediction studies using conventional tests, and the development of new assessment devices (Crook, 1986; Eisdorfer, 1986; Little et al., 1986). For all the criticism of the tests, very few studies have actually examined the relationships of memory function to everyday skills. Most test the relationship of memory skill self-report to memory test performance. These indicate that tests are moderately related to self-report (Gilewski & Zelinski, 1986). However, one study cast considerable doubt on the reliability and validity of self-report as a measure of everyday ability. Little et al. (1986) discovered that certain areas of memory function are better observed by elderly adults than others. For example, subjects were much better at assessing their own memory for reading material than their memory for phone numbers or new names. Most subjects underestimate their ability to remember names and other common information, presumably because errors in memory for this material are often noticed in everyday life. Consequently, subjects reported that their ability level was poor. Williams, Little, Scates, and Blockman (1987) also discovered that memory self-report is also strongly influenced by depression.

When other criteria are used, such as actual everyday skills (e.g., a test of memory for names and faces), the correlations between tests and everyday abilities rise (Little et al., 1986). However, most everyday skills cannot be formatted into a test as such, and when they are, they appear more like memory tests and not like their everyday referents. For example, once a name and faces memory test is constructed, it appears more like a paired associates memory test rather than the ecologically rich, complex task it is in everyday life.

SUMMARY OF EVERYDAY SKILL STUDIES

The general findings of these studies has been restated throughout. The relationship of everyday skills to neuropsychological tests is low to moderate. Typical Pearson correlations range from .2 to .5. Although this area suffers from too few studies and other methodological shortcomings, this overall characterization has been repeatedly sustained. There is no study which indicated that neuropsychological tests were strongly predictive of any everyday functional skill. Certainly patients who do very poorly, or are untestable, will have great problems at home and may not be able to function in any job. However, we do not have the clinical or experimental evidence to support predictive statements for patients who score higher. For patients who score in the borderline to normal ranges on our tests, available research suggests our predictions are essentially guesses. Until the measurement situation improves, we will continue to reason under extreme uncertainty.

Although a trend has developed in the overall findings, these studies suffer from methodological problems and considerable gaps in the conceptualization and coverage of everyday skill areas. First, and most important, are the conceptualization and design of what are termed the everyday skills. Most researchers and clinicians probably have a very reliable conceptualization of everyday skills. These are the skills used in home, school, and occupational environments. Such abilities include remembering new names and faces, driving a car, washing the clothes, and using the telephone. There is little controversy over defining these skills as in the province of the "everyday," and any test measuring or predicting them would certainly embody "ecological validity."

There are currently grave problems in translating this simple idea into a clinical assessment strategy or research study. On the clinical application side, most clinical neuropsychologists wish to keep their tried and true assessment batteries, either ones they individually compiled or the formal batteries. The idea of altering the tests is unpalatable. Such clinicians would certainly prefer to see prediction studies which show that their tests predict everyday skills at moderate to high levels. If such were demonstrated, then the clinicians would keep their tests intact and feel confidant in their clinical predictions.

On the side of research, it is very difficult to construct an everyday task which actually assesses the full complexity of everyday performance. For example, suppose an experimenter wishes to construct a name and faces memory test. One simple, straight-forward strategy would be to show subjects unfamiliar faces and pair them with names. Recall can be tested by later showing the subject the faces and requesting them to produce the name. Another strategy would be to present the subject with a videotape of someone giving a name and an introduction. The subject could then be showed the videotape without the sound and asked to recall the associated name and other pertinent information about the person on the tape. It is apparent that such tasks do not completely represent the full complexity and richness of the memory for names and faces which exist in the everyday world. The more one attempts to create a "test" of everyday function, the less ecological relevance is embodied in the task.

This problem of objectifying everyday tasks in order to design a test varies from task to task. Some everyday skills are more amenable to direct measurement than others. For example, a name and faces test is relatively easy to construct and is similar enough to the task in everyday life. However, a test of many everyday social skills required of certain occupations would probably be impossible or impractical to develop, both because they are too specific and complex; any test would consequently be very different than the real-life tasks. For example, many skills required of a factory supervisor would be very difficult to standardize and still have the test resemble the everyday activities.

Another approach to gathering information pertinent to success in everyday tasks is to use self-report or significant other questionnaires of everyday abilities (Little et al., 1986; McDonald, 1986; Williams, Davis, Little, & Haban, 1987; Williams, Klein, Little, & Haban, 1986). They rely on observations and inferences made either by the patient or a reliable observer of the patient (e.g., a family member). These measures are attractive because of their ease of administration. They are constrained by the relative unreliability of such observations and the limited coverage of possible content areas. Many everyday skills are difficult for patients or family members to rate. Many occupational tasks have not even been attempted at the time the questionnaire is administered.

A PROSPECTUS FOR NEW TESTS

There are two possible mechanisms by which ecological validity may influence the development of new tests. The first is by compelling test designers to build test batteries based upon traditional tasks and rating scales and then use them to predict everyday abilities. The advantage of this approach is that current tests need not change remarkably and new tests can have the comfortable look and feel of the older tests. Test developers and publishers must simply include studies of ecological validity as well as reliability and normative studies. If a test is represented by developers as an instrument for the prediction of rehabilitation outcome or independence among the elderly and the like, then these validity studies should be conducted as part of test development.

The second approach is to actually modify tests to include everyday tasks whenever possible. For example, the Memory Assessment Scales (Williams, 1991) includes a test of memory for names and faces. The Rivermead Behavioral Memory Test (Wilson, Cockburn, & Baddeley, 1985) also includes a variety of everyday memory tasks. Such innovations would probably result in a great increase in the ability of clinical evaluations to predict everyday functioning. Many content areas can be directly assessed using tasks which are very similar to their everyday referents. Some of these have been already invented but only a few have been incorporated into commercially available test batteries. The development of new everyday tasks should be part of a creative new movement in the invention and marketing of psychological tests.

The major constraint on the incorporation of everyday skills into clinical batteries is the specificity of many skills needed for occupational and everyday living environments. This problem will probably not be completely overcome by developing new and better tests. The format of present tests is just too limited to assess many of these skills. Such specific skills as supervisory ability, skilled craftwork, and the like are either far too complex or logistically impossible to assess directly. Most of the logistical problems arise because the examiner cannot construct a facsimile of the environment in which the skill is conducted. However, many everyday skills, such as memory for reading or everyday arithmetic skills, can be easily measured using a test. The ideal test battery would consequently include a mix of traditional and everyday tasks.

REFERENCES

Acker, M. B. (1986). Relationship between test scores and everyday life functioning. In B. Uzzell & Y. Gross (Eds.), *Clinical neuropsychology of intervention*. New York: Martinus Nijhoff.

Anchor, K., Sieveking, N., Peacock, C., & Presley, B. (1979). Work behavior sampling in vocational assessment: Applications for neuropsychological methodology. *Clinical Neuropsychology, 1*, 51-53.

Baltes, P. B. (1973). Prototypical paradigms and questions in life-span research on development and aging. *Gerontologist, 13*, 458-467.

Binet, A., & Simon, T. (1916). *The development of intelligence in children*. (E.S. Kit, trans.), Baltimore, MD: Williams and Wilkins.

Buckout, R. (1974). Eyewitness testimony. *Scientific American, 231*, 23-31.

Chelune, G., & Moehle, K. (1986). Neuropsychological assessment and everyday functioning. In D. Wedding, A. M. Horton & D. Webster (Eds.), *The neuropsychology handbook*. New York: Springer.

Crook, T. (1986). Overview of memory assessment instruments. In L. Poon (Ed.), *Handbook for clinical memory assessment of older adults*. Hyattsville, NM: American Psychological Association.

Dikman, S., & Morgan, S. F. (1980). Neuropsychological factors related to employability and occupational status in persons with epilepsy. *Journal of Nervous and Mental Disease, 168*, 236-240.

Eisdorfer, C. (1986). Conceptual approaches to the clinical testing of memory in the aged: An introduction to the issues. In L. Poon (Ed.), *Handbook for clinical memory assessment of older adults*. Hyattsville, MD: American Psychological Association.

Erickson, R. C., & Scott, M. L. (1977). Clinical memory testing: A review. *Psychological Bulletin, 84*, 1130-1149.

Gilewski, M. J., & Zelinski, E. M. (1986). Questionnaire assessment of memory complaints. In L. Poon (Ed.), *Handbook for clinical memory assessment of older adults*. Hyattsville, MD: American Psychological Association.

Golper, L., Rau, M., & Marshall, R. (1980). Aphasic adults and their decision on driving: An evaluation. *Archives of Physical Medicine and Rehabilitation, 61*, 34-40.

Gouvier, W. D., & Warner, M. S. (1987). Treatment of visual imperception and related disorders. In J. M. Williams & C. J. Long (Eds.), *The rehabilitation of cognitive disabilities*. New York: Plenum.

Gouvier, W. D., Webster, J. S., & Blanton, P. D. (1986). Cognitive retraining with brain damaged patients. In D. Wedding, A. M. Horton, & D. Webster (Eds.), *The neuropsychology handbook*. New York: Springer.

Hart, T., & Hayden, M. E. (1986). The ecological validity of neuropsychological assessment and remediation. In B. Uzzell & Y. Gross (Eds.), *Clinical neuropsychology of intervention*. New York: Martinus Nijhoff.

Heaton, R. K., & Pendelton, M. G. (1981). Use of neuropsychological tests to predict adult patients' everyday functioning. *Journal of Consulting and Clinical Psychology, 49*, 807-821.

Heaton, R. K., Chelune, G. J., & Lehman, R. A. (1978). Using neuropsychological and personality tests to assess likelihood of patient employment. *Journal of Nervous and Mental Disease, 166*, 408-416.

Kahneman, D., Slovic, P., & Tversky, A. (1982). *Judgment under uncertainty: Heuristics and biases*. New York: Cambridge University Press.

Little, M. M., Williams, J. M., & Long, C. J. (1986). Clinical memory tests and everyday memory. *Archives of Clinical Neuropsychology, 1*, 323-333.

Loftus, E. F., & Palmer, J. C. (1974). Reconstruction of automobile destruction: An example of the interaction between language and memory. *Journal of Verbal Learning and Verbal Behavior, 13*, 585 - 589.

McDonald, R. S. (1986). Assessing treatment effects: Behavior rating scales. In L. Poon (Ed.), *Handbook for clinical memory assessment of older adults.* Hyattsville, MD: American Psychological Association.

Neisser, U. (1979). The concept of intelligence. *Intelligence, 3*, 217-227.

Newnan, O. S., Heaton, R. K., & Lehman, R. A. (1978). Neuropsychological and MMPI correlates of patient's future employment characteristics. *Perceptual and Motor Skills, 46*, 635-642.

Poon, L. W. (1986). *Clinical memory assessment of older adults.* Washington, DC: American Psychological Association.

Prigatano, G. P., Fordyce, D. J., Zeiner, H. K., Roueche, J. R., Pepping M., & CaseWood, B. (1984). Neuropsychological rehabilitation after closed head injury in young adults. *Journal of Neurology, Neurosurgery, and Psychiatry, 47*, 505 -513.

Salthouse, T. A. (1985). *A theory of cognitive aging.* Amsterdam: North Holland.

Schaie, K. W. (1983). *Longitudinal studies of adult psychological development.* New York: Guilford.

Sternberg, R. J. (1977). *Intelligence, information processing, and analogical reasoning: The componential analysis of human abilities.* Hillsdale NJ: Erlbaum.

Sternberg, R. J. (1985). *Beyond IQ: A triarchic theory of human intelligence.* New York: Cambridge University Press.

Sternberg, R. J., & Wagner, R. K. (1986). *Practical intelligence.* New York: Cambridge University Press.

United States Department of Labor. (1970). *Manual for the USES General Aptitude Test Battery.* Washington, DC: U. S. Government Printing Office.

Wechsler, D. (1958). *The measurement and appraisal of adult intelligence* (4th ed.). Baltimore, MD: Williams and Wilkins.

West, R. (1985). *Memory fitness over 40.* Gainesville, FL: Triad Publishing Company.

Wilson, B., Cockburn, J., & Baddeley, A. (1985). *The Rivermead Behavioral Memory Test.* Reading, England: Thames Valley Test Company.

Williams, J. M. (1987a). The neuropsychologist's personal model of cognition. Paper presented at the annual meeting of the Tennessee Psychological Association, Nashville, TN.

Williams, J. M. (1987b). The role of cognitive retraining in comprehensive rehabilitation. In J. M. Williams & C. J. Long (Eds.), *The rehabilitation of cognitive disabilities.* New York: Plenum.

Williams, J. M. (1988). Everyday cognition and the ecological validity of intellectual and neuropsychological tests. In J. M. Williams & C. J. Long (Eds.), *Cognitive approaches to neuropsychology.* New York: Plenum.

Williams, J. M. (1991). *The Memory Assessment Scales.* Odessa, FL: Psychological Assessment Resources.

Williams, J. M., Klein, K., Little, M., & Haban, G. (1986). Family observations of everyday cognitive impairment in dementia. *Archives of Clinical Neuropsychology, 1*, 21-28.

Williams, J. M., Davis, K., Little, M., & Haban, G. (1987). *The Cognitive Behavior Rating Scale.* Odessa, FL: Psychological Assessment Resources.

Williams, J. M., Little, M., Scates, S., & Blockman, N. (1987). Memory complaints and abilities among depressed older adults. *Journal of Consulting and Clinical Psychology, 55*, 595-598.

8

WALKING AND CHEWING GUM:
The Impact of Attentional Capacity on Everyday Activities

Kimberly A. Kerns, Ph.D.
Catherine A. Mateer, Ph.D., A.B.P.P./A.B.C.N.

Attention is an important cognitive capacity. Everyday life is filled with examples of individuals trying to get people's 'attention.' Advertising campaigns compete for our attention. Educators and parents are well aware of the importance of having children "pay attention" within an educational setting in order to learn what is being said or demonstrated. Yet, in spite of the everyday use of the word and concept of attention, it is still not a well understood cognitive capacity.

Attention is defined in layman's terms by Webster's dictionary as "the act or state of attending especially through applying the mind to an object of sense or thought; a condition of readiness ... especially a selective narrowing or focusing of consciousness and receptivity." Though attention is a general term, within the realm of clinical and research psychology "attention" has been more technically defined and explored as a theoretical construct. Experimental psychologists have been exploring the nature of attentional processes for decades. Most theoretical interpretations of attention equate it with the amount of information that can be attended and responded to in some finite amount of time. Historically there have been many experimental models of attention. These have included the concepts of selectivity in attention (Triesman, 1969), automatic versus effortful processing (Shiffrin & Schneider, 1977), vigilance (Broadbent, 1958), and working memory (Baddeley, 1981). More recently there has been a tendency to incorporate these notions into larger schemes of attention which view this process area as multidimensional and having several dissociable components. Along with this development has been the generation of specific hypotheses about the brain mechanisms underlying these components.

CLINICAL MODELS OF ATTENTION

The shift to more componential theories of attention appears, at least in part, to have emerged out of the increasing linkage between cognitive psychology and neuropsychology and the detailed analysis of cognitive function in neurologically impaired patients. Sohlberg and Mateer (1987), for example, described what they termed a clinical model of attention derived by examining cognitive theories of attention in concert with clinical observations from the assessment and rehabilitation of individuals who had sustained traumatic brain injuries. Attention was considered to be a multidimensional cognitive capacity which directly impacts new learning, memory, communication, problem solving, perception, and all other dimensions of cognition. In the Sohlberg and Mateer model, attention was divided hierarchically into five dimensions: focused attention, sustained attention, selective attention, alternating attention, and divided attention.

Focused attention, in their model, was defined as the ability to respond to specific sensory information. Generally, this information is presented in the visual, auditory, or tactile modality. This type of attention is disrupted in metabolic disorders affecting level of consciousness, in the early stages following some brain trauma and during emergence from coma, when an individual may initially be responsive primarily to internal stimuli and only gradually regain the ability to respond to specific external events.

Sustained attention referred to the ability to maintain a consistent behavioral response for a period of time during continuous and repetitive activity. Sustained attention incorporates the notion of vigilance and involves both persistence on an activity over time, as well as the consistency with which that behavior is maintained. Patients with disruption in sustained attention ability may only be able to focus on a task for a few seconds or minutes, or may dramatically fluctuate in the accuracy of their performance over even brief periods. Sustained attention, at perhaps a higher level, also includes the constructs of "mental control" or "working memory," involving the ability to maintain and manipulate more than one piece of information in mind.

Selective attention was described as the ability to maintain a behavioral or cognitive set when other distracting or competing stimuli are present. It incorporates the ideas of "freedom from distractibility" and the ability to ignore irrelevant information. Individuals who have deficiencies in this area are easily drawn off task by extraneous or irrelevant stimuli including both external sights and sounds (the "cocktail party phenomena") and internal distractors (worries, ruminations, sensations, or thoughts). Clinical examples include individuals with the inability to perform tasks in noisy environments, such as a homemaker who after a head injury is unable to prepare a meal if her children are playing in the kitchen. Children with attention deficit disorders also experience considerable difficulty with this skill; for example, they have problems attending to a teacher's lecture when others are whispering in the classroom.

The construct of alternating attention referred to the capacity for mental flexibility that allows individuals to shift their focus of attention. Alternating attention involves switching between tasks having different cognitive demands or requiring different behavioral responses. For example, a student in class must shift between listening to the lecture and writing notes. Similarly, a secretary may have to quickly shift between answering phones, typing, and responding to questions. The individual must monitor which information will be attended to or which responses are appropriate. Individuals with difficulty in this area have problems changing tasks quickly or shifting their attention to new stimuli. They may continue with an old behavior which is no longer appropriate, or may need extra cues to initiate a new task.

Divided attention was described as the ability to respond simultaneously to more than one task or stimuli. Either more than one behavioral response is required, or more than one stimuli may need to be monitored. The capacity for divided attention is required whenever multiple simultaneous demands must be managed (e.g., driving a car while drinking coffee). Some tasks requiring divided attention but involving overlearned behavior patterns are easily accomplished by most individuals (e.g.,"walking and chewing gum"), while others require a higher attentional capacity (e.g., driving a car while trying to find your way on a map). A striking clinical example of this was seen in a brain-injured patient who appeared to have difficulty maintaining postural control, primarily when he was challenged by a potentially competing cognitive task. When given a task of grating cheese, for example, he was noted to progressively slump down and forward until his forehead nearly touched the counter as he lost postural integrity. The divided attentional demands of simultaneously maintaining his posture and grating cheese appeared to be beyond his capacity.

Similarly, in a pilot study, Shumway-Cook, Kerns, and Woollcot (1993) investigated the impact of performing a cognitive task on balance as indicated by postural sway. They found that postural stability was relatively compromised, even in control subjects, when they were required to engage in a demanding cognitive task. In a group of subjects with mild head injury, this compromise was exaggerated, particularly when the demands on postural control were increased by having to stand on a pliant foam rubber surface (thus providing less consistent kinesthetic feedback).

FACTOR ANALYTIC MODEL OF ATTENTION

In contrast to a clinical approach which considers theory but is based primarily on clinical observations and reports, the construct of attention has also been examined psychometrically. Similar to the factor analytically derived models of intelligence (i.e., Guilford [1967]; Wechsler [1958]), Mirsky, Anthony, Duncan, Ahearn, and Kellam (1991) derived a model of attention based upon factor analysis of several tests thought to assess attention. In their model, attention is seen as entailing four separate components. Psychometrically, these factors were derived using both varimax (deriving factors which are statistically non-correlated) and oblique (factors which can be correlated) rotational procedures. The results of both procedures produced a model of attention with essentially the same four factors. In addition to finding the same four factors regardless of the factor analysis procedure, the same structure was noted both in a sample of adults and of children, suggesting that this model of attention is applicable regardless of developmental level.

The four factors which Mirsky et al. (1991) derived are labeled as follows: 1) focus-execute, 2) sustain, 3) encode, and 4) shift. This multicomponent view of attention is in keeping with both information processing and clinical models which, as indicated earlier, incorporate a variety of functions including selectivity, vigilance, and shifting of set.

The "focus-execute" element represents the ability to select target information from an array for enhanced processing. It entails the idea of being able to selectively attend and pick out specific information. Tasks which loaded highly on this factor included Digit Symbol (from the *Wechsler Adult Intelligence Scale - Revised* [Wechsler, 1981]), *Talland's Letter Cancellation Test* (Talland, 1965), the *Trail Making Test* (Reitan & Davidson, 1974), and *the Stroop Word Color Interference Test* (Stroop, 1935). These tasks have in common the requirement to selectively attend to a certain piece of information in an array. This factor appears to include concepts of both sustained and selective attention as defined in the previous model.

The second factor Mirsky et al., (1991), defined was the "sustain" component of attention. This is defined as the capacity to maintain focus and alertness over time. This vigilance or sustained attention capacity is a factor which, as was seen earlier, has been recognized clinically and in cognitive studies. The task which defined this factor in Mirsky's study was the Continuous Performance Test (originally developed by Rosvold, Mirsky, Sarason, Bransome, & Beck, 1956). In this task, the subject is required to watch a visual display for periods of seven to 10 minutes and to press a button in response to a "target" stimuli. Examples include pressing a button when the letter "X" appears, or the more demanding task of responding only when the sequence of stimuli meets a certain condition (e.g., only when "X" is followed by an "A").

Mirsky et al. (1991) defined the third element of attention as the ability to change attentive focus in a flexible and adaptive manner, or shift. Incorporated within this element is the idea that attention is not only involved in selecting (i.e., monitoring or filtering) the relevant input, but also in selecting the proper or relevant output or response. Inability to change the output is one aspect of what is called "perseveration." This flexibility or shift component of attention was defined by measures on the *Wisconsin Card Sorting Test* (Grant & Berg, 1948), including the number of categories achieved, the number of correct responses, and the number of errors. The shift component is probably related most closely to the clinically derived concept of alternating attention.

The final element of Mirsky's attention model was labeled "encoding." This factor was not originally hypothesized as part of the model, but was a factor which was found consistently throughout the factor analyses. Tests which load on this factor included the Arithmetic and Digit Span subtests from the *WAIS-R*. The definition of the encode element is rather vague, but appears to be related to both memory and the ability to manipulate retrieved information in mind. This appears reminiscent of Baddeley's (1981) working memory model. Within a clinical model, this would most likely be incorporated under the rubric of higher level sustained attention, involving mental control.

The shift to viewing attention as having separable and measurable components appears to be a useful and productive one. As the boundaries of what constitutes attention broaden, however, one is struck with the pervasiveness of the constructs. Almost every cognitive ability or task one might imagine will have underlying attentional requirements and the distinctions between the attentional components and other information processing or motor requirements of a task can easily blur. Therefore, it is important to thoroughly evaluate the integrity of all involved processing systems when an attention deficit is hypothesized.

NEUROANATOMICAL SUBSTRATES OF ATTENTION

In the previous sections, attention was described as a complex set of processes which can be divided into a number of distinct components or functions. Research in neuropsychology and neurophysiology further supports that these functions are subserved by different brain regions. Several brain regions appear to have specialized roles in different aspects of attention, although some regions will share more than one aspect of attention. The regions and their functions, however, appear to be organized into a coordinated system. Considerable evidence indicates that performance on particular tests of attention may be impaired selectively by lesions of different brain areas. The following is a model for conceptualizing the neural organization of attentional mechanisms.

The tectal and mesopontine regions of the reticular formation and brain stem have been well established as essential to the maintenance of consciousness and the regulation of arousal. These structures comprise the basic, fundamental, and phylogenetically most primitive component of the attention system in the brain. These structures are believed to be critical to the maintenance of vigilance and sustained attention (Mirsky, Bakay Pragay, & Harris, 1977; Moruzzi & Magoun, 1949). There also appears to be a role of midline thalamic structures in sustained attention or maintenance of vigilance, through modulation of reticular activity (Yingling & Skinner, 1975). The brain stem reticular formation, mesencephalic region, and portions of the nonspecific reticular thalamus are believed to act in concert with certain cortical regions to provide the basis of awareness and modulate such factors as readiness to respond and reaction time.

The thalamus has probably been the brain structure most closely associated with the notion of selectivity. Not all of the myriad external sensory information or internally available input potentially available to the nervous system can be processed. The thalamus has been modeled as a gating system that "selects" and then filters information which will or will not go on for further processing (Mateer & Ojeman, 1983). It is believed to function through modulation of both downstream (brainstem and mesencephalon) and upstream (primarily cortical) systems (Yingling & Skinner, 1975).

The capacity to "shift" or "alternate" attention has traditionally been considered to involve the dorsolateral prefrontal cortex. This has been primarily on the basis of clinical studies of response patterns on tests such as the *Wisconsin Card Sorting Test* (Milner, 1963). Based on work in monkeys, cells associated with this capacity are equally represented in the medial frontal cortex and the anterior cingulate (Bakay Pragay, Mirsky, Ray, Turner, & Mirsky, 1978). In some respects the "shift" element of attention is but one component of an overarching classification of behaviors— the so-called executive functions— rather than that of attention, per se. The boundaries between higher levels of "attention" or "attentional control" and "executive function" are often indistinct, and it is probably most useful to think in terms of multiple and somewhat overlapping functional systems.

As discussed previously, impaired attention is often identified with poor performance on such measures as Digit Symbol from the *WAIS-R, Letter Cancellation*, the *Stroop Test,* and the *Trail Making Test.* These very complex tasks involve, in addition to sustained, selective, and/or shifting attention, abilities such as visual scanning, visual perception and recognition, speed of processing, and a more or less complicated motor response. Multiple cortical and subcortical regions are clearly involved in completion of these tasks, and they must act in concert with the regions described more specifically for the various attentional components. The neural circuitry to support such interactions is well established. The inferior parietal and superior temporal regions both have multimodal sensory convergence areas; these areas, in turn, have corresponding connections to sensory, limbic (i.e., cingulate cortex), thalamic, and brain stem reticular areas as well as motor and frontal cortices (Mesulam, 1987). Given the wide distribution of brain regions associated with attention and its various components, it is not unexpected that there would be a variety of different sites and sources of neurological injury that would disturb attention. For example, neurological disruption resulting from traumatic injury can affect a variety of brain regions, including brain stem, midbrain, diencephalic, and anterior cortical, many of which are involved in one or more aspects of attention.

COGNITIVE PROCESSING MODELS OF ATTENTION

The construct of attention has also been examined from a cognitive processing perspective. Models from this perspective are generally based on information from normal individuals versus clinical samples. The clinical and psychometric models of attention described earlier have primarily focused on measurement of attention through performance on specific tasks. Cognitive theorists, in contrast, have largely focused on the effect of varying attentional demands on performance of specific tasks. Though these tasks may be ecologically valid, there is no attempt made to measure the attention capacity which would allow an evaluation of individual differences. Major areas of investigation utilizing a cognitive processing approach include studies of vigilance, perceptual selection, dual task performance, and automaticity (see Baddeley, 1991 for review).

Research on "vigilance" has had some practical significance in that it has looked at the sustained attention necessary for such tasks as monitoring a radar screen or inspecting items on an industrial production line (Broadbent, 1958). Parasuraman's (1979) research demonstrated that performance on tasks in which some form of short-term storage is required is more difficult to sustain than on tasks without this requirement. For example, tasks which require comparisons between items show decrement in performance over trials whereas tasks in which each item is judged on its own merits do not.

"Selective attention" has been the subject of a great deal of theoretical and experimental interest. Early studies tended to focus on understanding how individuals could identify particular perceptual characteristics or features from background noise (e.g., a friend's voice at a party) (Broadbent, 1958; Treisman, 1969). Much of this work and later work on the processes of attentional selection involved language processing. These studies largely viewed attention as a system with a limited capacity.

Since the early 1970s "dual task" paradigms have been prominently used in the studies of attention and the broader area of "attentional control." Although most of the studies have involved experimental paradigms of a more laboratory nature, several researchers have used what might be considered more ecologically valid approaches. Brown, Tickner, and Simmonds (1969) studied driving performance in association with concurrent verbal reasoning tasks. They found that spatial judgment errors and slowed performance were significantly more common when the subject was engaged in the concurrent verbal task. The work of Schneider and Shiffrin (1977) suggested important factors which would limit interference effects. Their work showed that with sufficient practice on a task the behavior would acquire "automaticity." Repeated pairings of stimulus and response result in progressively less demand on attentional resources and thus the behavior is less interfered with by competing tasks. Although the phenomena of automaticity is important, it does not fully explain attentional control during complex or dual tasks.

Norman and Shallice (1986) proposed a model of attention and the control of action. Much of their thinking comes from observing everyday mental lapses or from observations of the breakdown of control of behavior seen in neuropsychological patients. The model assumes that actions or behaviors are controlled in two separate ways. The first way is behaviors which are well-learned (or overlearned) skills which occur rather automatically and require little conscious control or attention. Occasionally, however, two ongoing activities will come into conflict, requiring that priority be given to one. Norman and Shallice suggested that these cases are handled by a relatively automatic process called "contention scheduling," whereby some rules are built into the system and operate automatically. For example, if an individual were driving and talking with a passenger, and an event occurred requiring a higher level of attention (e.g., a car broken down on the road which needed to be navigated around), the driver would pay less attention to conversation (probably stopping talking) and contend with the demands of the driving. Little conscious or attentional control demands would be made for this scheduling of behaviors to occur.

In addition to these relatively automatic processes, Norman and Shallice (1986) also hypothesized that there was a "supervisory activating system" (SAS), which allowed for interrupting and modifying ongoing behavior. This system allowed for conscious control over behaviors and explained phenomena such as human will and choice overriding automatic behavior. Shallice (1982) suggests that patients suffering from frontal lobe syndrome have a deficit in this supervisory activating system. For example, perseverative behaviors are explained as an inability to interrupt or change a behavior once a strategy has been adopted. Likewise, distractibility can be explained as the system being captured by whatever stimulus the environment presents with no ability to monitor or inhibit the behaviors.

Reason (1984) also proposed a model of cognitive control involving attention to explain absent-mindedness and "cognitive failures" in everyday life. Cognition failures included a wide variety of behaviors such as forgetting to do things one intended to do, or performing the wrong action. It was noted that cognitive failures often occur in situations which would not appear to require a high attentional capacity. In fact, Reason's studies of cognitive failures suggested that they are likely to occur in highly familiar surroundings or during frequently performed behaviors.

A large portion of these failures involve strong "habit" intrusion. Other situations which are likely to increase the number of slips of action include changing a behavior from a well-established routine (e.g., forgetting and putting salt on your food when you had intended to cut down), a change in circumstances requiring modification of an established behavioral sequence or habit (e.g., repeatedly attempting to use electrical utensils when the power is out), and entering a familiar environment in a reduced state of "intentionality" (e.g., going into a room to get something, performing another action in the room, and then leaving the room without the desired object). Though everyone experiences cognitive failures, Reason (1984) notes that there are individual differences in the frequency of such failures.

Reason's (1984) model of cognitive control includes three closely related components; schemata, the intention system, and the attentional control resource. Schemata are similar to "automatic" behaviors and are defined as relatively permanent knowledge structures which provide the detailed guidance for largely automatic sequences of speech, thought, action, or perception. Activation of schemata occurs when some threshold level is met. Reason hypothesized two primary activating factors: domain-specific receive their primary activation from particular intentions to do or say things; universal factors exert influence across all cognitive domains, including the environmental context, current need states, influences from other schemata (especially those which share common operations), and the recency and frequency with which the schemata is activated (i.e., the more recently or frequently it has been performed, the lower the threshold for activation).

The intention system component is theorized as being comprised of a central processor and a storage unit. The main function is assembling plans for future actions, monitoring and guiding ongoing actions, coping with changes in circumstances, and detecting and recovering from errors. The storage unit for the intention system provides time extension to the central processor. Its contents, however, are limited, prone to interference, and may be short-lived. The attentional control system in Reason's (1984) model is selective and a limited commodity. Although this attentional capacity is very important in the *learning* of new behaviors after schemata are established attentional demands decrease.

Reason (1984) uses the notion of a "cognitive board," which can be conceptualized as a matrix with separate squares each representing individual schema which have different activation levels. All, however, can be affected by universal activating factors and each schema is potentially linked with one or more others by a complex nexus running throughout the "board." Using this level of the model alone, the control of actions or behaviors would be dominated by the schemata with the highest activation levels. Since activation is increased by recency/frequency factors, these behaviors would continue to dominate the system and actions would become increasingly repetitive (or perseverative) without some higher level of control to break the positive feedback. In addition, universal activating factors would be insufficient to elicit more complex cognitive processing capabilities (i.e., problem-solving, or forming new schemata). Thus, the concept of the attentional control system, referred to as the attentional "blob" by Reason is necessary.

Reason (1984) envisions the attentional "blob" as an additional control device. It is described as having several properties such as being highly mobile, having a limited and fixed quantity, and only being able act upon a minute proportion of all the possible schemata at a time. The specific function of the "blob" is to selectively energize or suppress activation of the schemata. The extent to which it carries out these modulating functions is dependent on the volume or amount of attention resource.

The amount of attention resource determines the level of processing and state of consciousness about that process. Low amounts of attention resource may produce behaviors in which there is no direct awareness of the detailed operations. Intermediate amounts of attention resource are affiliated with "pre-attentional" processes, and high amounts of attention resource are needed for higher mental functions such as problem-solving, decision-making, deliberate information retrieval, concept formation, planning, and the acquisitions of skills or creation of new schemata. It is with high levels of attention resources that the intention system comes into play.

Reason (1984) suggests movement of the attention "blob" is affected by several factors. Although guided by intentional activity it has a tendency to return to pressing concerns (even if they are not intended), making it both active and reactive. It can also be directed by the schema it has activated lowering the threshold of other schema through the complex of connections. Attentional resources also seem to be drawn toward "hot spots" on the board, or schema which have been energized by universal activating factors, significant changes in sense data, or by earlier activation. This tendency to be drawn to "hot spots" might explain intrusive ruminations which plague many individuals. Though one may resolve to not think about something anymore, the tendency to return to these thoughts may dominate the mental state.

The relevance of examining theories of cognitive control and the role of attention in these theories is made clear when trying to examine the correlations between psychometric measures of attention (or at least the theoretical construct of attention) and everyday life. The existence of schemata, their interaction with attention, and the ability to modulate behavior allows for explanation of how it is possible to have brain-injured individuals score low on tests of attention, yet be able to perform many daily functions with little disruption. A common criticism of neuropsychological measures of cognitive abilities is that they tend not to be ecologically valid or meaningful for everyday demands. Individuals may have impaired abilities on formal tests of attention, yet go on to successfully perform seemingly complicated behavioral tasks (e.g., driving, cooking). Alternatively, it is possible for individuals to do well on tests of attention, yet have difficulty in everyday tasks requiring conscious control or new learning of schemata. This may be particularly true if sampling of attentional skill is not broad or rigorous. To get a better understanding of how everyday life and measures of attention relate, it is imperative to know what different tests of attention may actually measure.

NEUROPSYCHOLOGICAL MEASURES OF ATTENTION: THE PSYCHOMETRIC APPROACH

Despite a vast experimental and cognitive psychology literature on attention as a cognitive process, the examination of attentional processes within a standard clinical neuropsychological assessment has remained quite poorly developed. The classical attention triad derived from the Wechsler adult and child intellectual assessment batteries (Digit Span, Arithmetic, and Digit Symbol or Coding), measure a number of different abilities; some tests have a speed component, while others don't; some involve working memory or holding information in a short-term memory store, while in others information remains present for ongoing processing; and some involve access to other learned information or skills (e.g., mathematical abilities). This same problem can be seen with the subtests that make up the Attention and Concentration Index of the Wechsler Memory Scale—Revised. Crossen and Wiens (1988) for example, described limited construct validity for the index in a group of individuals who had sustained moderate to severe head injury.

The following is a list of different theoretically based areas of evaluation which researchers have included under the rubric of attention and specific tests which could potentially sample the skills; 1) tests involving working memory and mental control (e.g., mental arithmetic, digit span backwards, *Seashore Rhythm Test* (Reitan & Davidson, 1974); 2) timed or paced measures requiring rapid processing of new information (e.g., *Paced Auditory Serial Addition Test*) (Gronwall, 1977); *Attentional Capacity Test* (Weber, 1988); Brief Attention Test (Schretlen & Bobholz, 1992); 3) measures of visual or auditory target detection Continuous Performance Task (Rosvold et al., 1956); Gordon Diagnostic System (Gordon, 1988); the Cancellation Test (Mesulam, 1987), 4) measures requiring the overriding of distracting information or competing response tendencies (Stroop Color Word Interference Test [Stroop, 1935]; Auditory Selective Attention Test [Goldman, Fristoe, & Woodcock, 1970]), 5) measures requiring rapid visuomotor responses involving quick shifts of visual attention (e.g., Symbol Digit Modalities Test [Smith, 1982]; Trail Making Test [Reitan & Davidson, 1974]), 6) measures requiring the maintenance or shifting of conceptual or motor response such as measured on the Wisconsin Card Sorting Test (Heaton, 1981), and 7) measures requiring the maintenance of information in immediate or short-term memory. These may include a period of delay or distraction such as the Consonant Trigrams Test (Peterson & Peterson, 1959) or have not such elements (digit span forward).

Unlike the development of language batteries and memory batteries, there have been few systematic attempts to develop sets of attentional tests that would work together to evaluate different theoretically based components of attention. In addition, there have been very few tests which require attention to auditory input, although this is clearly an important modality. Mateer, Sohlberg and Bene (1986) developed an attention battery called the Attention Process Training Test (APT-Test), which was modeled on a set of materials developed to train attentional skills (Attention Process Training or APT), (Sohlberg & Mateer, 1989). The APT-Test is made up of five subtests. All require responses to auditory input presented via tape so that the rate of stimulus presentation is fixed and the information is available only at the time of presentation. Results are presented in Figure 1 for a group of control subjects made up of family members of head-injured individuals and a group of mildly head-injured/ (MTBI) subjects. The patient group performed as well as controls on the measure of simple auditory sustained attention (sustained I; target detection) and on this same task done concurrently with a number cancellation task (divided attention). However the MTBI group demonstrated significantly lower scores on measures sampling higher level mental control (sustained II), distractibility (selective), and alternating attention. Results are consistent with other studies suggesting significant compromise of processing efficiency and auditory attention in individuals with concussion (Gronwall, 1977).

Another recent attempt to formally evaluate attentional capacity particularly with respect to real-life attentional demands can be seen in the The Rivermead Everyday Attention Test being developed by Wilson and Robertson (1993, personal communication). This test has a number of subtests measuring different aspects of attention using ecologically valid materials. Undoubtedly the field will see the development of new and more comprehensive measures of attention. Until that happens, clinicians should endeavor to use as broad and comprehensive a review of attentional functions as possible.

NEUROPSYCHOLOGICAL CORRELATES OF EVERYDAY FUNCTION

NEUROPSYCHOLOGICAL MEASURES AND OUTCOME STUDIES

In the last several years, there has been an increasing interest in applied issues in neuropsychology. There are many questions regarding the relationship between neuropsychological test results and everyday behaviors in dynamic real-world contexts. Heaton and Pendleton (1981) pioneered work in this field suggesting that complex, multifunctional neuropsychological tasks were good

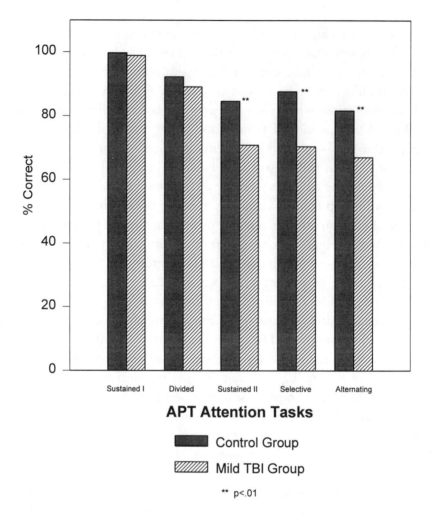

Figure 1. Mean percent correct responses on the 5 subtests of the APT-Test in a mild TBI group (N=127) and a control group (N=30).

predictors of overall functioning whereas more specific tasks served as better predictors of more narrow dimensions of everyday functioning. In another study, McSweeney, Grant, Heaton, Prigatano, and Adams (1985) also found neuropsychological status to be predictive of everyday life functioning in a clinical population (individuals with cardio-obstructive-pulmonary disease). They did not, however, find such relationships in a control sample of normal individuals.

Acker (1990) reviewed literature from studies done in the fields of rehabilitation, developmental disabilities, and corrections. These studies reported statistical correlations between various neuropsychological or psychological tests and ratings of function and outcomes. She divided the review of rehabilitation-based studies into studies focused on prediction during the early, intermediate, and late stages of recovery. Although problems with this kind of research were recognized, she concluded that a respectable amount of variance in outcome (up to 85%), could be accounted for using a multivariate approach with a number of predictors provided by these tests. Almost half of a list of potentially "robust prognostic indicators of outcome" were neuropsychological in nature. Other useful indicators included personality inventories, psychiatric instruments, tests of general abilities, and a variety of outcome and predictor scales.

In more extensive review of the individual studies (Acker, 1990) it was noted that outcome measures usually consisted of functional skills evaluations or disability ratings which were very general in nature. Usually, these global measures were being predicted by a battery of tests, or tests which supplied a measure of overall functioning (such as an overall IQ or memory quotient). There were few studies which predicted specific functional capabilities from neuropsychological test results, and most studies which attempted to utilize single tests to predict overall or specific functioning resulted in minimal correlations.

One area in which there has been a keen interest in developing predictor variables is that of driving a motor vehicle. This issue obviously has great practical import as many patients seen for neuropsychological assessment may have impairments that would cause such activity to be dangerous to themselves or others. Heaton and Pendleton (1981) hypothesized that tests such as the Trail Making Test and Category Test would predict complex behaviors such as driving, because they tap functions of decision-making, mental flexibility, analysis/organization of novel material, abstraction, problem-solving, and complex visuomotor responding. Indeed, Hale (1986) found that Trail Making (B), Digit Symbol and the Driver Performance Test were among the best predictors of automobile driving among brain-injured drivers. Despite such reports, there is reason to be cautious in overinterpreting or overgeneralizing this data. Based on their review of the driving literature, Hopewell and Van Zomeren (1990) indicate that previous driving and accident/violation history, general personality and attitudinal factors, pattern and severity of alcohol/substance abuse, and the nature and extent of psychiatric disturbance all exceed basic psychomotor abilities in their contribution to accident risk in both normal and disabled drivers. They suggest that though some neuropsychological markers may be viewed as limiting (or even disqualifying), emotional, social, and psychiatric factors must be incorporated into practical decision-making about recommendations for driving.

NEUROPSYCHOLOGICAL TESTS AND MEASURES OF EVERYDAY FUNCTIONING

Another approach to understanding the relationship between neuropsychological abilities and functional capacities involves examining the nature and frequency of naturally occurring cognitive failures. Several experimental approaches have been developed in this area. The "tip-of-the-tongue" phenomenon in which a person is temporarily unable to retrieve a specific word that subsequently returns to them, or the "slip-of-the-tongue" in which words or letters are transposed are two examples.

ERRORS OF ACTION

A system for measuring and describing errors of action for everyday activities has been proposed by Mayer, Reed, Schwartz, Montgomery, and Palmer (1990). They describe a coding system by which simple activities of daily living (ADLs) can be examined in patients who have suffered traumatic brain injury. Using this system they noted that brain-injured individuals often demonstrated errors of action in which parts of the intended action are substituted or compounded with other actions. They use an example of a brain-injured patient who while preparing his morning coffee, put sugar into an empty paper cup instead of his mug, and then began to spoon oatmeal into his coffee. His behavior suggests that he had the ability to complete several of the required actions (or schemas), but was unable to appropriately control or sequence them. This type of difficulty with attentional or executive control systems are common sequelae of head injury.

To more fully understand errors of action such as these, a coding system was developed in which activities of daily living are broken down into simple "action units." These basic action units are simple motor activities which are described as action primitives and include taking (i.e., an object that is nonpossessed becomes possessed), giving, moving, altering (i.e., changing the state of an object), and locomoting (i.e., moving oneself). Basic action units are not sufficient to describe larger ADLs such as a person brushing their teeth or drinking a cup of coffee. Rather, several of the basic units are organized into aggregates to describe more complex action sequences. Mayer et al. (1990) gives the example of brushing teeth, which is made up of several basic units including taking the cap off the toothpaste tube, placing the toothpaste on the brush, and placing the brush in your mouth, and brushing.

The coding system proposed breaks these actions down into key and non-key elements, provides an ecologically valid method for quantifying errors of action, seen secondary to traumatic brain injury. These errors are often severe enough to be debilitating to the affected individual. The data collected by this coding appear to be clinically useful and relevant, in that as individuals recover, changes in both the number and type of action errors are evident. Though this coding system is time consuming (requiring videotaping, coding, and a great deal of review) it does provide a wealth of information and may provide insight into understanding errors of action.

Analysis of actual cognitive failures can place taxonomic constraints on the theories proposed to account for such failures. Theories representing action sequences as involving schemes and sub-schemes (Norman & Shallice, 1986; Reason, 1984) and utilizing the idea of an attentional control or executive systems may be examined through the use of comprehensive behavioral analysis systems such as that proposed above.

QUESTIONNAIRE MEASURES OF COGNITIVE FAILURES

Another approach to the analysis of cognitive failures in everyday life is through the use of questionnaire data. Self-report instruments can produce indices of an individual's susceptibility to cognitive failure, rather than a detailed description of particular occasions on which such failures occurred. Herrmann and Neisser (1978), for example, using a questionnaire study identified eight different underlying factors in everyday forgetting, suggesting that this kind of data may be helpful in elucidating components of what appears to be more general behaviors. A number of self-report measures have been developed and reported.

Mateer, Sohlberg, and Crinean (1987) described a questionnaire in which individuals with traumatic brain injury rated the frequency of a variety of different kinds of forgetting experiences. Family members with no known history of neurologic compromise served as a control group. Factor analysis revealed four separable factors (anterograde memory, retrograde memory, autobiographical memory, attention/prospective memory). In both the brain-injured and control groups the frequency of forgetting was highest on items related to attention and prospective memory. Though both groups reported failures in this area, the brain-injured group had a significantly higher frequency.

The Cognitive Failures Questionnaire (CFQ) described by Broadbent, Cooper, Fitzgerald, and Parkes (1982) contains items that cover a variety of possible cognitive lapses. Examples of items that probe for failures of everyday perception, memory, and action respectively are "Do you fail to notice signposts on the road?"; "Do you find you forget whether you've turned off a light or locked the door?"; and "Do you bump into people?" Respondents indicate for each question the frequency with which the relevant event has occurred for them within the last six months on a five-point ordinal scale ranging from "never" to "very often."

Martin devised the Everyday Attention Questionnaire (EAQ) (1986) and the Everyday Memory Questionnaire (EMQ) (1983) to provide comparable but explicitly differentiated measures of these two components of cognitive activity. The EAQ consists of 18 probes designed to assess how easy people find it to pay attention in different everyday activities (e.g., "Imagine that you are carrying out some task you find easy [perhaps peeling potatoes or knitting]. What is the effect of humming or whistling to yourself on your ability to do this sort of task?"). Responses were scaled from "very distracting" to "very helpful." The EMQ consists of 37 relatively simple memory probes for different kinds of information (e.g., "The words of songs or poems"). Individuals judge how good they are at remembering such information relative to other people on a five-point response scale from "very poor" to "very good."

Martin (1983) examined the intercorrelations between several of these measures. Her study indicated a correlation between results on the CFQ and the EMQ, but no significant relationship between the EAQ and either of the other two measures. The EAQ appeared to be measuring an aspect of cognitive performance that was either weakly or not at all related to other measures. Self-reported questionnaire data have also been compared to actual performance on experimental tasks, in the hope that systematic associations between these two types of measures would increase our understanding of the generation of cognitive failures in everyday life.

Martin and Jones (1983) reviewed research which investigated whether individual differences in self-reported susceptibility to cognitive failure are related to the objective ability to distribute attention. Several studies indicated that the efficiency with which a person can distribute attention (or do more than one thing at a time) is linked with the occurrence of cognitive failures. They found a significant relationship between reports of cognitive failures on the CFQ and the ability to perform detection and reading tasks when these tasks were done concurrently, but not when either was performed in isolation. Wakeford, Clements, Biner, and Whay (1980) found that young children who reported many cognitive failures were also less efficient at concurrently counting backwards and mirror-drawing, though their performance on either of these tasks in isolation did not differ significantly from those reporting few cognitive failures.

Harris and Wilkins (1982) found that CFQ scores were related to a task requiring distributed attention. In this study, distributed attention was measured in a task in which subjects were required to watch a film about which they would be tested. Concurrently, subjects also signaled when a particular time setting was reached on a clock. Harris and Wilkins found that the score on the CFQ was correlated with the correct signaling of times. These studies suggest that high self-reported susceptibility to cognitive failures is associated with relatively poor objective performance on tasks that make strong demands on the ability to distribute attention. Martin and Jones (1983) suggest that this is not a general cognitive limitation, but one involving the ability to correctly maintain the goals appropriate to several different independently active tasks.

In contrast to distributed attention tasks that assess the ability to do more than one thing at a time, focused attention tasks assess how well one can do only one thing at a time. For such tasks, the relationship between performance and the CFQ is very different. Martin (1983) found no significant relationship between CFQ scores and the magnitude of the interference effect on a Stroop Test or speed of performance on the Embedded Figures Test. Martin (1978) also found no relationship between CFQ scores and recall of attended versus unattended words in a dichotic listening task. She did find, however, a significant negative correlation between the EAQ and recall of attended words. She proposed that the EAQ may have been assessing the degree to which people prefer to divide their attention, which is negatively related to their objective ability to focus attention. Martin goes on to suggest that the degree to which people prefer concurrent inputs in everyday life may relate to the degree of difficulty they experience in focusing their attention, but not to their actual ability to perform in dual-task situations.

SUMMARY AND CONCLUSIONS

Attention is a critical ability, important to a broad range of everyday life functioning. The construct of attention is currently conceptualized quite broadly, sometimes referring to a very specific capacity and at other times referring to a complex hierarchy of interdependent functions incorporating elements of working memory and executive control.

Current test instruments and test philosophy often mirror this confusion; few tests in current use in clinical settings are based on any particular theory or construct of attention. Additionally, by its very nature, psychometric assessment systematically reduces just those variables that challenge attentional resources and capacities in real-life situations (e.g., reducing noise in testing rooms, having subjects focus on just one task, structuring the environment). There has been a movement towards development and use of more demanding, higher level, and theoretically based measures of attention; these probably have more potential to tap some of the requirements of everyday functioning.

Measurement of everyday functioning also remains a challenge. There has been research on some specific skill areas (e.g., grooming, dressing and driving), but it is on just such familiar, overlearned, and practiced tasks that attentional demands are minimized. Even an individual with significant higher level attentional problems might drive uneventfully for an extended period of time, but have a critical failure if circumstances were such that competition for, or demand on, attentional processing exceeded some threshold level. Thus, correlations between simple attention measures and real-life functioning are likely to be minimal. Indeed, it is on tasks which demand new learning or place demands on several systems that higher levels of mental control and attention are required. Consequently, activities which require these abilities may more readily reflect deficits in attention and attentional control.

The analysis of spontaneous errors of action may prove fruitful in elucidating the nature of attentional functioning in everyday activities, yet such approaches rely on detailed observations during natural tasks, or on self-report. By nature, these are more difficult to quantify and to incorporate into assessment batteries. The data derived from such studies could, however, lead to the development of tests which more closely approximate the complex and changing attentional demands of everyday functioning.

Despite the difficulty in adequately assessing either attention or everyday functioning, evidence from both the "cognitive failures" and "error of action" literature suggests that inefficient distribution of attention between two or more concurrent tasks (on alternating or divided attention tasks) is a significant cause of failure. Such failures appear to be the consequence of attempting to perform adequately two or more tasks whose joint requirements interact to exceed temporarily the resources available. There is little evidence, however, that intact or even above average simple sustained or selective attention abilities can prevent or even reduce failures in everyday life.

As is the case with any true hierarchical model, some basic level of ability is required for operation of the system. Thus, in individuals with significant limitations in basic arousal and sustained attention, predictions of poor performance in functional contexts is clearly easier and more accurate. It is when the base rate of cognitive failures is relatively low and when they occur intermittently that predictions based on psychometric measures will be less robust. For patients who basic arousal and sustained attention systems are intact, test instruments that sample higher levels of attentional capacity may be more useful in predicting functional capacities. In normal individuals, tasks which require distribution of attention over more than one channel will probably provide a higher potential for predicting the relatively infrequent and unstable occurrences of cognitive failure than tests which require focusing of attention upon a single channel of information. As higher levels of attention are addressed, investigators, theory builders, and clinicians will have to address the indistinct boundaries between attentional control, executive function, working memory, and myriad other higher-level cognitive control functions and their implications for everyday functioning.

REFERENCES

Acker, M. B. (1990). A review of the ecological validity of neuropsychological tests. In D. E. Tupper & K. D. Cicerone (Eds.), *The neuropsychology of everyday life: Assessment and basic competencies.* Boston: Kluwer Academic Publishers.

Baddeley, A. D. (1981). The concept of working memory: A view of its current state and probable future development. *Cognition, 10,* 17-2

Baddeley, A. (1991). *Human memory: Theory and practice* (pp. 117-125). London: Lawrence Erlbaum Associates.

Bakay Pragay, E., Mirsky, A. F., Ray C. L., Turner, D. F., & Mirsky, C. V. (1978). Neuronal activity in the brain stem reticular formation during performance of a "go-no go" visual attention task in the monkey. *Experimental Neurology, 60,* 83-95.

Broadbent, D. E. (1958). *Perception and communication.* London: Pergamon.

Broadbent, D. E. (1982). Task combination and the selective intake of information. *Acta Psychologica, 50,* 253-290.

Broadbent, D. E., Cooper, P. F., Fitzgerald, P., & Parkes, K. R. (1982). The Cognitive Failures Questionnaire (CFQ) and its correlates. *British Journal of Clinical Psychology, 21,* 1-16.

Brown, I. D., Tickner, A. H., & Simmonds, D. C. V. (1969). Interference between concurrent tasks of driving and telephoning. *Journal of Applied Psychology, 53,* 419-424.

Crossen, J. R., & Wiens, A. N. (1988). Residual neuropsychological deficits following head-injury on the Wechlser Memory Scale - Revised. *The Clinical Neuropsychologist, 2(4),* 393-399.

Goldman, R., Fristoe, M., & Woodcock, R. W. (1970*). Goldman-Fristoe-Woodcock Test of Auditory Discrimination.* Circle Pines, NM: American Guidance Service.

Grant, D. A., & Berg, E. A. (1948). A behavioral analysis of degree of reinforcement and ease of shifting two new responses in a Weigl-type card sorting problem. *Journal of Experimental Psychology, 38,* 404-411.

Gronwall, D. M. A. (1977). Paced Auditory Serial Addition Task: A measure of recovery from concussion. *Perceptual and Motor Skills, 44,* 367-373.

Guilford, J. P. (1967). *The nature of human intelligence.* New York: McGraw Hill.

Hale, P. N., Jr. (1986). *Rehabilitation engineering center for personal licensed vehicles.* (Annual Report). Ruston, LA: The Center for Rehabilitation Science and Biomedical Engineering.

Harris, J. E., & Wilkins, A. J. (1982). Remembering to do things: A theoretical framework and an illustrative experiment. *Human Learning, 1,* 123-136.

Heaton, R. K. (1981). *A manual for the Wisconsin Card Sorting Test.* Odessa, FL: Psychological Assessment Resources.

Heaton, R. K., & Pendleton, M. G. (1981). Use of neuropsychological tests to predict adult patients' everyday functioning. *Journal of Consulting and Clinical Psychology, 49*, 807-821.

Herrmann, D. J., & Neisser, U. (1978). An inventory of everyday memory experiences. In M.M. Gruneberg, P. E. Morris, & R. N. Sykes (Eds.), *Practical aspects of memory*. London and New York: Academic Press.

Hopewell, C. A., & Van Zomeren, A. H. (1990). Neuropsychological aspects of motor vehicle operation. In D. E. Tupper & K. D. Cicerone (Eds.*), The Neuropsychology of everyday life: Assessment and basic competencies*. Boston: Kluwer Academic Publishers.

Martin. M. (1978). Retention of attended and unattended auditorily and visually presented material. *Quarterly Journal of Experimental Psychology, 30*, 187-200.

Martin, M. (1983). Cognitive failure: Everyday and laboratory performance. *Bulletin of the Psychonomic Society, 21*, 97-100.

Martin, M. (1986). Ageing and patterns of change in everyday memory and cognition. *Human Learning, 5*, 63-74.

Martin, M., & Jones G. V. (1983). Distribution of attention in cognitive failure. *Human Learning, 2*, 221-226.

Mateer, C. A., & Ojeman, G. A. (1983). Thalamic mechanisms in language and memory. In S. J. Segalowitz (Ed.), *Language functions and brain organization*. New York: Academic Press.

Mateer, C. A., Sohlberg, M. M., & Bene, J. (1986). *Attention Process Training Test*. Puyallup, WA: Association for Neuropsychological Research and Development.

Mateer, C. A., Sohlberg, M. M., & Crinean, J. (1987). Focus on clinical research: Perceptions of memory function in individuals with closed head injury. *Journal of Head Trauma Rehabilitation, 2*, 74-84.

Mayer, N. H., Reed, E., Schwartz, M. F., Montgomery, M., & Palmer, C. (1990). Buttering a hot cup of coffee: An approach to the study of errors of action in patients with brain damage. In D. E. Tupper & K. D. Cicerone (Eds.*), The neuropsychology of everyday life: Assessment and basic competencies*. Boston: Kluwer Academic Publishers.

McSweeny, A. J., Grant, I., Heaton, R. K., Prigatano, G. P., & Adams, K. M. (1985). Relationship of neuropsychological status to everyday functioning in healthy and chronically ill persons. *Journal of Clinical and Experimental Neuropsychology, 7(3)*, 281-291.

Mesulam, M. M. (1987). Attention, confusional states and neglect. In Mesulam, M. M. (Ed.), *Principles of behavioral neurology*. Philadelphia: Davis.

Milner, B. (1963). Effects of different brain lesions on card sorting. *Archives of Neurology, 9*, 90-100.

Mirsky, A. F., Anthony, B. J., Duncan, C. C., Ahearn, M. B., & Kellam, S. G. (1991). Analysis of the elements of attention: A neuropsychological approach. *Neuropsychology Review, 2*, 109-145.

Mirsky, A. F., Bakay Pragay, E., & Harris, S. (1977). Evoked potential correlates of stimulation-induced impairment of attention in Macaca mulatta. *Experimental Neurology, 57*, 242-256.

Moruzzi, G., & Magoun, H. W. (1949). Brain stem reticular formation and activation of the EEG. *Electroencephalography and Clinical Neurophysiology, 1*, 455-473.

Parasuraman, R. (1979). Memory load and event rate control sensitivity decrements in sustained attention. *Science, 205*, 924-927.

Peterson, L. R., & Peterson, M. J. (1959). Short-term retention of individual verbal items. *Journal of Experimental Psychology, 58*, 193-198.

Reason, J. T. (1984). Absent-Mindedness and Cognitive Control. In J. E. Harris & P. E. Morris (Eds.), *Everyday memory, actions, and absent-mindedness*. London: Academic Press Limited.

Reitan, R. M., & Davidson, L. A. (eds). (1974). *Clinical neuropsychology: Current status and applications.* Washington, DC: V.H. Winston and Sons.

Rosvold, H. E., Mirsky, A. F., Sarason, I., Bransome, E. D., Jr., & Beck, L. H. (1956). A continuous performance test of brain damage. *Journal of Consulting Psychology, 20,* 343-350.

Schretlen, D., & Bobholz, J.H. (1992). Standardization and initial validation of a brief test of executive attentional ability. *Journal of Clinical and Experimental Neuropsychology, 14,* 77.

Schneider, W., & Shiffrin, R. M. (1977). Controlled and automatic information processing I: Detection, search and attention. *Psychological Review, 84,* 1-66.

Shallice, T. (1982). Specific impairments of planning. *Philosophical Transactions of the Royal Society London B, 298,* 199-209.

Shiffrin, R. M., & Schneider, W. (1977). Controlled and automatic human information processing II: Perceptual learning, automatic attending and a general theory. *Psychological Review, 84,* 90-190.

Shumway-Cook, A., Kerns, K. A., & Woollacot, M. (1993). *The interacting effect of cognitive demand and postural control following T.B.I.* Presented at The West Coast Conference on Attention: Eugene, OR.

Smith, A. (1982). *Symbol Digit Modalities Test.* Los Angeles: Western Psychological Services.

Sohlberg, M. M., & Mateer, C. A. (1987). Effectiveness of an attention training program. *Journal of Clinical and Experimental Neuropsychology, 9,* 117-130.

Stroop, J. R. (1935). Studies of interference in serial verbal reactions. *Journal of Experimental Psychology, 18,* 643-662.

Talland, G. A. (1965). *Deranged memory.* New York: Academic Press.

Triesman, A. (1969). Strategies and models of selective attention. *Psychological Review, 76,* 282-299.

Wakeford, F., Clements, K., Viner, J., & Whay, J. (1980). "An investigation into the incidences and causes of absent-minded behavior," British Broadcasting Corporation "Young Scientist of the Year" report.

Wechsler, D. (1958). *Measurement and appraisal of adult intelligence.* Baltimore: Williams and Wilkins.

Wechsler, D. (1981). *Wechsler Adult Intelligence Scale-Revised.* Cleveland: The Psychological Corporation.

Weber, A. M. (1988). A new clinical measure of attention: The Attentional Capacity Test. *Neuropsychology, 2.*

Yingling, C. D., and Skinner, J. E. (1975). Regulation of unit activity in nucleus reticularis thalami by the mesencephalic reticular formation and the frontal granular cortex. *Electroencephalography and Clinical Neurophysiology, 39,* 635-642.

9

THE ECOLOGICAL VALIDITY OF EXECUTIVE FUNCTION TESTING

Lloyd I. Cripe, Ph.D., A.B.P.P.

*The real history of science is a maze, in which most paths lead to
dead ends and all are littered with the broken crockery of error and
misconception*

Timothy Ferris

INTRODUCTION

Experienced clinicians witness the adaptive devastation of frontal brain damage and executive dysfunction. The knowledge of this real-world devastation
typically comes more from observing the patient and the reports of significant
others than from neuropsychological test scores. In fact, there is often a notable
discrepancy between test performances and the reported or observed adaptive
problems of the patient. Why?

The first patient the author examined who had severe bilateral frontal brain
damage was a 42-year-old high school graduate who was the victim of a fire
fighting accident on a large boat. He and a partner were fighting their way into
a section of the boat when suddenly an iron hatch cover blew off. The partner
was decapitated and the patient suffered bilateral frontal depressed skull fractures. Images of the brain shortly after the accident revealed severe bilateral
frontal pole damage.

He was in a coma for about a month and suffered post-traumatic amnesia
for three months. Neuropsychological examination occurred five months post-
injury. He thought he had made a good recovery. When asked what problems
he had, he stated, "Maybe I'm a little slow, but I want to go back to work."

Table 1 summarizes his test performances five months post injury. Most neuropsychologists would probably agree that the test scores indicate impairment of neurobehavioral functioning and would predict problems with adaptation in life. There is a notable discrepancy between the patient's reported problems and his impaired performances on tests. He appears more impaired on tests than he realizes.

TABLE 1
NEUROPSYCHOLOGICAL TEST DATA OF BILATERAL FRONTAL POLE DAMAGE FIVE MONTHS POST-INJURY

Test	Score
WAIS FSIQ	86
VIQ	88
PIQ	86
INF	7
DSP	10
VOC	8
ART	6
COM	8
SIM	7
PC	9
PA	8
BD	6
OA	6
DS	6
WRAT READING	81 PERCENTILE
WRAT SPELLING	73 PERCENTILE
WRAT ARITHMETIC	30 PERCENTILE
HALSTEAD IMPAIRMENT	0.6
CATEGORY	95 ERRORS
WISCONSIN CARD SORTING	
CATEGORIES	0
PERSEV. ERRORS	94
TPT TOTAL	11.5
DOMINANT	4.2
NONDOMINANT	4.3
MEMORY	7
LOCALIZATION	3
SEASHORE RHYTHM	23
SPEECH SOUNDS	6 ERRORS
GRIP DOMINANT	31.0 KG
GRIP NONDOMINANT	30.0 KG
TAPPING DOMINANT	40.8

(Continued)

(Continued from previous page)

TABLE 1

NEUROPSYCHOLOGICAL TEST DATA OF BILATERAL FRONTAL POLE DAMAGE FIVE MONTHS POST-INJURY

Test	Score
TAPPING NON DOMINANT	41.4
TRAILS A	42 SECONDS (0 ERRORS)
TRAILS B	133 SECONDS (0 ERRORS)
STROOP I (DODRILL)	98 SECONDS
STROOP II	323 SECONDS
SENSORY PERCEPTUAL	
RIGHT	2 ERRORS
LEFT	4 ERRORS
FORM DISCRIMINATION	
RIGHT	8 SECONDS (NO ERRORS)
LEFT	8 SECONDS (NO ERRORS)
WECHSLER MEMORY SCALE	
STORIES INITIAL	16
STORIES DELAYED	15
VISUAL INITIAL	3
VISUAL DELAYED	2
MMPI CODE: 89"7652-140/3: L/F"K:	

The patient was stopped about half way through administration of the Wisconsin Card Sorting Test because he was continually sorting by number of objects on the card with no consideration of the feedback given to him. He was taught the three different sorting possibilities. He clearly understood the three possibilities and testing was continued. He again continued matching by number of objects, still oblivious to the feedback. He could discuss the different ways of categorizing, but could not adjust his sorting behavior. It was a most impressive display of perseveration.

It was recommended that the patient not return to work. He needed time to recover plus certain rehabilitation interventions before it would be appropriate to return to the demands of gainful employment.

He was re-evaluated three and one-half years. Later, he had no complaints and he wanted to return to his former employment responsibilities. His wife complained that he did nothing unless she initiated and structured it.

Table 2 summarizes the re-evaluation test scores. The results indicate improvement in test performances in most regards since the first evaluation. While some variabilities in test performances are seen, suggesting some weaknesses in functioning, the test data do not predict the severity of impairment. This is a man who when left on his own, just sits around all day and does nothing! It is believed he never returned to gainful employment. There is a marked disparity between relative good test performances and very poor real-world adjustment. Why?

TABLE 2
NEUROPSYCHOLOGICAL RE-EVALUATION TEST DATA OF BILATERAL FRONTAL POLE DAMAGE FOUR YEARS POST-INJURY

Test	Score
WAIS FSIQ	104
VIQ	99
PIQ	111
INF	9
DSP	10
VOC	9
ART	10
COM	10
SIM	10
PC	11
PA	10
BD	9
OA	12
DS	8
WRAT READING	63 PERCENTILE
WRAT SPELLING	66 PERCENTILE
WRAT ARITHMETIC	58 PERCENTILE
HALSTEAD IMPAIRMENT	0.3
CATEGORY	31 ERRORS
WISCONSIN CARD SORTING	
CATEGORIES	2
PERSEV. ERRORS	24
TPT TOTAL	10.9
DOMINANT	4.1
NONDOMINANT	4.4
MEMORY	6
LOCALIZATION	1
SEASHORE RHYTHM	24
SEASHORE TONAL MEMORY	29
SPEECH SOUNDS	3 ERRORS
GRIP DOMINANT	39 KG
GRIP NONDOMINANT	40 KG
TAPPING DOMINANT	52.4

(Continued)

(Continued from previous page)

<table>
<thead>
<tr><th colspan="2" align="center">TABLE 2
NEUROPSYCHOLOGICAL RE-EVALUATION TEST DATA OF BILATERAL FRONTAL POLE
DAMAGE FOUR YEARS POST-INJURY</th></tr>
</thead>
<tbody>
<tr><td align="center">Test</td><td>Score</td></tr>
<tr><td>TAPPING NON DOMINANT</td><td>46.2</td></tr>
<tr><td>TRAILS A</td><td>25 SECONDS (0 ERRORS)</td></tr>
<tr><td>TRAILS B</td><td>81 SECONDS (0 ERRORS)</td></tr>
<tr><td>STROOP I (DODRILL)</td><td>103 SECONDS</td></tr>
<tr><td>STROOP II</td><td>247 SECONDS</td></tr>
<tr><td>SENSORY PERCEPTUAL</td><td></td></tr>
<tr><td>   RIGHT</td><td>1 ERROR</td></tr>
<tr><td>   LEFT</td><td>0 ERRORS</td></tr>
<tr><td>FORM DISCRIMINATION</td><td></td></tr>
<tr><td>   RIGHT</td><td>8 SECONDS (0 ERRORS)</td></tr>
<tr><td>   LEFT</td><td>9 SECONDS (0 ERRORS)</td></tr>
<tr><td>WECHSLER MEMORY SCALE</td><td></td></tr>
<tr><td>   STORIES INITIAL</td><td>22</td></tr>
<tr><td>   STORIES DELAYED</td><td>14</td></tr>
<tr><td>   VISUAL INITIAL</td><td>7</td></tr>
<tr><td>   VISUAL DELAYED</td><td>7</td></tr>
<tr><td>REY AVLT TRIAL V</td><td>11</td></tr>
<tr><td colspan="2">MMPI CODE: 8"9'7250-64/13: L/F'K#</td></tr>
</tbody>
</table>

Another unforgettable clinical case involved a 35-year-old male with 18 years of formal education. He was in a motor vehicle accident that caused a severe closed head injury with two weeks of coma and at least one month of post-traumatic amnesia. He was evaluated throughout his recovery and completed a comprehensive neuropsychological testing one year post-injury.

Table 3 summarizes his test findings. Although some inefficiencies in test performances are noted, it is highly improbable that a neuropsychologist would look at these test scores and declare this man as having "the most impaired executive functions they have ever seen." However, a year later, a very reputable brain injury treatment center that had seen the patient daily for over a year, made this statement. The author saw the patient three years post-injury for re-evaluation and he still was not gainfully employed. He had been relieved from several volunteer positions. Although he had few complaints, his wife reported many real-life problems. The treatment staff and the patient's wife were seeing something that the tests were missing.

TABLE 3
NEUROPSYCHOLOGICAL TEST ONE-YEAR POST SEVERE HEAD TRAUMA

Test	Score
W-R FSIQ	101
VIQ	105
PIQ	97
INF	12
DSP	10
VOC	12
ART	9
COM	10
SIM	12
PC	10
PA	10
BD	9
OA	6
DS	9
WRAT READING	91 PERCENTILE
WRAT SPELLING	77 PERCENTILE
WRAT ARITHMETIC	68 PERCENTILE
HALSTEAD IMPAIRMENT	0.3
CATEGORY	22 ERRORS
WISCONSIN CARD SORTING	
CATEGORIES	6
TOTAL ERRORS	10
TPT TOTAL	18.3
DOMINANT	6.3
NONDOMINANT	7.8
MEMORY	6
LOCALIZATION	2
SEASHORE RHYTHM	28
SPEECH SOUNDS	3 ERRORS
GRIP DOMINANT	54 KG
GRIP NONDOMINANT	55 KG
TAPPING DOMINANT	57.4
TAPPING NON DOMINANT	49.2
TRAILS A	25 SECONDS (0 ERRORS)
TRAILS B	52 SECONDS (0 ERRORS)
STROOP I (DODRILL)	85 SECONDS
STROOP II	276 SECONDS

(Continued)

(Continued from previous page)

TABLE 3
NEUROPSYCHOLOGICAL TEST ONE-YEAR POST SEVERE HEAD TRAUMA

Test	Score
SENSORY PERCEPTUAL	
RIGHT	2 ERRORS
LEFT	7 ERRORS
FORM DISCRIMINATION	
RIGHT	9 SECONDS (0 ERRORS)
LEFT	9 SECONDS (0 ERRORS)
WECHSLER MEMORY SCALE	
STORIES INITIAL	24
STORIES DELAYED	21
VISUAL INITIAL	11
VISUAL DELAYED	5
MMPI CODE: 9-5432/0781:6# L:F-K/	

Eslinger and Damasio (1987) published the case of EVR. He was a man in his thirties with extreme adaptive problems, graphically imaged massive frontal orbital and mesial lesions, and statistically normal neuropsychological test scores. A summary of EVR's test scores is presented in Table 4.

Although we can quibble over whether the "right battery" of tests was administered, the obvious finding is how well the patient performed on neuropsychological tests. The tests miserably fail to predict the severe real-world dysfunction.

These cases grab our attention. There is such an obvious disparity between the reality of test scores and the reality of the patient's maladaptation. How can persons with so much maladaptive behavior due to frontal brain damage and executive dysfunction be so misclassified on neuropsychological tests? These cases cast deep shadows on the ecological validity of tests predicting executive dysfunctions.

It is hoped this chapter stimulates thought which will guide us into a deeper understanding of the limits and possibilities of our technology. What are executive functions? What do we know about the ecological validity of tests used to measure executive functions? Why do executive functions pose such a challenge to measurement and prediction? What are the limits of tests in imaging reality? What can we do to more accurately assess executive functions?

TABLE 4
NEUROPSYCHOLOGICAL TEST DATA OF CASE EVR

Test	Score
WAIS-R	
VIQ	129
PIQ	135
SHIPLEY VOCABULARY	37/40
SHIPLEY ABSTRACT	40/40
WECHSLER MEMORY	
QUOTIENT	143
DIGIT SPAN	14
LOGICAL	18.1
PAIRED ASSOC.	16.3
REY AUDITORY VERBAL	
TRIAL V	14
RECOGNITION	14
DELAYED RECALL	11
BENTON VRT	
CORRECT	9
ERRORS	1
REY COMPLEX FIGURE	
COPY	36/36
DELAYED RECALL	32/36
VISUAL NAMING	64 (89 PERCENTILE)
SENTENCE REPETITION	15 (89 PERCENTILE)
DIGIT REPETITION	10 (85 PERCENTILE)
WORD FLUENCY	49 (89 PERCENTILE)
ORAL SPELLING	11 (70 PERCENTILE)
WRITTEN SPELLING	10 (39 PERCENTILE)
TOKEN TEST	44 (89 PERCENTILE)
AURAL COMPREHENSION	18 (71 PERCENTILE)
READING COMPREHENSION	10 (+2 Z-SCORES)
WRITING	NORMAL
DICHOTIC LISTENING	NORMAL
FACIAL RECOGNITION	43 (32 PERCENTILE)
JUDGMENT OF LINE	30 (74 PERCENTILE)
3-D CONSTRUCTION	29 (INTACT)
WAIS-R BLOCK DESIGN	16 (98 PERCENTILE)
WISCONSIN CARD SORTING	
CATEGORIES	6
PERSEV. ERRORS	6

(Eslinger & Damasio, 1985)

WHAT ARE EXECUTIVE FUNCTIONS?

Few subjects in neurology have been associated with as much enigma and paradox as the behavioral afflictions of the prefrontal cortex
Marsel Mesulam

Many prominent neuropsychologists, such as Hebb, Tueber, Halstead, Hecaen, Luria, Benton, and Pribram, have researched and discussed the frontal brain system and the associated neuropsychological functions.

Luria (1980) offered one of the more detailed and comprehensive clinical descriptions and theories of the neurobehavioral problems associated with frontal brain dysfunctions. The problems he described could be called executive functions. He taught that a number of neurobehavioral syndromes are associated with impairments to the frontal brain depending upon the geographical sites. He noted problems with energy, motivation, initiation of actions, formulation of behavioral goals and programs, and the self-monitoring of behavior associated with frontal lesions. His theory of higher cortical functioning included a special executive role for frontal brain systems. His descriptions convey the concept of executive functions although the term is never specifically mentioned (Luria, 1973):

> There is thus conclusive evidence that the prefrontal regions of the cortex are tertiary cortical structures, in intimate communication with nearly every other principal zone of the cortex, and if it were necessary to mention any particular feature distinguishing the prefrontal regions of the brain from the tertiary zones of the posterior regions, it would be that the *tertiary portions of the frontal lobes are in fact a superstructure above all other parts of the cerebral cortex, so that they perform a far more universal function of general regulation of behavior* than that performed by the posterior associative center...*destruction of the prefrontal cortex leads to a profound disturbance of complex behavioral programmes* and to *marked disinhibition of immediate responses to irrelevant stimuli*, thus making the performance of complex behavioral programmes impossible...*the frontal lobes not only perform the function of synthesis of external stimuli, preparation for action, and formation of programmes, but also the function of allowing for the effect of the action carried out and verification that it has taken the proper course...* (pp. 89-93)

Lezak (1983) defined executive functions as "those capacities that enable a person to engage in independent, purposive, self-serving behavior successfully." In another publication (1982) Lezak provides the following definition:

> The executive functions comprise those mental capacities necessary for formulating goals, planning how to achieve them, and carrying out the plans effectively. They are at the heart of all socially useful, personally enhancing, constructive, and creative activities. With the executive functions intact, a person can suffer many different kinds and combinations of sensory, motor, and cognitive deficits and still maintain the direction of his own life and be productive as well. Impairment or loss of these functions compromises a person's capacity to maintain an independent, constructively self-serving, and socially productive life no matter how well he can see and hear, walk and talk, and perform tests...The definition of executive functions... provides a framework for conceptualizing them in terms of four major classes or functional categories of executive capacities. These are (1) capacities necessary for formulating goals; (2) capacities involved in planning; (3) capacities having to do with carrying out plans to reach goals; and (4) capacities for performing these activities effectively. These classes involve distinctive sets of behavior. All are necessary for appropriate, socially responsible, and effectively self-serving adult conduct. (pp. 281-285)

Stuss and Benson (1986) proposed a hierarchy of brain functions with the frontal brain systems associated with the highest levels. Deficits with these higher levels are called "metacognitive deficits." Figure 1 graphically summaries their concept of executive functions as metacognitive.

Stuss (1987) made the following comments regarding the frontal brain:

> The human frontal cortex attends, anticipates, plans, executes, oversees, modifies, and judges all nervous system activities. Most human functions, based on posterior brain systems, can run without frontal participation. However, the control of behavior, the decision making "I" at the base of the highest human functions, appears to depend on the frontal lobes. (p. 33)

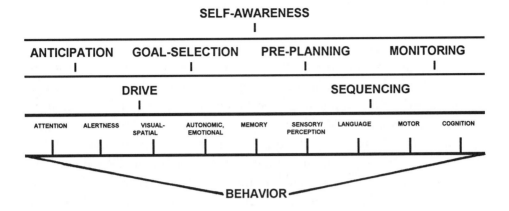

Figure 1. Hierarchy of Brain Functions (Stuss & Benson, 1986). This figure illustrates the proposed model of brain functioning. External behavior is dependent upon various organized integrated fixed functional systems such as attention, alertness, and so on, hypothesized to be based, in relation to the frontal lobes, in more posterior/basal brain regions. The next three levels are all more intimately associated with the frontal lobes with self-awareness (self-consciousness, self-reflectiveness) hypothesized as the highest attribute of the frontal lobes.

All of these persons have conceptualized a higher order system which orchestrates mental functions. They have used terms like "superstructure, supramodal, and metacognitive" in an attempt to describe these complex functions. Executive functions involve how mental resources are utilized. They involve the management of the system: Planning, Organization, Direction, and Control. Executive functions are process-oriented involving how things get done rather than just what gets done. Executive functions are process as well as outcome-oriented.

We also know that these phenomena exist within ourselves and others. These definitions, however, are difficult to operationalize. There has never been a collective professional effort to derive a consensual operational definition of executive functions to guide research and clinical investigation.

WHAT DO WE KNOW?

> *In all scientific fields theory is frequently more important than experimental data. Scientists are generally reluctant to accept the existence of a phenomenon when they do not know how to explain it. On the Other hand, they will often accept a theory that is especially plausible before there exists any data to support it.*
>
> Richard Morris

EXECUTIVE FUNCTION ASSESSMENT AND ECOLOGICAL VALIDITY

Based on research, we know enough to know how little we know. A computer literature search of the PSYCINFO data base of studies from 1967 to March 1992 yielded no studies of executive functions and everyday functioning, or executive functions and real-world functioning. A search for executive functions and validity yielded one study (Bayless, 1987). The same search using "frontal lobes" instead of "executive functions" yielded one study (McKay & Golden, 1979). There are no studies that have substantially validated the concept of executive functions and no studies that have explored the ecological validity between the testing of executive functions and real-world adaptation.

In a book titled *Reliability and Validity in Neuropsychological Assessment* (Franzen, 1989), there is no chapter on executive functions. In fact, the term is not even indexed. There is a chapter titled Tests of Higher Cognitive Functions (pp. 225-235) which discusses the Porteus Maze Test, Elithorn's Perceptual Maze Test, the Verbal Concept Attainment Test, and the Weigl Color-Form Sorting Test, but this is a discussion of these tests with no mention of the measurement of executive function and its validity.

In a book titled *The Neuropsychology of Everyday Life: Assessment and Basic Competencies* (Tupper & Cicerone, 1990) there is no chapter on executive functions. The term is, however, indexed. A clear definition is not given and the issue of validity is not adequately discussed. In one of the chapters "Review of the ecological validity of neuropsychological tests," Acker mentions Newcombe's (1987) concerns that gross IQ measures may not reflect the sequelae of head injury and in particular frontal lobe functions, but there is no discussion of the validity of executive functions and their assessment.

Chelune and Moehle (1986) do not mention executive functions in their review and discussion of "Neuropsychological assessment and everyday functioning." In their "Tentative Guide for Clinical Interpretation of Everyday Activities" they suggest using various tests to determine if the patient's behavior is appropriate in routine or complex situations, but there is no discussion of ecological validity.

FRONTAL LOBE ASSESSMENT AND ECOLOGICAL VALIDITY

Since there is little validation of the concept of executive functions, the testing of these functions, or their ecological validity, can we find studies of frontal lobe assessment that have validated specific tests to assess frontal brain functioning and their ecological validity?

Stuss and Benson's (1984) review of neuropsychological studies of the frontal lobes discusses various functions associated with frontal lobe functioning but never establishes the validity of various tests. No mention is made as to how well tests predict adaptive difficulties. They conclude that we have much to learn about this geographical area of the brain:

> Although this article has outlined a number of apparent frontal lobe functions, it is obvious that the functions of this massive and phylogenetically novel prefrontal cortex are complex, interrelated, and as yet incompletely understood. Part of the riddle of the frontal lobes derives from the size and complexity of the cortical area in question, but knowledge has also been hindered by inadequate test procedures and inability to obtain control of such variables as lesion size, location, and even lateralization. Consequently, current explanations of apparent frontal lobe malfunction remain limited and vague. (p. 22)

Wang (1987) discusses a number of concept formation tests that attempt to identify frontal brain dysfunction. He presents data regarding the correct identification, but the classification rates are weak. He suggests guidelines for the development of new procedures and recommends that qualitative analysis should be incorporated. He does not discuss ecological validity.

Varney (1988) studied anosmia in closed head injuries and demonstrated a possible correlation between frontal-orbital brain damage and vocational problems. Varney found that 93% of patients with complete anosmia had vocational disability (employed less than 25% of the time). Persons with partial anosmia had problems with vocation (54%) but less than the total anosmics. He reasoned that this may validate the notion that patients with frontal-orbital brain damage have a higher probability of psychosocial dysfunction. While this is a probable hypothesis, it was not rigorously verified.

A most interesting aspect of Varney's (1988) study is the lack of correlation between the neuropsychological tests administered and the vocational disability. The sign of anosmia, as reported by the patient was more predictive than the tests. Varney also found that interviewing relatives and employers was necessary because the cognitive measures did not seem to manifest the patients' real problems. This suggests poor ecological validity from the test results alone.

Lhermitte, Pillon, and Serdaru (1986) present evidence of *imitation behavior* and *utilization behavior* in frontal brain lesion patients. The methods of their studies included some neuropsychological testing and examiner gesture tasks. The 50 normal controls "never imitated the examiner." Seventy-five patients demonstrated imitation behavior. Ninety-six percent of the patients with focal lesions of the frontal lobes demonstrated this behavior. Twenty-six of 29 of the patients with focal frontal lesions demonstrated involvement of the "inferior half of the anterior part of one or both frontal lobes." Lhermitte (1986) studied real-world behavior of several of these patients in the doctor's office, a lecture room, a car, a garden, an apartment, and if possible, a gift shop. He describes the observed behavior and demonstrates with photographs. He finds a real-world manifestation of the imitation and utilization behaviors. He coins the term environmental dependency syndrome.

In the Lhermitte (1986) studies, results of neuropsychological tests were variable and all groups contained patients with normal test scores. Direct observations inside and outside the clinic were more revealing than traditional tests. These studies suggest the unpredictable nature of tests alone and demonstrate innovative methods for validating the ecological validity of frontal brain and executive function disorders. The Lhermitte studies are unique and represent one of the only studies of frontal disordered patients and ecological validity.

WHAT DO WE KNOW ABOUT EXECUTIVE FUNCTION TESTS?

The behavioral changes associated with frontal cortex damage introduce additional difficulties as they tend to be exceedingly complex, variable, difficult to define in technical terms, and almost impossible to quantitate by available tests.

Marsel Mesulam

Neuropsychologists use a variety of tests to assess frontal brain and executive function problems (Bayless, Varney, & Roberts, 1989; Bornstein & Leason, 1985; Lezak, 1983). The list includes: The Halstead-Reitan battery, Wisconsin Card Sorting Test, Category Test, Verbal Concept Attainment Test, Controlled Oral Word Association Test, Thurston Word Fluency Test, Design Fluency Test, Ruff Figural Fluency Test, Austin Maze Test, Porteus Maze Test, Tinker Toy Test, Stroop Test, Trail Making Tests, Rey Complex Figure, and various motor tests such as the Finger Tapping Test, Purdue Pegboard Test, and the Grooved Pegboard Test.

While these tests have some sensitivity to frontal brain dysfunction, none of the so-called frontal brain tests mentioned above have proven to be *specific* measures of the frontal brain or executive dysfunction (Bigler, 1988). Their validity as frontal brain measures is not well established. Some patients with frontal brain problems do very well on these measures (Heck & Bryer, 1986), while others do poorly. Patients with brain lesions in nonfrontal areas may do either poorly or well on the same measures. Additionally, there is considerable variation among normal controls on many of these tests. Base rates in normals is not studied. Almost nothing is known about the ecological validity of these tests.

The Wisconsin Card Sorting Test (WCST) is often used to make judgments regarding a person's frontal brain system and executive functions. The author commonly sees evaluation reports that rely solely upon the results of this test to make statements about executive functions. This belief in the validity of the WCST as a measure of executive functions is unmerited.

A recent study by Anderson, Damasio, Jones, and Tranel (1992) demonstrates the fallacy of heavily relying on this test as a measure of frontal brain functioning. They examined 91 patients with stable MR- and CT-verified focal brain lesions (49 frontal, 24 nonfrontal, 18 with frontal but not limited to frontal areas) and found no significant differences between the groups on WCST performances. Several of the patients with extensive frontal damage performed normally on the test. Cutoff scores (Perseverative Response = 19 or greater and Perseverative Error = 16 or greater) only gave a 62% accurate classification rate. Analysis of frontal subregions was unproductive. The author cautions against interpreting performance on the WCST as an index of frontal lobe damage.

Bigler (1988) accurately and succinctly summarizes the present status of frontal brain assessment:

> Damage to the frontal lobes can alter behavior and cognition in a multifaceted fashion and, in terms of current understanding and test usage, no one clinical syndrome can encompass all the potential signs and symptoms ascribed to frontal damage. Similarly, because of this complexity, no current neuropsychological battery of tests is going to be uniformly sensitive to frontal lobe impairment. Thus, the current status of assessment will require the clinician to continue to use a broad spectrum of neuropsychological measures. Fortunately, we now have available neuroimaging techniques that better specify the size and extent of the frontal brain lesion. This will allow the clinician to focus primarily on the behavioral and cognitive changes that accompany such frontal damage. Careful observation and family/spouse interviewing appears to be indispensable in quantifying personality/emotional changes as traditional psychological measures appear to be generally insensitive to alterations in these

areas and frontal lobe patients are a poor judge of and lack insight into the changes that have occurred. Since many neuropsychological tests and tests thought to tap frontal lobe function are not uniformly affected by frontal damage, we are still lacking appropriate methods to specifically assess the full constellation of deficits that accompany damage to the frontal regions. Hopefully this will change in the future. (p. 295)

To summarize, there is very little systematic validation of the ecological validity of neuropsychological tests in assessing frontal brain and executive dysfunction. At times, persons with very significant frontal brain dysfunction and the related real-world problems will do very well on testing procedures. At other times, the tests seem to have some sensitivity. This variability in discrimination plays havoc with ecological validity.

WHY ARE TESTS LIMITED IN OBSERVING EXECUTIVE FUNCTION?

> *What we call reality consists of a few iron posts of observation between which we fill in by an elaborate papier-mache construction of imagination and theory.*
>
> John Archibald Wheeler

Despite the dearth of research evidence, *based upon direct observations* (clinical and real-world), astute neuropsychologists know that impaired executive functions exist and can have drastic effects upon a patient's adaptive behavior. Why does such a chasm exist between our tests and reality?

Executive functions eluding test scores is not new to neuropsychology (Kolb & Whishaw, 1985). Early in the history of neurology and neuropsychology, the frontal brain was often thought of as the "silent area" of the brain because deficits in it were not clearly evident in many patients with frontal brain damage. Test performances were often adequate. This was puzzling because persons who knew the patient saw obvious problems in real-life functioning even though the testing was unrevealing.

A number of neuropsychology scholars addressed the problem of assessing executive functions and offered possible explanations (Bigler, 1988; Eslinger & Damasio, 1987; Lezak, 1982; Mesulam, 1986; Newcombe, 1987; Stuss & Benson, 1984; Stuss, 1987).

Lezak (1982) reviewed the problems in assessing executive functions and offers explanations. She suggests that executive defects tend to be *supramodal.* She thinks the structure of the examination process makes it "difficult if not impossible" to observe these problems. She states, "Breakdown in the capacity to carry out purposive behavior is often not seen in the usual structured examination because traditional examinations rarely give the patient an opportunity to do much more than he is told to do...."

Lezak (1982) argues that the examination situation is too controlled and structured to allow the manifestation of executive problems. Lezak's argument is a common one which leads researchers to try and develop *less structured* tests like the Wisconsin Card Sorting Test and Lezak's Tinker Toy Test. These tests offer the patient a less structured challenge which will hopefully place a heavier demand on self-regulated executive abilities. While these special tests may demonstrate some sensitivity for frontal brain problems, they are not specific to frontal dysfunction. There is poor validation for these instruments as measures of frontal brain functions.

Mesulam (1986) discusses problems of in-the-office assessment of frontal brain dysfunction:

> ...quantifiable deficits in standard tests are not always impressive. In fact, some patients with sizable frontal lobe lesions may have routine neurological and neuropsychological examinations that are quite unremarkable. This creates a problem in the assessment of these patients, especially since the behavioral derangements—which sometimes constitute the only salient features—are also too complex to test in the office. This paucity of "objective" findings is sometimes responsible for overlooking the possibility of brain damage in some patients with frontal lesions. Even if some of the relevant behaviors could be reduced to testable, non trivial components, there is reason to believe that the performance in the office may not necessarily reflect daily behavior. It is not uncommon to find patients with a history of major behavioral difficulties who behave impeccably in the office. This is in keeping with the notion that these patients are most impaired under circumstances with minimal external control of behavior; the office setting may introduce sufficient external structure to suppress some of these behavioral tendencies. Furthermore, the same patient who gives perfect answers to questions about hypothetical social or moral dilemmas may act with a total lack of judgment when faced with the real situ-

ation. The clinical adage that judgment and complex comportment cannot be tested in the office is particularly pertinent to the evaluation of patients with frontal brain damage. (pp. 321-322)

Acker (1990) nicely summarizes the differences between "task demands of assessment in clinical settings and those imposed by everyday life."

Based upon the above authors, several factors seem to contribute to the problem of measuring executive functions:

1. The complexity of frontal lobe structure and function;
2. The nature and complexity of executive functions;
3. The heterogeneity of frontal lobe problems;
4. Poor definitions of executive functions;
5. Structure of the tests and testing situations.;
6. The push for maximum performance;
7. A focus upon outcome scores and a neglect of process.

Clinical Setting:	Everyday life:
Structured by examiner	Unstructured
Assisted in task focus by examiner	Little task focus provided
Nonpunitive setting	Negative feedback on errors
Planning aided by examiner	Planning by individual
Motivation aided by examiner	Self-motivation necessary
Persistence encouraged	Persistence up to individual
Failure not emphasized	Fear of failure
Protected environment	Minimally protective milieu
Inadequacies not exposed	Inadequacies visible to others
Competition absent	Competition present

Figure 2. Differences between clinical setting and real life (Acker, 1990).

THE FUNDAMENTAL PROBLEM

While all of these factors and possibly others contribute to the difficulty of measuring executive function problems, the author proposes that there is a more fundamental reason. The reason is a very basic metaphysical and epistemological problem which the author calls *the mind-data problem*. The basic thesis is that test scores are reductionistic symbolic representations of real events and as real events become more complex, interactive, and dynamic, the reductionistic symbols become a poorer representation of the reality.

If we want to measure a fixed or static object like a simple glass container, we can very easily observe it, take measurements, describe its dimensions, numerically record the information obtained, and make statements regarding it's features. "It is 4 inches tall, it is round at the top having a diameter of 2.5 inches and a circumference of x." These descriptive statements have considerable public agreement although we would have some error of measurement due to the nature of our measuring devices and the variability of persons taking the measures.

Our oral or written statements about this object would be descriptive or interpretive. To say, "the container is round at the top with a 2.5 inch diameter" is *descriptive*. To say the object is very beautiful because of its design and symmetry is *interpretive*. Descriptive statements, "*What* statements", generally have more public agreement while interpretive statements, "*Why* statements", are generally more variable among observers vulnerable to speculation.

If we try to measure a more complex fixed or static object, the measurement becomes more complicated. A glass container with multiple facets and curves is more difficult to measure and more difficult to describe. It requires multiple measures. The description is more difficult and is more vulnerable to interpretive statements. However, with more effort, challenging complex objects can be measured and accurately described.

These facts lead to some basic propositions:

1. Simple static objects can be measured with a reasonable degree of accuracy and reliability.
2. The measures obtained are not the object. They are only a symbolic representation of the object.
3. As static objects become more complex in their design and structure, measurement becomes more difficult.

When movement, a dynamic property, is added to the objects, measurement becomes much more difficult. Motion requires more data points. The description of moving objects is much more difficult. How would we thoroughly and accurately measure and describe a merry-go-round? If multiple objects are moving and interacting the measurement problem becomes even more difficult. How can we measure and describe all of the rides and activities at a carnival? Can we reduce it to a single number?

4. Moving objects are more difficult to measure and describe than static ones, requiring more data and more complex methods of measurement.
5. Multiple objects moving and interacting as a dynamic system(s) are extremely difficult to measure and describe.
6. More complex dynamic actions require multiple measures over time to best understand their effects and outcomes.
7. Reducing complex dynamic realities to single measures results in limited and incomplete information about complex realities.
8. The realities of dynamic systems are best understood when as much information as possible is observed and the maximum amount of information is considered in the description and interpretation of the phenomenon.
9. Single test scores exclude too much reality to allow accurate predictions of the behavior of complex dynamic systems.

The human mind and its resultant actions constitute a very complex, dynamic, and interactive system. Because of this complexity, observation and measurement of mind and behavior requires methods that will be sensitive to this complexity. The measurement of mind is extremely difficult. Probably because of the complexity and difficulty involved, we avoid being overwhelmed and resort to a reductionistic process which tries to reduce to single numbers very complicated things. Unfortunately, this reduction excludes information that is often essential to understand and predict the phenomenon. The end result is an oversimplification which cannot reflect the complex realities. Description and prediction become impossible.

In neuropsychology, our reductionism requires a person to perform a structured task over time. The tasks are often complex (multifactorial). The task is often timed and the task outcome is assigned a number or score. This number is a symbol of the performance and this number reduces the multiple complex dynamic system outputs to a single abstraction which is a symbolic representation of the reality which has occurred. *The number is not the reality, it is only an abstract symbol of some part or aspect of the reality measured.* The number is a reduction of many events into a single symbol. The reality was the complex dynamic performance.

Once this number is obtained, a description is made regarding what the examiner thinks the number represents. The analysis of what the number means is an attempt to describe the real-world referent. It is often more interpretive than descriptive. A reification often occurs where it is believed that the number means something whether there has or has not been verification or validation with the referent. Statements and beliefs become attached to the numbers. These statements and beliefs about what the numbers mean often displaces the actual reality. The numbers are vulnerable to losing their connections to the real objects and become connected to the interpretative abstractions which are even farther removed from the original real events.

The reduction of complex human actions to a numerical index or symbol limits or excludes much of the reality which produced the number. It results in a loss of information. To further complicate things, test scores are particularly vulnerable to manipulation, distortion, and misinterpretation. They allow an apparent but artificial control which potentially leads to many maneuvers that can further remove the symbols from reality. Statistics often generate a "significance" which lacks clinical meaning.

Most psychologists were told in graduate school, "If *it* cannot be reduced to numbers, *it* doesn't exist." They should have been taught, "If *it* can be reduced to numbers, *it* exists, but the number is not *it!*"

Because the human mind is the product of multiple, complex, interacting systems and is a dynamic process, it's measurement requires very complex methods which are capable of detecting and integrating multiple pieces of information into accurate and meaningful descriptions and interpretations.

We cannot directly observe the mind. We can only observe the mind in process and the multiple outcomes or effects of this process. The dynamic nature of the mind cannot be adequately understood by single test scores. Such scores reduce complex realities into oversimplified symbolic representations that are extremely limited in understanding the underlying processes. These reductions are extremely vulnerable to misinterpretation and speculation.

Looking only at test scores (symbolic reductions of dynamic processes) results in limited if not inadequate understanding of the realities from which the scores were extracted, especially when the real objects are complex and dynamic. By relying solely on test scores, we are excluding too much information. The exclusion of information, when studying complicated things, often results in misunderstanding and ignorance. When people lack information, while needing to understand, they become inventive in trying to fill the information gaps.

Their inventiveness can range from cautious hypotheses to crazed speculations. A lack of information at best results in ignorance and at worst mythical delusions. Perhaps this is why we hear many speculative interpretations of test scores which seem to defy the realities of a person's real-world functioning (either over- or under-estimations).

Luria (1980) surely had this in mind when he commented on the use of the tests in the Halstead-Reitan Battery for trying to understand complex higher cortical functions:

> ...at best these tests can provide only an overall picture compiled from the results of investigation of widely different processes; it is almost impossible to interpret the significance of these observations as part of the concrete picture of lesions...the application of these tests to the diagnosis of circumscribed brain lesions has completely failed to justify the confidence placed in them. (p. 390)

There are serious limitations imposed upon complex realities when we attempt to reduce complex phenomenon to single symbolic abstractions. The reduction of complex phenomenon results in a loss of information regarding the real object. It is a general problem with the assessment of dynamic systems and is particularly a problem with the assessment of more complex brain functions. This is the mind-data problem.

Since executive functions are very complex (metacognitive) dynamic processes, their observation is particularly limited by symbolic reductions (single test scores). This is why executive functions often elude test scores. Too much data is excluded from the evaluation process.

Think of the difference between being there versus just getting a report of an event. The report may reveal some or many aspects of the actual experience, but the report is not equal to being there throughout the experience. The report will be missing a lot of the data of the experience. We have all heard the reports of the astronauts' moon walks, but do the reports really equal the reality of actually setting foot on it?

Think of the difference between a still photograph and a videotape of an event. A picture in the sports section of the newspaper regarding the Super Bowl may reveal a certain amount of information but hardly communicates as much of the reality of the game as a video of the entire scenario. The final score will tell us something, but exclude a real understanding of the game.

The Dow-Jones index tells something about the reality of the stock market, but it cannot accurately predict how any particular individual's investment portfolio may have behaved on a particular day. Poor ecological validity?

Think of trying to understand the dynamics of a family system by looking at each individual's MMPI profile versus sitting down with the family in a room and asking them to solve a problem together as you sit back and observe the multiple interactions. Which would be more revealing of what really goes on in that complex family system?

What does a Category Test score of 66 errors really tell you about a person? Does it tell you what went on during the 30+ minutes the test was administered? Does it tell you how the person learned to form concepts as a child and how they now form them as an adult? Does it give you enough information to decide if the person is having problems forming concepts due to brain damage versus the inefficiency of an obsessive or impoverished thought process? Does it really tell you how they will behave in "novel problem-solving" situations?

Complex, multisystem phenomenon are difficult to quantify. Attempting to reduce this complexity to a single number results in a constriction and loss of information. While some information may be garnered from this quantitative reduction, there is too much information missing to render an accurate image of the total reality. Because executive functions are very complex dynamic multisystem phenomenon, the attempt to study these functions with summary test scores results in missing information, a limited understanding of the realities, and poor ecological validity.

HOW CAN WE BETTER ASSESS EXECUTIVE FUNCTION?

> *A purely quantitative approach to the measurement of brain disturbance of behavior that uses a test battery with a cut-off score as a performance criterion is insufficient to yield rich data for a comprehensive neuropsychological interpretation. The blind method of interpretation of standardized tests without prior knowledge of the patient's history and clinical test data can hardly serve in providing a complete and sound analysis for the diagnosis of brain lesions and for treatment recommendations.*
>
> Luria & Majovski

The mind-data problem poses a significant challenge to measurement. The assessment of the mind through summary test scores is extremely limited. Since test scores are the outcomes of complex realities, some references to the causative event can be made from the scores, but the information is very limited. That is, we can learn something about the realities of mind from summary test data, but because so much information is excluded through this method, it limits understanding of the underlying realities. This is true for all functions of the mind, but especially true when assessing the complex higher order mental processes like executive functions.

Summary test scores typically reveal little about the process of task performance and are very insensitive to "meta process" issues. Test outcome scores will always be limited in the amount of information they convey regarding the realities of complex dynamic realities. Additional methods are needed.

To best understand complex dynamic realities, multiple pieces of data from multiple methods need to be observed, analyzed, and integrated. Observing the dynamic process in action is essential. At present, the human mind is best equipped to do this parallel interactive processing. The phenomenon must be observed in action. Perhaps in the future computers can aid this process, but presently the programs offer limited assistance.

The study of executive functions and their effects can best be understood by a complex evaluation process that incorporates objective quantitative as well as objective qualitative methods of observation. The heavy use of quantitative procedures (test scores) with the minimum use of qualitative procedures (direct observations of the processes) greatly limits the observation of these complex functions of mind. In the case of "metacognition" such an approach virtually insures that the phenomenon will not be detected or observed.

Even though qualitative methods of observation are poorly understood, they are utilized by many neuropsychologists. Now, considerable thought and application of these procedures are being developed in educational, sociological, and anthropological research (Depoy, 1992; Taylor & Bogdan, 1984)

Some neuropsychologists mistakenly confuse the terms subjective and qualitative. Qualitative methods are not necessarily subjective. They can be conducted very objectively. The use of direct observation, description, and deductive analysis of themes can contribute significantly to an objective understanding of complex human phenomenon. This approach adds significant data to the assessment process which cannot result from test scores alone. For example, in the case of EVR, discussed earlier in this chapter, the patient's severe executive dysfunction would not have been missed if the "data" included the results of qualitative analysis. We need to study these methods more carefully and incorporate them into our assessment process.

Our best hope of accurately and thoroughly observing and measuring the reality of complex dynamic human mental events lies in a comprehensive assessment approach which utilizes multiple objective qualitative and quantitative methods. These include:

- Use of both *objective qualitative* and *objective quantitative* observations.
- Thorough interviews of the patient and significant others obtaining a clear understanding of the patient's history, onset, course, and pattern of problems.
- Careful observations of the patient in interview and in the process of handling various structured and unstructured problems.
- Observations of the patient in other settings where demands and problems are less structured and place a heavier demand upon dynamic mental processes. *People who live with a patient observe more data and are more likely to see the real-world realities of impairments. Before discounting their reports, consider living with the patient for a day or more.*
- Use of a comprehensive, well-validated battery of tests which have demonstrated an ability, at some level, to discriminate between brain-impaired and nonimpaired groups.
- Use of tests that have demonstrated some sensitivity to the executive functions and the frontal brain areas realizing the tests will never be specific to these issues.
- Careful study of the process of a test performance by close direct observation.
- Closer examination of a specific task observing and documenting more points of data during the performance of the task. For example, instead of just getting a summary Category Test score after 30 or more minutes, have a computer document reaction times and many other variables. This will deliver more complete data of the process.
- Analysis of *all* the data from all the observations (the tests and the person) noting interactions, themes, and patterns which would be indicative of a break down in complex dynamic processes.
- Look for convergence of evidence across functions. Since executive functions are "metacognitions" or like "shell-programs," dysfunction should manifest itself across multiple functions and various situations. A single indicator (e.g., WCST score or a single error on a test like Trail Making) may mean nothing other than a normal variation while a pattern of converging data from quantitative and qualitative observations signals executive dysfunction.

The least accurate way to observe executive dysfunction is to engage in "blind analysis" relying solely upon summary test scores from a data sheet collected by someone else without spending time directly observing the patient in action. This approach insures darkened perceptions and isolation from all the important data needed to accurately detect the reality of executive problems. We should spend less time observing test scores and spend more time directly observing patients. If we don't, we will miss too much information and end up with a partial picture of the reality of executive functions.

CASE ILLUSTRATION

M.B. is a 32-year-old-left-handed male with a high school education. Four years prior to neuropsychological evaluation, he suffered severe facial and head injuries when he was catapulted from a truck, fell down a bank, and landed face-first on a railroad iron. He has no memory of the accident or the one-month hospitalization following the accident. He was in a coma for 13 days. Upon regaining consciousness, he noted problems with his memory and marked confusion. He took notes to aid his memory. He made a good recovery and returned to work four months after the accident. His wife noted that his personality seemed to change after the accident. He "offended people with a surly attitude." At the time of evaluation, the patient reported a change in his appearance from the facial fractures and a loss of smell. He was totally anosmic. He also reported other people seeing him as changed, "They say my personality is changed." He reportedly seemed "shorter fused" with his temper.

Table 5 presents the patient's test scores. Some variabilities are present, but generally the summary scores are unremarkable. If all we had were these test scores, we would have difficulty predicting any significant adaptive problems, but analysis of additional data is revealing.

On the Stoop Test (Dodrill Version), the patient performed well within normal limits on the first part which requires simply reading the words. On the second part (saying the color of the ink in which the words are printed), he had difficulty inhibiting the impulse to say the word. He made numerous errors and performed slowly. On verbal memory tasks he made some interesting errors. On the Rey Auditory Verbal Learning Test, he made many intrusion (coming up with words not on the list) and contamination errors (confusing words of the two lists). On the recognition portion of this test he circled 23 words although he clearly knew there could only be 15. He never counted the words to check how many he had circled. When asked how many words were on the list, he responded with "15." He was surprised that he had circled 23. On the Wechsler Memory Scale stories he both simplified and confused information. He confused information within and between stories. After he heard the first story, he said, "Anna Thompson, who worked as a scrubwoman in Boston, was robbed of $15.00....The police officers felt compassionate and made up a purse for her." I pressed him for more information and he stated, "That's it...I used to listen to these stories, but also took notes." I then cued him by asking if he

TABLE 5
NEUROPSYCHOLOGICAL TEST DATA OF CASE M.B.

Test	Score
WAIS FSIQ	98
VIQ	100
PIQ	96
INF	10
DSP	14
VOC	11
ART	7
COM	11
SIM	10
PC	12
PA	8
BD	11
OA	10
DS	7
WRAT READING	63 PERCENTILE
WRAT SPELLING	50 PERCENTILE
WRAT ARITHMETIC	12 PERCENTILE
HALSTEAD IMPAIRMENT	0.1
CATEGORY	50 ERRORS
WISCONSIN CARD SORTING	
CATEGORIES	6
PERSEV. ERRORS	5
TPT TOTAL	8.3
DOMINANT	3.3
NONDOMINANT	3.1
MEMORY	8
LOCALIZATION	2
SEASHORE RHYTHM	28
SPEECH SOUNDS	2 ERRORS
GRIP DOMINANT	51.5 KG
GRIP NONDOMINANT	41.5 KG
TAPPING DOMINANT	50.6
TAPPING NON DOMINANT	54.6
TRAILS A	17 SECONDS (0 ERRORS)
TRAILS B	53 SECONDS (0 ERRORS)
STROOP I (DODRILL)	79 SECONDS
STROOP II	239 SECONDS
SENSORY PERCEPTUAL	
RIGHT	0 ERRORS
LEFT	0 ERRORS

(Continued)

(Continued from previous page)

TABLE 5	
NEUROPSYCHOLOGICAL TEST DATA OF CASE M.B.	
Test	Score
FORM DISCRIMINATION	
RIGHT	8 SECONDS (0 ERRORS)
LEFT	9 SECONDS (0 ERRORS)
WECHSLER MEMORY SCALE	
STORIES INITIAL	16
STORIES DELAYED	12
VISUAL INITIAL	13
VISUAL DELAYED	13
MMPI CODE: 9'534817/260: L/F/K/	

recalled anything about her circumstance. He stated, "She was working when this happened and I think she was working on the fourth floor." He apparently came up with the fourth floor from the four children. When I read the second story, he repeated, "Whew!...the American Liner Boston, while steaming to a port in Liverpool, struck an iceberg and was rescued by a steamship and towed into port...that's it." He confused a word from the first story and put it into the second. On the WAIS-R Digit Span subtest, his overall score was adequate (14) but he had significant difficulty with digit backwards (14 Forward and 8 Backward). On the second trial of digit backwards he confused the order of the numbers. Picture arrangement was weak (Scaled Score 8). Concept formation seemed weak. Abstractions were poorly formed. When asked, "What does this saying mean? 'Shallow brooks are noisy'?, he responded, "I don't know...never heard of it before...Hum...the only way I see that...even though something is beautiful, like a brook, it has its bad side to it...not everything is as beautiful as it seems." The patient's motor operations seemed inefficient.

Upon further investigation, the patient's wife reported "insidious changes in his personality....He was a very mellow person before all of this...his bubble was always up and he saw everything through rose-tinted glasses....everything was always fine...he was easy going...was good at his job and knew what he wanted to do for a career....he now seems to have changed....It seems like there is a bomb in there waiting to explode....He sometimes has a belligerent manner which is very unlike him....other people say he has changed since the accident....he seems to be hard on himself...he gets ticked at himself for forgetting things...he agues about things he thinks he said when he didn't....he seems unreasonable....he turns things around....he thinks we, the family, are confused....if I write a note to him, he will not get it right....it is like I didn't even write the note....he will argue that it is not what I said....his memory seems to work, but he gets it all twisted around in the wrong sequence."

She reported the following real-world incident. About two months before the evaluation, they were expecting important business visitors. The patient and his family raised and sold purebred pygmy goats. Before she left for her nursing job, she instructed her husband to have the son when he got home from school, to "Put new straw in the sheds, wash the twin goats, and trim the hooves" of one particular goat. She told him, "We really have to get this done today." He assured her that he would make sure it got done. When she came home late that night, she noticed that the job wasn't done. She confronted the son who said, "I did everything that Dad told me to do." He indicated that he had put a great deal of time into this project. Upon further questioning, she discovered that the son had been told, *"Put new alfalfa in the mangers and trim all the goats hooves."* He had trimmed 32 hooves and put many hours into it! Her husband denied any miscommunication. She stated, "This type of incident is quite common!"

She further reported that her husband was quick to anger over very little things. "He blows little disappointments into big things...he never did this before." He seemed to have a "hair-triggered temper and swears a lot." He was able to function sexually, but never initiated sexual activity. She stated, "He has no problem performing...he has no problem when he gets involved....he just doesn't initiate it....he doesn't get the urge....he forgets its a part of the program until he is reminded."

The patient's wife is reporting definite changes in the patient's functioning. The types of problems she reports are personality changes, dyscontrol of emotions, unreasonableness, lack of initiative, confusion and poor regulation of memory. These problems are often reported by significant others living with frontal-impaired patients and are known to result from frontal brain dysfunction.

It is the convergence of all the information from all the methods utilized in this evaluation that leads to the conclusion of frontal brain and executive dysfunction. No single piece of data is sufficient. The realities of the accident; the medical facts; frontal fractures; anosmia; onset, course and type of symptoms; real-world reports of significant others; test findings (especially qualitative data); direct observations; and a knowledge of frontal brain problems. No single piece of data adequately confirms this conclusion, but the constellation of data from the multiple observational methods forms a solid platform to conclude—this man has a frontal brain syndrome with practical implications. Ecological validity comes into focus.

CONCLUSION

> *Pure logical thinking cannot yield us any knowledge of the empirical world; all knowledge of reality starts from experience and ends in it…because Galileo saw this, and particularly because he drummed it into the scientific world, he is the father of modern physics—indeed, of modern science altogether.*
>
> Albert Einstein

The frontal lobes are complicated. As the saying in neuroanatomy goes, "The frontal lobes are connected to everything!" The functions associated with this complex area of the brain are no less complicated. The most elaborate of its functions is executive function. Research of this complex phenomenon reveals limits in using psychometric measures. The ecological validity of tests is variable and limited, because complicated dynamic interactive realities cannot be reduced to single numbers. This reductionistic method for understanding this elaborate reality is just too simplistic. Single numbers leave too few "iron posts" on which to anchor a direct knowledge of this complicated reality.

None of the cases presented in this chapter, including the case of EVR, lack ecological validity if multiple methods of observation are utilized. We cannot see the complete reality and make accurate predictions when we rely solely upon test scores. There are too many gaps in the information. We come closest to seeing the reality of complicated things when we use multiple observation methods—both qualitative and quantitative.

With a comprehensive observational approach, having our eyes wide open, we stand the best chance of seeing, understanding, and describing executive function and dysfunction. Looking at test scores in isolation drastically limits the possibility of perceiving these complex dynamic phenomenon. Blind test analyses most often lead down blind interpretation alleys. Such an approach constrains, excludes and limits the potential information necessary to perceive the complex realities. Test scores are only shadows of the reality which confront us, we see most by studying the full light of the reality passing by. With our eyes fully open we can see the real- world effects of executive dysfunction. Ecological validity then becomes possible.

REFERENCES

Acker, M. B. (1990). A review of the ecological validity of neuropsychological tests. In Tupper, D. E., & Cicerone, K. D. (Eds.), *The neuropsychology of everyday life: Assessment and basic competencies* (pp. 19-56). Boston: Kluwer Academic Publishers.

Anderson, S. W., Damasio, H., Jones, R. D., & Tranel (1992). Wisconsin Card Sorting Test performance as a measure of frontal lobe damage. *Journal of Clinical and Experimental Neuropsychology, 13*, 909-922.

Bayless J. D., Varney, N. R., & Roberts, R. J. (1989). Tinker toy test performance and vocational outcome in patients with closed-head injuries. *Journal of Clinical and Experimental Neuropsychology, 11*, 913-917.

Bayless, J. D. (1987). Self-directed constructional performance in brain-injured persons: Evaluation of a proposed assessment technique for executive functions. *Dissertation Abstracts International, 47*(12A), 4289.

Bigler, E. D. (1988). Frontal lobe damage and neuropsychological assessment. *Archives of Clinical Neuropsychology, 3,* 279-297.

Bornstein, R. A., & Leason, M. (1985). Effects of localized lesions on the verbal concept attainment test. *Journal of Clinical and Experimental Neuropsychology, 7,* 421-429.

Chelune, G. J., & Moehle, K. A. (1986). Neuropsychological assessment and everyday functioning. In *The neuropsychology handbook: Behavioral and clinical perspectives* (pp. 489-525). New York: Springer Publishing Company.

Depoy, E. (1992). A comparison of standardized and observational assessment. *Journal of Cognitive Rehabilitation, 10,* 30-32.

Eslinger, P. J., & Damasio, A. R. (1987). Severe disturbance of higher cognition after bilateral frontal lobe abbation: Patient EVR. *Neurology, 35,* 1731-1741.

Franzen, M. D. (1989). *Reliability and validity in neuropsychological assessment.* New York: Plenum Press.

Heck, E. T., & Bryer, J. B. (1986). Superior sorting and categorizing ability in a case of bilateral frontal atrophy: An exception to the rule. *Journal of Clinical and Experimental Neuropsychology, 8,* 313-316.

Kolb, B., & Whishaw, I. Q. (1985). *Fundamentals of human neuropsychology (2nd ed.).* New York: W. H. Freeman and Company.

Lezak, M. D. (1982). The problem of assessing executive functions. *International Journal of Psychology, 17,* 281-297.

Lezak, M. D. (1983). *Neuropsychological Assessment (2nd ed.).* New York: Oxford University Press.

Lhermitte, F., Pillon, B., & Serdaru, M. (1986). Human autonomy and the frontal lobes. Part I: Imitation and utilization behavior: A neuropsychological study of 75 patients. *Annals of Neurology, 19,* 326-334.

Lhermitte, F. (1986). Human autonomy and the frontal lobes. Part II: Patient behavior in complex and social situations: The Environmental dependency syndrome. *Annals of Neurology, 19,* 335-343.

Luria, A. R. (1973). *The working brain: An introduction to neuropsychology.* New York: Basic Books, Inc.

Luria, A. R. (1980). *Higher cortical functions in man (2nd ed.).* New York: Basic Books, Inc.

McKay, S., & Golden, C. J. (1979). Empirical derivation of experimental scales for localizing brain lesions using the Luria-Nebraska Neuropsychological Battery. *Clinical Neuropsychology, 1,* 19-23.

Mesulam, M. M. (1986). Frontal cortex and behavior: Editorial, *Annals of Neurology, 19,* 320-325.

Newcombe, F. (1987). Psychometric and behavioral evidence: Scope, limitations, and ecological validity. In H. S. Levin, J. Grafman, & H. M. Eisenberg (Eds.), *Neurobehavioral recovery from head injury* (pp. 129-145). New York: Oxford University Press.

Stuss, D. T., & Benson, F. D. (1984). Neuropsychological studies of the frontal lobes. *Psychological Bulletin, 95,* 3-28.

Stuss, D. T., & Benson, F. D. (1986). *The Frontal Lobes.* New York: Raven.

Stuss, D. T. (1987). The neuropsychology of the frontal lobes. *Barrow Neurological Institute Quarterly, 3,* 28-33.

Taylor, S. J., & Bogdan, R. (1984). *Introduction to qualitative research methods: The search for meanings (2nd. ed.).* New York: John Wiley & Sons.

Tupper, D. E., & Cicerone, K. D. (Eds.) (1990). *The neuropsychology of everyday life: Assessment and basic competencies.* Boston: Kluwer Academic Publishers.

Varney, N. R. (1988). Prognostic significance of anosmia in patients with closed-head trauma. *Journal of Clinical and Experimental Neuropsychology, 10,* 250-254.

Wang, P. L. (1987). Concept formation and frontal lobe function: The search for a clinical frontal lobe test. In Perecman, E. (Ed.), *The frontal lobes revisited* (pp. 189-205). New Jersey: Lawrence Erlbaum Associates, Publisher.

10

THE ECOLOGICAL VALIDITY OF PERCEPTUAL TESTS

Barbara Ann Cubic, Ph.D.
William Drew Gouvier, Ph.D.

INTRODUCTION

To what extent are neuropsychological instruments useful in predicting patients' behavioral deficits in their everyday environments? Do clinical interventions actually lead to meaningful functional changes in patients' lives? Facing these issues will require conceptual dismantling of comprehensive batteries and programs into areas of specific functioning, and a more discrete analysis of each component.

This chapter focuses on existing perceptual assessment techniques and interventions, and discusses their applicability to various remediation procedures. In recent decades, increased attention to perceptual disorders has lead to a number of reports of successful interventions. These interventions are viewed in terms of the type of processing ("rule-oriented" versus "rote behavioral strategies") required for successful application. The argument is made that perceptual remediation is dependent, in part, on both rote behavioral and rule-oriented strategies. Suggestions are made as to how clinicians can tailor specific treatment programs to individualized cases based on the level of behavioral and cognitive abilities the patients have in their repertoires.

THE ECOLOGICAL VALIDITY OF PERCEPTUAL TESTS

Early developments in the field of neuropsychology centered around assessment issues. First, attempts were made to develop and validate assessment instruments to detect and localize cerebral lesions. Second, these tests were used to delineate the behavioral consequences of identified lesions. Third, these assessments served to predict the impact that the behavioral deficits would have on the patient's functioning in their everyday environment.

In recent decades, a new focus in the field of neuropsychology has shifted from clarifying diagnostic issues to supporting rehabilitative attempts. The identification of behavioral deficits and strengths lead neuropsychologists more directly into the realm of treatment. As neuropsychological interventions were more frequently proposed and provided to patients, the ecological validity or practical applicability, of the techniques used was called into question.

The ecological validity of perceptual remediation is of considerable importance as perceptual disorders are frequent sequelae of neurological trauma (Gouvier, Webster, & Warner, 1986). Furthermore, the impact a perceptual disability has on functioning can often be debilitating (Sundet, Finset, & Reinvang, 1988). For example, visuoperceptual disturbances such as neglect often reduce the patient's employability, driving capability, or even independent mobility of any sort, and ability to complete many ordinary activities of daily living. Given the degree of functional interference caused by perceptual disorders, the emerging research in this area is well represented with intervention studies. The initial treatment studies are encouraging, which should challenge clinicians to continue to use and develop treatments with the highest ecological validity and, therefore, the greatest practical impact on patients' lives.

This chapter explores ecological validity issues in the assessment and treatment of disturbed perceptual functioning. Following a brief review of common perceptual disorders, assessment techniques used in the area are described. A theoretical model for understanding perceptual remediation is presented and current intervention studies are reviewed within the context of this model.

PERCEPTUAL DISORDERS

VISUOPERCEPTUAL DISORDERS

Visuoperceptual disorders most commonly occur following insults involving the right hemisphere (Hier, Mondlock, & Caplan, 1983), and can range from partial blindness to subtle alterations in complex visual organization and processing. The degree of disturbance will depend on the nature, site, and extent of the damage, as well as the age of the injured individual (Hughes, 1990).

Commonly occurring visual disorders include visual field cuts, unilateral neglect, agnosias, gaze and movement disorders, and disorders of perception. Visual field cuts lead to blindness in the affected areas. These cuts can range from small areas of blindness, or scotomas, to the loss of a quadrant or side of the visual field to total cortical blindness. Patients with unilateral visual neglect fail to report, attend, or orient to stimuli in the visual field contralateral to the cerebral lesion. This disorder is often viewed as an attentional deficit, as the sensory capabilities of that visual field are intact. When the patient is directed to focus on stimuli in the neglected hemispace visual functioning remains. In extreme cases of neglect the patient reacts as if an entire side of their world has been deleted. Even mild cases of neglect often leave the patient at risk for accidents and decrease the rehabilitative potential (Denes, Semenza, Stoppa, & Lis, 1982). Patients with visual agnosia fail to recognize sensory information although sensory input is present. For example, in object agnosia the patient can see an object (i.e., visual sensation is intact) but not recognize the object. Agnosias for color, form, objects, and faces have been reported (Varney & Digre, 1983). Gaze disturbances may cause patients to have difficulty moving their eyes from one field to another, in tracking and visual pursuit, or in maintaining conjugate gaze. Lastly, disorders of perception are manifested in disturbed integration and processing of complex stimuli.

DISORDERS OF AUDITORY PERCEPTION

Disorders of auditory functioning have received relatively little attention when compared to visual perceptual disorders. Disturbances in this realm involve imperception of both verbal and nonverbal auditory stimuli. Dysfunction of nonverbal auditory perception is usually associated with cerebral damage in the right temporal region (Kolb & Whishaw, 1985). Nonverbal disturbances are often manifested as poor recognition, comprehension, and discrimination of sounds, rhythms, patterns, or music. Inability to detect the spatial location of a sound would also fall into this category.

Auditory dysfunction regarding verbal material often results from left temporal damage (Dean, 1986). These disorders are characterized by comprehension difficulties or an inability to understand symbolic information such as language. Assessment of such difficulties might include use of the Speech Sounds Perception Test from the Halstead Reitan Battery (Reitan & Davison, 1974), the Wepman Auditory Discrimination Test (Wepman, 1973), dichotic listening tasks (Roberts, Paulsen, Richardson, & Varney, 1990; Springer, Varney, Garvey, & Roberts, 1991), or monaural/binaural listening tests such as the Auditory Comprehension Test (Green, 1978).

BODY SCHEMA DISTURBANCES

Disorders of body schema include alterations in somatic sensations of touch, pressure, temperature, pain, and limb position or movement. Patients with tactile deficits often do not report feeling tactile stimulation, or report alterations in their sense of "normal" feeling. In other cases, the patient is capable of identifying one tactile stimuli at a time, but is unable to divide attention between and correctly identify two or more competing stimuli. When the two points are adjacent to one another, this is a measurement of two point sensory threshold which involves establishing the minimum distance at which two points are felt as two as opposed to a single point of stimulation. When opposite sides of the body are stimulated this is referred to as simultaneous extinction, which is tested by touching the patient with alternating unilateral and simultaneous bilateral stimulation to separate body parts (e.g., the right and left hand). Thresholds for pain, touch, and pressure often are altered after neurological trauma and the intensity of the stimuli must be increased for detection.

Somatoperceptual disorders also include astereognosia and asomatognosia. Astereognosia refers to an inability to recognize the tactile qualities of an object. When a patient demonstrating astereognosia is not allowed to see a familiar object they can hold the object, but not be able to identify the object in their hand. Asomatognosia is defined as a loss of knowledge about one's own body. For example, the patient may be unable to point out or name their own body parts. This condition can be limited to isolated parts of the body, or can affect the entire body. In milder cases, patients may demonstrate poor correspondence between where they have been touched and their perceptual locus of that touch. A protocol for assessment and treatment of body schema disorder has been described by Weinberg et al. (1979).

ASSESSMENT INSTRUMENTS

VISUAL FUNCTIONS

Visuoperceptual skills. A variety of neuropsychological assessment techniques are available to identify visuoperceptual disorders. The most direct measure of visual dysfunction is an optometric examination which includes techniques to monitor the patient's eye positions, sensitivity to light, and direct reaction to stimuli. The instrumentation necessary for these types of assessment are often unavailable to the neuropsychologist, forcing the clinician to rely heavily on the sensory-perceptual examination. During the sensory-perceptual examination the visual fields can be assessed for field cuts or neglect through supplemental perimetric field testing while the patient maintains central fixation. Stimuli are presented using an ascending and descending method of limits at points along several planes in the visual fields, and the patient is asked to respond when a stimulus is noted to enter and leave the field of vision.

Cancellation tasks are commonly used to identify hemispatial scanning deficits. These assessments present the patient with an array of stimuli such as lines placed in various orientations on a piece of paper. The page is centered on the sagittal midline of the patient's trunk and the patient is asked to draw a line through all of the target stimuli on the page. These tasks may be varied by placing the lines in different orientations, using geometric symbols, words, numbers, or mixtures of stimuli to assess finer gradients of discriminatory ability. Albert's (1973) line cancellation procedure and the Visual Search for Parallel Lines (Vilkki, 1989) are examples of this type of procedure. When omissions commonly occur on one side this is viewed as a sign of neglect; omissions evenly distributed on both sides might suggest carelessness, inattention, or acuity deficits. Variations on presentation and scoring also allow detection of differences in the upper or lower visual quadrant (Halligan & Marshall, 1989).

The ecological validity for cancellation tasks has been partially supported. Diller and Weinberg (1977) studied recorded accidents on a rehabilitation unit and compared them with the cancellations scores obtained by left (LBD) or right (RBD) brain-damaged stroke patients. The scores on this simple digit cancellation task were predictive of the number of accidents sustained by the patients. Errors on the cancellation measure were correlated with the number of multiple accidents for both groups. However, the time required to complete the task differentially predicted accidents across the two groups. RBD patients who completed the task quickly were more accident prone, whereas, slowness on the cancellation measure predicted more accidents for the LBD patients. The authors attributed the quick performances of RBD patients to neglect and believed the slowness seen in the LBD patients was due to decreased processing ability for graphic lexical stimuli.

Matching tasks in which the patient has to chose among items to match a centrally presented stimuli have also been studied. The possible matches are displayed in different areas of the visual field to increase visual scanning for the correct match. The most commonly used matching task is the Raven's Coloured Progressive Matrices (Raven, 1965). The Lateral Asymmetry in Visual Attention Test (LAVA) (Piasetsky, 1981) is another figure match test which permits the assessment of finer grained aspects of spatial attention, as the right and left edges of the matching pieces are subtly altered.

Techniques such as the cancellation and matching tasks have also been computerized. Computerized versions may allow finer degrees of discrimination and allow the tester to have more precise control of the presentation of stimuli. The basic concept is the same, but in this instance the patient is to push a button when a light or predetermined stimuli is presented on different areas of the computer screen. An example of a computerized visuoperceptual task is the Searching for Shapes program designed by Gianutsos and Klitzner (1981). This program displays a complex pattern in the center of the screen. The patient is to find an exact match out of a large array of shapes around the central stimuli. When the match is located the space bar is pressed and the computer records the amount of time required.

Perimeter testing has also been computerized (Anton, Hershler, Lloyd, & Murray, 1988). The patient sits in the midst of an array of lights located on a semicircular grid. He or she fixates on a central light in the middle of the computer screen and holds a box with two buttons (left or right). When the patient sees the light he or she is instructed to push the correct button. For more detailed information regarding computerized programs the reader is referred to more comprehensive sources (Bracy, 1982; Gianutsos, Vroman, & Matheson, 1983; Gianutsos & Klitzner, 1981).

Visual word recognition should be assessed when one suspects visual field deficits. One method to test word recognition was developed by Battersby, Bender, Pollak, and Kahn (1956) and presents patients with 10 cards with four-word phrases. Omissions suggest the existence of a visual defect which can be further examined by other techniques. Picture recognition can be informally assessed through simple tasks such as presenting symmetrical magazine pictures and asking the patient to verbally describe or recall various elements of detail (Battersby et al., 1956).

Prosopagnosia, or the inability to recognize familiar faces, can be measured through presentation of familiar photographs or having the patients family and friends participate in the assessment. The distinction between prosopagnosia and memory loss must be clearly differentiated. The ability to recognize unfamiliar faces must be assessed separately as there are not significant correlations between familiar and unfamiliar facial recognition (Warrington & James, 1967) The Test of Facial Recognition (Benton & Van Allen, 1968) was developed to further assess recognition of unfamiliar faces. This task requires individuals to match photographs of unknown individuals to photographs of the same person under several different conditions. The Recognition Memory Test (RMT) (Warrington & James, 1967) can also be used to assess recognition of memory for faces.

Color perception or color blindness can be tested through a variety of means. The Ishihara Color Blind Test (Ishihara, 1964) is the most commonly used method. This test provides cards printed with different color dots forming a recognizable figure against a background of dots of a second color. Color agnosia, the inability to identify a color, can be measured by having the subject arrange colors based on varying hues or asking the subject to sort material based on color as in the Color Sorting Test (Goldstein & Scheerer, 1953). De Renzi and Spinnler (1967) have developed an entire color perception battery if the reader requires a more detailed assessment.

Several assessment techniques have been designed specifically to mimic visuoperceptual skills needed in the everyday environment. Caplan (1987) developed the Indented Paragraph Reading Test, to identify subtle incidences of neglect. The patient is asked to read 30 lines of text in which the left side margin indention changes from line to line. This format prevents the patient from anchoring their visual scanning on the margin. The applicability of this measure to everyday reading and the potential for detecting subtle visual problems suggests it may be a useful instrument.

The Rivermead Behavioral Inattention Test (RBIT) (Wilson, Cockburn, & Halligan, 1987) also assesses daily living skills requiring visuoperceptual functioning. The subject performs nine tasks: simulating eating a meal, making a phone call, reading a menu, setting a clock and telling time, sorting coins, copying an address, and following a map. As the reliability of these measures is still being investigated, the ecological validity has yet to be established. Measures such as the Indented Paragraph Reading Test and the RBIT do have the advantage of appearing face valid.

Visuoconstructive skills. Most assessment techniques falling under this rubric assess constructional dyspraxia. This term refers to difficulty in drawing or reproducing objects or simple geometric designs. Constructional dyspraxia is often assessed through several subtests of the Wechsler Adult Intelligence Scale-Revised (WAIS-R) (Wechsler, 1981) such as Block Design, Object Assembly, and Picture Completion. Studies have shown that poor performance on these perceptual measures predicted problems in daily living such as decreased ability for self-care skills including dressing and grooming (Lorenze, Cancro, & Sokoloff, 1961; Lorenze & Cancro, 1962). This appears to substantiate the ecological validity of using these instruments as predictors of functioning among the neurologically impaired.

The Bender-Gestalt test (Bender, 1938) is also a measure which requires complex visual processing and the reconstruction of geometric designs, and, thus, has been widely used with the neurologically impaired as a measure of constructional abilities. To enhance the sensitivity of this test and to assess the

distraction created by interference Canter (1966) developed a Background Interference Procedure. When this procedure is applied, the patient first draws
the designs on a blank sheet of paper and then reproduces them a second time
on a page printed with irregularly shaped, wavy lines.

Another variation of the Bender-Gestalt is the Minnesota Perceptuo-Diagnostic Test. The Minnesota Perceptuo-Diagnostic Test (Fuller, 1969) uses two
of the Bender figures and presents each of them in three different orientations.
The patient is asked to draw each of the variations of the figures and the degree
of rotation in the patient's reproduced drawings is assessed. Draw-a-Person,
House-Tree-Person, and the Bicycle Drawing Test have also been used as
visuoconstructive techniques, but these tests have not been studied to determine their predictive ability regarding everyday functioning.

Tests created specifically for the measurement of constructional skills include the Benton Visual Retention Test (BVRT) (Benton, 1974) and the Rey-
Osterrieth Complex Figure Test (Rey, 1941). Both of these measures begin
with a direct copying procedure and then require the patient to reproduce the
drawings from memory with varying delay periods. The BVRT measures the
direct copying of 10 separate figures whereas the Rey complex figure is one
drawing with numerous complex details within the design. An even more sophisticated task involving an added dimension of complexity is the Three Di-
mensional Constructional Praxis Test (Benton, Hamsher, Varney, & Spreen,
1983).

Specific studies relating these various visuoconstructive measures with situations in the naturalistic environment are rare. At least one study (Williams,
1967) has suggested that poor perceptual scores on a number of measures correlated with deficits in dressing, but this study did not report other psychometric scores nor the relation of poor scores to other activities of daily living. Thus,
it is not clear whether cognitive or memory deficits would have also predicted
poor performance in self care.

Visuospatial skills. Visuospatial skills require a more complex integration of
visual information than simple copying or construction skills. Deficits in this
area are often manifested in an inability to perform tasks in which spatial relationships must be determined or organized visual processing is needed.

Benton, Varney, & Hamsher (1978) developed a brief test to assess a patient's
visuospatial judgment. The Judgment of Line Orientation test consists of an
array of 11 lines which form a semicircular design. Each line is separated by an
18° angle. The patient is then presented a card with two of the 11 lines and is
asked to chose the two lines on the master card which match the lines presented
on the test card.

Closure tests are also commonly used. These tests require the individual to fill in a missing part or section from a picture. Although these tests may provide useful information, Lezak (1983) asserts that they are not as sensitive to perceptual problems as most of the other measures discussed. Common closure tasks include the Street Completion Test (Street, 1931), Mooney's Closure Test (Mooney & Ferguson, 1951) and the Gestalt Completion Test (Ekstrom, French, Harman, & Dermen, 1976). The Hooper Visual Organization Test (Hooper, 1958) requires more organizational skills as the person views an object which has been fragmented and presented on various parts of the page. Then, the patient must decide what the pieces would make if placed back into their correct positions. The Minnesota Paper Form Board Test (Likert & Quasha, 1970) uses geometric figures in much the same way. The patient is presented with a picture of a fragmented design and must decide what the design would be if the pieces were placed back together.

Visual gaze and tracking skills. Visual search and tracking techniques assess the patient's ability to follow a stimuli over a designated area. The patient may be presented with a pattern or a maze and asked to move from section to section. For example, the Trail Making Tests (Army Individual Test Battery, 1944) are considered tracking measures. First, the examiner presents the patient with a page that has an array of numbers and the patient draws a line from number to number in ascending order. The task is complicated later by having the patient alternate drawing lines between numbers and letters in a second sequence.

Other tasks purported to be useful in the assessment of visual tracking include the Digit Symbol subtest of the WAIS-R (Wechsler, 1981), the Symbol Digit Modalities Test (Smith, 1968), and several subtests of the MacQuarrie Test for Mechanical Ability (MacQuarrie, 1925,1953). This latter test, and particularly the Tracing and Pursuit subtests, are described in detail in Lezak (1983).

Driving skills. Rarely are only one or two visual tests used to predict complex behavioral functioning. More often, a battery is used to predict an ecologically significant skill and visuoperceptual tests are only one component. One such area which has received increasing attention is the integration of visual tests into batteries for predicting driving performance. The importance of driving is underscored by the fact that driving provides enhanced community independence and increases chances for employment. At the same time, the risks to the patient and the general public must be considered. Thus, assessments to predict driving need to be accurate and assess the coordination of both visual and motor skills.

With few exceptions (e.g., Colarusso & Hammill, 1972) most studies have found positive results in predicting driving skills from psychological assessment techniques. A comparison of the driving performance of head-injured patients, spinal cord patients, and controls showed the head-injured patients were the worst drivers (Sivak, Olson, Kewman, Won, & Henson, 1981), and the perceptual and cognitive assessments predicted the performance of the head-injured. These findings have been replicated by Gouvier et al., (1989) who also showed that driving skills could be predicted from performances on psychological assessments and driving simulators. Even more detailed assessment devices, such as specialized vehicles, have been developed to assess driving skills prior to allowing the patient on the highway (Hale, Schweitzer, Shipp, & Gouvier, 1987). Although these techniques are not specific to visuoperceptual functioning, visual processing is an essential component.

AUDITORY FUNCTIONS

Peripheral or cortical hearing loss will interfere with the ability to detect whether other perceptual problems exist. Decreased auditory acuity can be detected on an audiological examination and should be evaluated routinely after neurological trauma. Direct tests of auditory verbal perception can also be confounded by language deficits. Aphasia screening examinations will help the clinician establish the extent to which the deficit involves language functions vis a vis auditory perceptual functions.

Only a few techniques are available specifically to assess auditory perception. Auditory attention is tested on the sensory-perceptual examination. During the auditory portion of the exam a sound is presented behind either the right, left, or both ears. The patient acknowledges when a sound registers and this allows the clinician to assess for omissions and suppressions. Dichotic listening tasks, in which information is presented to both ears simultaneously through head phones, also allow an assessment of suppressions and even more subtle disorders of interhemispheric coordination (Roberts et al., 1990). The Auditory Comprehension Test (Green, 1978) can be used to identify lateralized ear superiority under more naturalistic listening conditions. The determination of significant unilateral ear advantage is clinically relevant. Green (1987) reports that auditory comprehension in various patient groups including schizophrenics, learning disabled children, and organic brain syndrome patients can be substantially improved by occluding the disadvantaged ear of those subjects who show marked performance discrepancies between left and right monaural conditions.

Tests of nonverbal perception are often presented via a tape recorder. For example, the Seashore Rhythm Test (Seashore, Lewis, & Saetveit, 1960) presents the patient with 30 pairs of rhythmic patterns and requires the listener to distinguish whether the pairs were the same or different. One test of auditory discrimination, the Speech Sounds Perception Test (Reitan & Davison, 1974), presents sets of four nonsense syllables which all have the "ee" sound in the center. The patient is then asked to chose the presented sound from four multiple choice possibilities. The task also assesses auditory attention as 60 of these words are presented over 20-minutes .

More simplistic assessments involve the examiner tapping out various rhythms on the table, humming or whistling a familiar melody, or having the patient discriminate between various pitches. Formalized batteries for exploration of nonverbal auditory perception are available. For further information the reader is referred to Benton (1977).

TACTILE FUNCTIONS

Before evaluation of tactile perception is conducted, the integrity of the sensory system should be assessed. Simple tests, such as touching the patient with a pin, applying varying degrees of pressure, or having the patient complete a two-point discrimination task, should be conducted with the patient's eyes closed. Touches should involve various areas of the body, hand, back of the leg, cheek, etc., as normal sensitivity in these areas differs. Once the ability to perceive touch is established the tactile portion of the sensory perceptual examination should be conducted. Either hands only or alternately the hand and face are touched unilaterally or bilaterally, and the patient states where a touch was felt. Alterations of this measure include allowing the patient to open their eyes or staggering the bilateral touches slightly to see if performance improves when the weaker side is stimulated first.

Further testing of tactual functioning almost always involves the hands. The absolute values of tactile thresholds for the hands or any other body areas can be established using a set of Von Frey Hairs, or the more sophisticated Pressure Aesthesiometer devices. These techniques are reviewed in Spreen and Strauss (1991). The Quality Distinction Test (Schwartz, Marchok, & Flynn, 1977) is used to assess whether the patient can make finer determinations between tactile stimuli. The patient is familiarized with a number of textures (velvet, sandpaper, wire, etc.) and then blindfolded. The textures are rubbed on the patient's hand and the patient is asked to identify the material. Tactile sensitivity can also be measured by a finger agnosia and fingertip number writing task. The patient places their hand in a shielded apparatus which hides the hand from their view. The examiner, using a pencil eraser, touches various fingers and the patient verbally or nonverbally (through pointing at a picture) recalls which finger was touched. In the number writing task the test is more difficult as the number 3, 4, 5, or 6 is written on the patient's finger and the patient identifies what was written. This task can be simplified by substituting x's and o's if necessary.

INTERVENTIONS

Intervention studies in the area of visuoperceptual disorders will be discussed, as the predominant amount of work regarding ecological validity in perception has centered around the visual system. Recovery of function involves spontaneous recovery, retraining, and development of compensatory strategies for remaining losses. The intervention techniques range from reliance on "bottom-up processing" such as behavioral interventions and recognition of deficits to reliance on "top-down processing" which is more rule-oriented and focuses on problem solving and cognitive self-regulation of directed behavior.

Several changes in the patient's functioning can be made through simplistic interventions. For example, visual neglect can be reduced when the patient is trained to use the hand contralateral to the lesion to point at or pick up items (Joanette, Brouchon, Gauthier, & Samson, 1986). Frequent reminders to look left and to trace words with the finger during reading may yield increased reading performances (Lawson, 1962). Cueing the patient to look left also increases performance on cancellation measures (Riddoch & Humphreys, 1983) although continued prompting may be needed. A simple position activated switch and buzzer system can be used to help patients overcome problems with somatosagnosia (Gruskin, Abitante, & Gorski, 1983). And, token reinforcements have been used to increase proper head posture and direct gaze (Wood, 1986).

Simple cueing and practice techniques can be used as compensatory techniques to retrain a patient to drive (Strano, 1989). These include slowing the speed of the vehicle to compensate for poorer visual acuity and recommending frequent head turns and relocating the mirrors in cases of neglect.

Psychometric approaches have been used in which deficits in visual perception are treated through training on a task that was originally designed to assess the impairment. The concept is based on the idea that successful repetitions can lead to amelioration of the initial deficit. Patients are trained to complete a psychometric procedure such as making perceptual discriminations between stimuli, or constructing geometric shapes. They continue to practice each item until they no longer demonstrate a deficit on the test. The hope is that the skill will then generalize to other areas requiring similar capabilities. Visual scanning training follows this rationale. The technique teaches the patient to scan the entire visual field prior to responding. Letter cancellation tasks and lightboards (Diller, et al., 1974; Diller & Gordon, 1981; Gouvier, Bua, Blanton, & Urey, 1987; Webster et al.,1984) and computer-generated stimuli (Gianutsos, Glosser, Elbaum, & Vroman, 1983; Gianutsos & Grynbaum, 1982) have been used. These training techniques reliably lead to better performance on the task, but often do not generalize well.

In other cases daily functioning is enhanced as two studies (Webster et al., 1984; Gouvier et al., 1984) showed the scanning tasks in combination with other methods improved wheelchair navigation. It is likely that the improvement in wheelchair navigation seen in these studies is more closely related to the additional training exercises (which more closely approximated the demands of the criterion task) than to the simple visual scanning training. Training on a double simultaneous stimulation testing procedure has also been shown to lead to improvements in identifying simultaneously presented stimuli, but no generalization to other skills was demonstrated (Goldman, 1966).

Psychometric techniques have also lead to enhanced driving skills among the brain-injured. Sivak et al., (1984) trained eight patients on paper-and-pencil perceptual, motor, and cognitive tests and found that the training improvements generalized to their driving skills. Structured practice on a simulated driving training course also lead to improvements in real driving in another study (Kewman et al., 1985).

Overall, the value of the psychometric approach for increasing everyday functioning is still unknown. This is largely because the standard for evaluating the outcome in such studies has been pre- and post-test scores on the psychometric measure used. In reality, changes in test scores may have no relation to functional and useful skills in everyday living.

Specialized interventions have also been applied. Patients with poor visual acuity, scotomas, visual field cuts, or cortical blindness can be taught to identify stimuli in the defective areas. In one study, the size of a patient's measured scotoma was reduced by presenting lights in an ascending and descending fashion at the margins of the visual field (Zihl & VonCramon, 1979). Hemianopic patients have been trained to identify stimuli in their blind half-fields through verbal feedback paired with the presentation of a stimuli (Zihl, 1980). A patient with total cortical blindness was trained to identify several shapes through verbal feedback, tracing cues, and the use of multiple choice response alternatives (Merrill & Kewman, 1986). But there is no evidence to document that any of these studies had any impact on the subjects' ability to function safely or with increased effectiveness in their everyday environments.

Systematic perceptual organization training may prove beneficial. Weinberg, Piasetsky, Diller, and Gordon (1982) provided right CVA patients with training in identifying spatial coordinates, organizing stimuli, and visual exploration in a rule-governed fashion. This training lead to improved visual analysis and organization. In a separate study, iconic memory training, letter span practice, and assisted reading increased reading comprehension and word identification in a set of patients (Parente, Anderson-Parente, & Shaw, 1989).

The creative application of computerized technology has lead to several advances in perceptual remediation. For example, Sivak, Hill, and Olson (1984) trained four patients with acquired brain damage on remedial programs which required diverse perceptual skills: right/left discrimination, color matching, visual scanning and search, judgment of line orientation, shape discrimination, visual memory, eye tracking, visuomotor coordination, and visual imagery. Ten hours of training lead to significant benefits for two of the patients and modest benefits for the other two patients on a variety of perceptual tasks. A recent multiple baseline study, however, suggests that the treatment gains from computerized training may be limited to computer tasks (Robertson, Gray, & McKenzie, 1988).

THEORETICAL MODEL OF PERCEPTION REMEDIATION

Rehabilitation is built on a framework in which a patient's behavioral strengths and deficits are identified. Torkelson, Jellinek, Malec, & Harvey, (1983) reported, in general, that the more intact a patient's abilities are at the beginning of rehabilitation, the more likely that patient will benefit from rehabilitation. It is also intuitively apparent (but largely unproven) that rehabilitative efforts will be enhanced when the training techniques capitalize on the patient's residual capabilities. The pursuit of maximal generalization of functioning requires that training be provided in a wide variety of settings and across various tasks related to the criterion behaviors.

Perceptual functioning can be viewed as relying on two overall processes: rule-governed behavior and specific behavioral strategies. One process is viewed as a "top down" organization where rules are developed first and then specialized behavioral strategies are used which fit the requirements of the cognitively mediated rules. From a "top down" framework, strategic interventions are formulated which rely on compensatory strategies developed through problem solving. The other process is "bottom up," as specific behavioral activities are "driven" by the sensory information that is received. At this level the task is to perceive, organize, and store sensory information as accurately and truly as possible, and interventions focus on insuring that this sensory information is made available in its entirety for the brain to process. To clarify this idea consider the role of perceptual functioning in reading. Numerous rules govern our reading behavior, most notably, that we read a page from left to right and top to bottom. Without these rules our ability to read would be disorganized as we would look haphazardly over a page of text. A functional analysis of reading skills further breaks down these overall rules into specific behavioral strategies. At the most elementary level each letter of each word has to be perceived, integrated with the other letters, organized into words and then put into a meaningful context. Successful reading is dependent on complete acquisition of the relevant stimuli ("bottom up") and guided in a rule-governed manner that allows the correct sequential processing of that information ("top down").

Clinicians need to be flexible in viewing perceptual remediation as a process requiring both types of processing. Many of our failures in remediation may be due to the fact that we often provide the patient with a task that either over- or underestimates their current level of functioning. Often the tasks do not balance the demands of "top down" versus "bottom up" processing. This might be altered simply by breaking complex tasks into functional units or by taking the basic tasks and creating the rules that tie the tasks together. Bolger (1982) suggests that therapists can manipulate a patient's strategy for executing tasks, their capacity for managing tasks, and the demand levels of the tasks. In the context of the "top down," "bottom up" dichotomy, improving strategies for task completion would be an application of "top down" processing. Rote behavioral practice in exercising a skill (e.g., memory span) would be an example of a "bottom up" approach. The factor of task demand can be manipulated in a manner to promote better generalization of the newly learned skill, particularly when the demand levels applied at the end of training actually exceed the customary demand levels encountered in the everyday environment.

Each case must be approached as an individual challenge, but general rules for structuring interventions do apply. Utilizing a systematic approach to intervention may be inherently therapeutic, as both patient and clinician learn more about the richness of strengths and weaknesses which exist. As in all areas the starting point is in a thorough assessment. Identifying the patient's strengths and limitations will be necessary before interventions can begin. During the assessment process the clinician should be evaluating the patient's higher cognitive capabilities as well as their remaining sensory-perceptual and motor skills. The goal is to determine the residual capacity for cognitive processing the client still has available. This information is used to determine whether the primary focus of training will be at the rote behavioral level, the cognitive problem solving level or both.

Prior to treatment the patient needs to be educated regarding the extent of their deficits. Creative ways of demonstrating the extent of the deficit are helpful. For example, the patient who is demonstrating left-sided neglect will have no awareness of this problem. One useful technique to make the deficit salient to the patient is to place dollar bills of various denominations on a table before the patient enters a room. The bills of highest denomination are placed in the neglected visual field area. When the patient sits at the table they are instructed to pick up all the money they see, but they often miss the bills on the extreme left. Demonstrating to the patient after completing the task that they have left most of the money on the table makes their neglect more of a reality.

The treatment plan needs to consider both processing dimensions: "top-down" and "bottom-up." In regards to "bottom-up" processing training should begin with tasks of low complexity designed to use rote practice in ameliorating deficits in acquiring and perceiving sensory information. The assessment will provide the clinician with a good starting point. If the clinician focuses on tasks the patient already has in their repertoire then the initial treatment trials will be successful. By structuring the tasks to allow for early success experiences the patient will be more motivated.

Once the patient has been able to perform the initial tasks with accuracy then the demands of the tasks should be increased incrementally. At the onset of training, the training environment should be controlled to eliminate distractions or any unnecessary stress. The therapist should provide the patient with structured activities at this point which require very little independent thought. A patient with left visual neglect would benefit from repeating a cancellation task in a quiet laboratory environment in which the clinician prompts the patient to look left as they scan each line. This task is structured, relatively stress-free, and likely in the patient's repertoire.

During early phases of treatment more verbal feedback from the therapist will be necessary. A beneficial way of gathering and presenting appropriate feedback to the patient is through behavioral monitoring. Presenting the patient with graphs or summarized data about their performance will help them more readily recognize improvements.

As the patient begins to demonstrate mastery of skills at the primary level then the expectations are elevated. Hart and Hayden (1986) recommend that the task demands increase across three dimensions: complexity, autonomy, and stress. The tasks become more difficult, less structured, and more environmental distractions such as noise, additional people, and alterations to the environment are added. These changes are made in an effort to approximate the patient's natural environment. At this point the patient with visual neglect might be trained to do a number of tasks at the intermediate level. Tasks could include having the patient enter a room on the rehabilitation unit and scan the room for a number of objects. Other tasks might include having the patient practice telling time, looking up a number in a phone book, making a telephone call, or reading a passage.

Lastly, the patient is trained to complete the skills in the criterion environment at home, work, or play. Then the patient with visual neglect should be able to rely on self-generated rules (i.e., "top down" processing) to remind them to scan their entire visual field and to be especially aware of the need to look left. These rules have been built on the earlier experiences with "bottom-up" behavioral practice. Efforts should be made to give the patient opportunities to practice these skills in the naturalistic setting prior to discontinuing treatment. At this point assignments can be based around real-life events like going to a restaurant and ordering from the menu, using a bank teller machine, or completing tasks at the home. As success in these areas occur more complex skills (e.g., driving) can be addressed.

CONCLUSION

Issues regarding ecological validity center around whether the demands of a therapy or rehabilitation setting approximate that of the real world. The use of artificial stimuli in a self-contained environment is far removed from everyday demands. Formal psychological testing situations provide the patient one-to-one attention, a quiet atmosphere, and structured tasks. The real world often offers the same patient overwhelming challenges, distraction, disorganization, and pressure. Psychometric tasks do not always allow the patient to display compensatory strategies, past experiences, individualized skills, or motivation. Testing situations also do not take into account the physical environment in which the patient will be living.

Actual research in the area of ecological validity and perceptual disorders is scarce. This is likely due to the realistic constraints involved in remediation. Cognitive functions are not independent entities which can be isolated into distinct units. Rather, any real-life task requires the integration of perceptual, motor, cognitive, and memory domains. Thus, attempts to dissect skills in order to establish their independent ecological validity would appear paradoxical.

Even with this theoretical paradox a few studies have been conducted which attempted to assess individual perceptual assessments and training techniques. Most of these studies have focused on visuoperceptual skills. The limited results at this time suggest that generalization is often poor unless several skills are targeted through various interventions, and the interventions are carried through to the criterion environment. The reason for this appears clear. To equate performances on perceptual tasks with everyday living requirements is difficult, and capturing the nuances of an ever-changing environment is not possible in the context of a typical psychological evaluation. Even approximating daily demands will require the development of sophisticated training tasks which resemble the skills needed in the real environment. Or, naturalistic techniques will be required which move the assessment out of the clinic and into the criterion environment. Conversely, tasks which have enhanced ecological validity may lose their ability to provide a functional analysis of a deficit at the more molecular level. Therefore, the virtue of an assessment instrument should not be only based on the ability to predict everyday functioning, but also on the ability to analyze specific deficits.

Despite the dearth of published studies it is likely that clinicians actually do create real-world assessments and treatments during rehabilitation. Publishing the results of this work may be difficult, as objective measures are not always obtained and quantifying the treatment gains may be difficult. Regardless of these problems, the available studies in the area of perceptual disorders and daily functioning are promising, but the ecological validity of most specific measures has yet to be established.

REFERENCES

Albert, M. L. (1973). A simple test of visual neglect. *Neurology, 23*, 658-664.

Anton, H. A., Hershler, C., Lloyd, P. , & Murray, D. (1988). Visual neglect and extinction: A new test. *Archives of Physical Medicine and Rehabilitation, 69*, 1013-1016.

Army Individual Test Battery. Manual of directions and scoring. (1944). Washington, DC: War Department, Adjutant General's Office.

Battersby, W. S., Bender, M. B., Pollack, M. , & Kahn, R. L. (1956). Unilateral "spatial agnosia" ("inattention") in patients with cortical lesions. *Brain, 79*, 68-93.

Bender, L. (1938). *A visual motor gestalt text and its clinical use.* New York: American Orthopsychiatric Associations.

Benton, A. (1974). *Revised visual retention test* (4th ed.). New York: The Psychological Corporation.

Benton, A. L. (1977). The amusias. In M. Critchley & R. A. Henson (Eds.), *Music and the brain.* London: William Heinemann.

Benton, A. L., Hamsher, K. D. S., Varney, N. R., & Spreen, O. (1983*). Contributions to neuropsychological assessment.* New York: Oxford University Press.

Benton, A. L., & Van Allen, M. W. (1968). Impairment in facial recognition in patients with cerebral disease. *Cortex, 4*, 344-358.

Benton, A. L., Varney, N. R., & Hamsher, K. D. S. (1978). Visuospatial judgment. A clinical test. *Archives of Neurology, 35*, 364-367.

Bolger, J. (1982). Cognitive restraining: A developmental approach. *Clinical Neuropsychology, 4*, 66-70.

Bracy, O. D. (1982). *Cognitive rehabilitation programs for brain injured and stroke patients.* Indianapolis: Psychological Software Services.

Canter, A. (1966). A background interference procedure to increase sensitivity of the Bender-Gestalt Test and organic brain disorder. *Journal of Consulting and Clinical Psychology, 30,* 91-97.

Caplan, B. (1987). Assessment of unilateral neglect: A reading test. *Journal of Clinical and Experimental Neuropsychology, 9,* 359-364.

Colarusso, R. P., & Hammill, D. D. (1972). *Motor-Free Visual Perception Test.* Novato, CA: Academic Therapy Publications.

Dean, R. (1986). Lateralization of cerebral functions. In D. Wedding, A. Horton, & J. Webster (Eds.), *The neuropsychology handbook: Behavioral and clinical perspectives.* New York: Springer Publishing Company.

Denes, G., Semenza, C., Stoppa, E., & Lis, A. (1982). Unilateral spatial neglect and recovery from hemiplegia: A follow-up study. *Brain, 105,* 543-552.

De Renzi, E., & Spinnler, H. (1967). Impaired performance on color tasks in patients with hemispheric damage. *Cortex, 3,* 194-217.

Diller, L., Ben-Yishay, Y., Gerstman, L., Goodkin, R., Gordon, W. A., & Weinberg, J. (1974). *Studies in cognition and hemiplegia* (Rehabilitation Monograph No. 50). New York: New York University Medical Center, Institute of Rehabilitation Medicine.

Diller, L., & Gordon, W. A. (1981). Interventions for cognitive deficits in brain-injured adults. *Journal of Consulting and Clinical Psychology, 49,* 822-834.

Diller, L., & Weinberg, J. (1977) Hemi-inattention in rehabilitation: The evoloution of a rational remediation program. In E. Weinstein & R. Friedland (Eds.). *Advances in neuropsychology* (Vol. 18) (pp. 63-82). New York: Raven Press.

Ekstrom, R. B., French, J. W., Harman, H. H., & Dermen, D (1976). *Manual for Kit of Factor-Referenced Cognitive Tests.* Princeton, N J: Educational Testing Service.

Fuller, G. B. (1969). *Minnesota Perceptuo-Diagnostic Test* (Rev. ed.). Brandon, VT: Clinical Psychology Publishing Company.

Gianutsos, R., Glosser, D., Elbaum, J., & Vroman, G. (1983). Visual imperception in brain-injured adults. Multifaceted measures. *Archives of Physical Medicine and Rehabilitation, 64,* 456-461.

Gianutsos, R., & Grynbaum, B. (1982). Helping brain injured people to contend with hidden cognitive deficits. *International Journal of Rehabilitation Medicine, 5,* 37-40.

Gianutsos, R., & Klitzner, C. (1981). *Handbook: Computer programs for cognitive rehabilitation.* Bayport, NY: Life Science Associates.

Gianutsos, R., Vroman, G., & Matheson, P. (1983). *Handbook: Computer programs for cognitive rehabilitation, Volume II.* Bayport, NY: Life Science Associates.

Goldman, H. (1966). Improvement of double simultaneous stimulation perception in hemiplegic patients. *Archives of Physical Medicine and Rehabilitation, 47,* 681-687.

Goldstein, K. H., & Scheerer, M. (1953). Tests of abstract and concrete behavior. In A. Weider (Ed.) *Contributions to medical psychology* (Vol. 2). New York: Ronald Press.

Gouvier, W. D., Bua, B. G., Blanton, P. D., & Urey, J. R. (1987). Behavioral changes following visual scanning training: Observations of five cases. *The International Journal of Clinical Neuropsychology, 9,* 74-80.

Gouvier, W. D., Cottam, G., Webster, J. S., Beissel, G. F., & Wofford, J. D. (1984). Behavioral interventions with stroke patients for improving wheelchair navigation. *International Journal of Clinical Neuropsychology, 4,* 186-190.

Gouvier, W. D., Maxfield, M. W., Schweitzer, J. R., Horton, C. R., Shipp, M., Neilson, K., & Hale, P. N. (1989). Psychometric prediction of driving performance among the disabled. *Archives of Physical Medicine and Rehabilitation, 70,* 745-750.

Gouvier, W. D., Webster, J. S., & Warner, M. S. (1986). Treatment of acquired visuoperceptual and hemiattentional disorders. *Annals of Behavioral Medicine, 8,* 15-20.

Green, P. (1987). Interference between the two ears in speech comprehension and the effect of an earplug in psychiatric and cerebral lesioned patients. In R. Takahashi, P. Flor-Henry, J. Gruzelier, & S. Niva (Eds.), *Cerebral dynamics, laterality, and psychopathology.* New York: Elsevier.

Green, P. (1978). Defective interhemispheric transfer in schizophrenia. *Journal of Abnormal Psychology, 87,* 472-480.

Gruskin, A., Abitante, S., & Gorski, A. (1983). Auditory feedback device in a patient with left sided neglect. *Archives of Physical Medicine and Rehabilitation, 64,* 606-607.

Hale, P. N., Schweitzer, J. R., Shipp, M., & Gouvier, W. D. (1987). A small-scale vehicle for assessing and training driving skills among the disabled. *Archives of Physical Medicine and Rehabilitation, 68,* 741-742.

Halligan, P. W., & Marshall, J. C. (1989). Is neglect (only) lateral? A quadrant analysis of line concellation. *Journal of Clinical and Experimental Neuropsychology, 11,* 793-798.

Hart, T., & Hayden, M. E. (1986). The ecological validity of neuropsychological assessment and remediation. In B. P. Uzzell & Y. Gross (Eds.), *Clinical neuropsychology of intervention.* Boston: Martinus Nijhoff Publishing.

Hier, B. D., Mondlock, J., & Caplan, L. R. (1983). Behavioral abnormalities after right hemisphere stroke. *Neurology, 33,* 337-344.

Hooper, H. E. (1958). *The Hooper Visual Organizational Test manual.* Los Angeles: Western Psychological Services.

Hughes, B. (1990). *Parenting a child with traumatic brain injury.* Springfield, IL: Thomas.

Ishihara, S. (1964). *Tests for color blindness* (11th ed.). Tokyo: Kanehara Shuppan.

Joanette, Y., Brouchon, M., Gauthier, L., & Samson, M. (1986). Pointing with left versus right hand in left visual field neglect. *Neuropsychologia, 24,* 391-396.

Kewman, D. G., Seigerman, C., Kintner, H., Chu, S., Henson, D., & Reeder, C. (1985). Simulation training of psychomotor skills: Teaching the brain-injured to drive. *Rehabilitation Psychology, 30,* 11-27.

Kolb, B., & Whishaw, I. Q. (1985). *Fundamentals of human neuropsychology* (2nd ed.). New York: W. H. Freeman and Company.

Lawson, I. R. (1962). Visual-spatial neglect in legions of the right cerebral hemisphere. *Neurology, 12,* 23-33.

Lezak, M. D. (1983). *Neuropsychological assessment* (2nd ed.). New York: Oxford University.

Likert, R., & Quasha, W. H. (1970). *The revised Minnesota Paper Form Board Test manual.* New York: The Psychological Corporation.

Lorenze, E. J., & Cancro, R. (1962). Dysfunction in visual perception with hemiplegia: Its relation to activities of daily living. *Archives of Physical Medicine and Rehabilitation, 43,* 514-517.

Lorenze, E. J., Cancro, R., & Sokoloff, M. A. (1961). Psychologic studies in geriatric hemiplegia. *Journal of the American Geriatrics Society, 9,* 39-47.

MacQuarrie, T. W. (1953). *MacQuarrie Test for Mechanical Ability.* Monterey, CA.: CTB/McGraw-Hill.

MacQuarrie, T. W. (1925). *MacQuarrie Test for Mechanical Ability.* Monterey, CA.: CTB/McGraw-Hill.

Merrill, M., & Kewman, D. (1986). Training of color and form identification in cortical blindness: A case study. *Archives of Physical Medicine and Rehabilitation, 67,* 479-483.

Mooney, C. M., & Ferguson, G. A. (1951). A new closure test. *Canadian Journal of Psychology, 5,* 129-133.

Parente, R., Anderson-Parente, J. K., & Shaw, B. (1989). Retraining the mind's eye. *Journal of Head Trauma Rehabilitation, 4,* 53-62.

Piasetsky, E. (1981). *A study of pathological asymmetries in visual-spatial attention in unilaterally brain-damaged stroke patients.* Unpublished doctoral dissertation, City of New York, NY.

Raven, J. C. (1965). *Guide to using the coloured progressive matrices.* London: H. K. Lewis.

Reitan, R. M., & Davison, L. A. (1974). *Clinical neuropsychology: Current status and applications.* New York: Hemisphere Press.

Rey, A. (1941). L'examen psychologique dans les cas d'encephalopathie traumatique. *Archives de Psychologie, 28,* 286-340.

Riddoch, N. J., & Humphreys, G. W. (1983). The effect of cueing on unilateral neglect. *Neuropsychologia, 21,* 589-599.

Roberts, R., Paulsen, J., Richardson, E., & Varney, N. (1990). Dichotic listening and complex partial seizures. *Journal of Clinical and Experimental Neuropsychology, 12,* 448-458.

Robertson, I., Gray, J., & McKenzie, S. (1988). Microcomputer-based cognitive rehabilitation of visual neglect: Three multiple-baseline single-case studies. *Brain Injury, 2,* 151-163.

Schwartz, A. S., Marchok, P. L., & Flynn, R. E. (1977). A sensitive test for tactile extinction: Results in patients with parietal and frontal lobe disease. *Journal of Neurology, Neurosurgery, and Psychiatry, 40,* 228-233.

Seashore, C. E., Lewis, D. & Saetveit, D. L. (1960). *Seashore measures of musical talents* (Rev. ed.). New York: The Psychological Corporation.

Sivak, M., Hill, C. S., & Olson, P. L. (1984). Computerized video tasks as training techniques for driving-related perceptual deficits of persons with brain damage: A pilot evaluation. *International Journal of Rehabilitation Research, 7,* 389-398.

Sivak, M., Hill, C. S., Henson, D. L., Butler, B. P., Silber, S. M., & Olson, P. L. (1984). Improved driving performance following perceptual training in persons with brain damage. *Archives of Physical Medicine and Rehabilitation, 65,* 163-167.

Sivak, M., Olson, P. L., Kewman, D. G., Won, H., & Henson, D. L. (1981). Driving and perceptual/cognitive skills: Behavioral consequences of brain damage. *Archives of Physical Medicine and Rehabilitation, 62,* 476-483.

Smith, A. (1968). The Symbol Digits Modalities Test: A neuropsychologic test for economic screening of learning and other cerebral disorders. *Learning Disorders, 3,* 83-91.

Spreen, O., & Strauss, E. (1991). *A compendium of neuropsychological tests.* New York: Oxford.

Springer, J., Varney, N., Garvey, M., & Roberts, R. (1991). Dichotic listening in dysphoric neuropsychiatric patients who endorse multiple seizure like symptoms. *Journal of Nervous and Mental Diseases, 179,* 459-467.

Strano, C. M. (1989). Effects of visual deficits on ability to drive in traumatically brain-injured populations. *Journal of Head Trauma Rehabilitation, 4,* 35-43.

Street, R. F. (1931). *A Gestalt Completion Test.* Contributions to education, No. 481. New York: Bureau of Publications, Teachers College, Columbia University.

Sundet, K., Finset, A., & Reinvang, I. (1988). Neuropsychological predictors in stroke rehabilitation. *Journal of Clinical and Experimental Neuropsychology, 10,* 363-37.

Torkelson, R. M., Jellinek, H. M., Malec, J. F., & Harvey, R. F. (1983). Traumatic brain injury: Psychological and medical factors related to rehabilitation outcome. *Rehabilitation Psychology, 28,* 169-174.

Varney, N. R., & Digre, K. (1983). Color amnesia without aphasia. *Cortex, 19*, 545-550.

Warrington, E. K., & James, M. (1967). Disorders of visual perception in patients with localized cerebral lesions. *Neuropsychologia, 5*, 253-266.

Webster, J. S., Jones, S., Blanton, P. D., Gross, R., Beissel, G. F., & Wofford, J. D. (1984). Visual scanning training with stroke patients. *Behavior Therapy, 15*, 129-143.

Wechsler, D. (1981). *Wechsler Adult Intelligence Test-Revised (WAIS-R) manual.* New York: The Psychological Corporation.

Weinberg, J., Diller, L., Gordon, W., Gerstman, L., Lieberman, A., Lakin, P., Hodges, G., & Ezrachi, O. (1979). Training sensory awareness and spatial organization in people with right brain damage. *Archives of Physical Medicine and Rehabilitation, 60*, 491-496.

Weinberg, J., Piasetsky, E., Diller, L., & Gordon, W. (1982). Treating perceptual organization deficits in non-neglecting RBD stroke patients. *Journal of Clinical Neuropsychology, 4*, 59-75.

Wepman, J. M. (1973). *The Auditory Discrimination Test.* Chicago: Language Research.

Williams, N. (1967). Correlation between copying ability and dressing activities in hemiplegia. *American Journal of Physical Medicine, 46*, 1332-1340.

Wilson, B., Cockburn, J., & Halligan, P. (1987). Development of a behavioral test of visuospatial neglect. *Archives of Physical Medicine Rehabilitation, 68*, 8-102.

Wood, R. (1986). Rehabilitation of patients with disorders of attention. *Journal of Head Trauma Rehabilitation, 1*, 43-53.

Zihl, J. (1980). "Blindsight:" Improvement of visually guided eye movements by systematic practice in patients with cerebral blindness. *Neuropsychologia, 18*, 71-77.

Zihl, J., & VonCramon, D. (1979). Restitution of visual functions in patients with cerebral blindness. *Journal of Neurology, Neurosurgery, and Psychiatry, 42*, 312-322.

11

THE ECOLOGICAL VALIDITY OF MEMORY TESTING PROCEDURES:
Developments in the Assessment of Everyday Memory

Glenn J. Larrabee, Ph.D., A.B.C.N., A.B.P.P.
Thomas H. Crook, III, Ph.D.

INTRODUCTION

Williams (1988) traces the roots of ecological validity and everyday cognition to three sources: 1) the study of practical intelligence in cognitive psychology (Neisser, 1982a), 2) the study of everyday cognition in gerontology (West 1986a), and 3) the prediction of everyday function in neuropsychological rehabilitation settings (Chelune & Moehle, 1986; Heaton & Pendleton, 1981). A major historical landmark in the consideration of ecological validity in memory assessment was the 1978 conference on "Practical Aspects of Memory" (Gruneberg, Morris, & Sykes, 1978; Neisser, 1982b). During the past decade interest has continued to grow; as has controversy as reflected in recent spirited exchanges in the *American Psychologist* (Banaji & Crowder, 1989; Loftus, 1991).

As the concept of ecological validity receives increased attention, a variety of procedures have been developed for evaluating everyday memory functioning. These procedures can be grouped into three major approaches: 1) behavioral rating scales (self-rated, family-rated, or clinician-related; Feher, Mahurin, Inbody, Crook, & Pirozzolo, 1991; Gilewski & Zelinski, 1986; Hermann, 1982; Williams, 1987); 2) direct measurement of the person in their environment (West, 1985; 1986b; Wilson, Cockburn, Baddeley, & Hiorns, 1989); and 3) specific performance tests or general batteries constructed to simulate everyday tasks (Crook & Larrabee, 1988; Delis, Kramer, Kaplan, & Ober, 1987). In the remainder of this chapter, the authors discuss these three methodologies for evaluating everyday memory.

RATING SCALES FOR EVALUATING EVERYDAY MEMORY FUNCTION

Extensive reviews of self-report scales of everyday memory are provided by Gileweski and Zelinski (1986) and Hermann (1982). Hermann, in his review of a variety of self-report memory scales, cautioned that although such approaches can yield useful information about memory beliefs, they should not be used as the sole means of evaluating memory because of the weak associations between memory report and actual performance.

Subsequently, Gilewski and Zelinski (1986) noted additional advantages of evaluating self-rated memory, including comparing self-rated and family-rated memory in the differential diagnosis of Alzheimer's Disease (AD) and depression. In AD, there may be relatively accurate awareness of memory abilities in the early stages of the disorder (van der Cammen et al., 1987), whereas in the middle and later stages, patients may overestimate memory abilities (Reisberg et al., 1986; Figure 12-1). Conversely, patients with depression tend to report poor memory, even though they may frequently have no measurable performance deficits (Williams, Little, Scates, & Blockman, 1987).

THE MEMORY FUNCTIONING QUESTIONNAIRE

Subsequent to their review, Zelinski and colleagues published data on the Memory Functioning Questionnaire (MFQ) (Gilewski, Zelinski, & Schaie, 1990; Zelinski, Gilewski, & Anthony-Bergstone, 1990). Gilewski et al. (1990) reported four factors for the 64-item MFQ: General Frequency of Forgetting, Seriousness of Forgetting, Retrospective Functioning (comparison of current with previous memory), and Mnemonics Usage. Factor structure was shown to be invariant across age, across samples, and across a three-year follow-up, demonstrating good reliability.

In a separate validation study, Zelinski et al. (1990) evaluated the concurrent validity of the MFQ. The General Frequency of Forgetting factor predicted immediate and delayed list recall, and Seriousness of Forgetting predicted list recognition, with modest R^2 values ranging up to .08. Of particular importance, the predictive relationship persisted after the effects of depression, health status, and educational attainment were partialled out. In a second sample, General Frequency of Forgetting significantly predicted acquisition performance on the Randt Memory Test (Randt, Brown, & Osborne, 1983). MFQ General Frequency of Forgetting and Seriousness of Forgetting predicted actual failures recorded in a daily memory failure diary. Finally, Zelinski et al. (1990), found that informant (spouse)-rated MFQ scores significantly predicted Randt test acquisition and delay, as well as Folstein Mini-Mental State score (Folstein, Folstein, & McHugh, 1975), and the prospective memory subtest score from the Rivermead Behavioral Memory Test (Wilson et al., 1989). Zelinski and colleagues (Gilewski et al., 1990; Zelinski et al., 1990) suggest that the MFQ would be useful in laboratory research on nondemented elderly subjects, although they do not recommend it as a substitute for traditional clinical memory or mental status tests.

Of particular interest, the MFQ scores showing the greatest concurrent validity are the General Frequency of Forgetting scale and the Seriousness of Forgetting scale. Although Zelinski et al. (1990) interpret this as consequent to the General Frequency of Forgetting factor representing the greatest amount of MFQ variance, it is also noteworthy that this factor and the Seriousness of Forgetting factor contain a variety of fairly specific everyday memory items. By contrast, the other MFQ factors (Retrospective Functioning; Mnemonics Usage) are more general dimensions, which are more representative of metacognitive awareness of memory function, rather than judgments about specific memory events. This suggests that self-report of specific everyday events in terms of frequency of failure or overall ability may have greater potential for yielding significant correlations with actual memory performance.

In general, the MFQ would seem to have additional utility beyond the evaluation of normal adults, if it is combined with an informant-rated MFQ. The comparison of self- and family-rated memory may be of particular interest in the clinical setting for differential diagnosis of depressive pseudo-dementia and dementia.

MEMORY ASSESSMENT CLINICS SELF- AND FAMILY-RATING EVERYDAY MEMORY SCALES

Another recently published instrument for evaluation of self-rated everyday memory is the scale published by Crook and colleagues (Crook & Larrabee, 1990; Crook & Larrabee, 1992a; Winterling, Crook, Salama, & Gobert, 1986). This scale, the MAC-S, consists of 49 items. Twenty-one items describe specific tasks or problems encountered in everyday life and are rated by the person in terms of perceived overall ability to perform the task (e.g., remember "the name of a person just introduced to you"). Twenty-four items are rated in terms of frequency of occurrence of specific memory problems (e.g., "forget what you intended to buy at a grocery store or pharmacy"). Finally, the MAC-S includes four global rating items assessing the person's overall rating of his or her memory. These items relate to global ability, speed of recall relative to the best their memory has been, overall function of memory compared to the best it has ever been, and degree of concern or distress over current memory function.

Factor analysis of the MAC-S yielded five factors for the Ability-rated items and five factors for the Frequency-of-occurrence-rated items. The Ability factors were: 1) Remote Personal Memory, 2) Numeric Recall, 3) Everyday Task-oriented Memory, 4) Word Recall/Semantic Memory, and 5) Spatial/Topographic Memory. The five Frequency factors were: 1) Word and Fact Recall/Semantic Memory, 2) Attention/ Concentration, 3) Everyday Task-oriented Memory, 4) General Forgetfulness, and 5) Facial Recognition. Factor structure did not vary as a function of age or gender. Also, Crook and Larrabee (1990) reported that MAC-S summary scores (e.g., Ability Total, and, particularly, Frequency Total) demonstrated higher correlations with self-rated depression (Geriatric Depression Scale or GDS); (Yesavage et al., 1983) than did MAC-S factor scores. This suggests that the MAC-S factor scores are less susceptible to potential confound with self-rated depression than are global summary ratings. Crook and Larrabee (1992a) report normative data on the MAC-S, based on 1,106 normal adults. They also report test-retest reliabilities which range above .80 for the different MAC-S factor scores on three-week inter-test intervals.

In a subsequent investigation, Larrabee, West, and Crook (1991) reported a significant association between several MAC-S factor scores and performance on a computer-simulated everyday memory battery in a sample of normal adults (Crook & Larrabee, 1988). Larrabee et al. (1991) reported a canonical variate which accounted for 27.9% of shared variance between the MAC-S factor scores and a computerized general memory factor, after initially controlling for the association of MAC-S scores with self-rated depression (GDS). MAC factor scores associated with actual performance included the Ability factors for Remote Memory, Everyday Memory, and Semantic Memory, as well as the Frequency factors for Concentration and Forgetfulness.

The MAC-S also exists in a parallel version, the MAC-F, which can be completed by the subject's family member or significant other. Feher et al. (1991), in an investigation of anosognosia, computed global MAC-S minus MAC-F difference scores for 38 AD patients and compared these scores with clinical measures of memory and dementia. The "denial" scores (MAC-S minus MAC-F) demonstrated a nonsignificant linear trend ($r = .27$, $p < .10$) with dementia severity. Significant correlations were demonstrated between the "denial" score and scores on Wechsler Memory Scale (WMS) (Wechsler, 1945) Logical Memory ($r = -.42$, $p < .01$) and Paired Associate Learning ($r = -.38$, $p < .05$) subtests. A trend was observed between greater awareness (smaller "denial" scores) and greater depression on the Hamilton Depression Scale ($r = -.29$, $p < .10$).

THE COGNITIVE BEHAVIOR RATING SCALES

Williams (1987) has published an omnibus rating scale to be used by family members and/or significant others in evaluating a patient's function. This instrument, the Cognitive Behavior Rating Scales (CBRS), consists of nine scales: Language Deficit, Apraxia, Disorientation, Agitation, Need for Routine, Depression, Higher Cognitive Deficits, Memory Disorder, and Dementia. Although the CBRS assesses more than memory, several of the subscales are directly related to memory function (Orientation, Need for Routine) or to conditions/problems that affect memory and other abilities.

Williams (1987) suggests that the greatest utility of the CBRS is in evaluating the cognitive sequelae of dementia, since many demented patients may refuse testing or be unable to complete conventional neuropsychological testing. Test-retest correlations on 31 dementia patients rated on the CBRS ranged from .61 to .94. Alpha coefficients for the CBRS scores of 400 normal subjects ranged from .78 to .92. The Memory Disorder Scale showed a high test-retest correlation (.80) and high coefficient alpha (.92). CBRS factor scores, with the exception of the Depression Scale, discriminated between moderately demented patients and age-and-education-matched control subjects. Williams cautions that further study is needed, including those among groups of mildly demented patients, depressed patients, and patients with various types of brain damage.

SUMMARY CONCERNING EVERYDAY MEMORY RATING SCALES

The rating scales reviewed demonstrate promise as tools in the evaluation of a patient's memory and related neuropsychological functions. Clearly, self-rating scales, such as the MFQ or MAC-S, or family rating versions, such as the MFQ family version, MAC-F, or CBRS, cannot be used as the sole means of evaluating memory in general or everyday memory specifically. However, combining these measures with formal objective assessment can enhance the yield of standardized neuropsychological evaluation. In particular, comparison of self- and family-ratings of everyday memory abilities on a particular patient can provide a useful means of quantifying awareness of deficits (cf. Feher et al., 1991; Prigatano & Schacter, 1991). Similarly, comparisons of self- and family-ratings of everyday memory function may yield useful information in the differential diagnosis of depressive pseudo-dementia.

DIRECT MEASUREMENT OF EVERYDAY MEMORY IN THE PATIENT'S ENVIRONMENT

THE RIVERMEAD BEHAVIORAL MEMORY TEST

Wilson and colleagues (Wilson, Cockburn, & Baddeley, 1985; Wilson, Cockburn, Baddeley, & Hiorns, 1989) have published the Rivermead Behavioral Memory Test (RBMT), a brief, portable measure of everyday memory function. The authors intended the RBMT to be "....a bridge between laboratory-based measures of memory and assessments obtained by questionnaire and observation" (Wilson et al., 1989, p. 856). There are 12 components of the RBMT, including remembering a *first and last name, remembering a hidden belonging* (an item of minimal value is requested from the subject and placed in a specified location*), remembering an appointment* (after 20 minutes), *picture recognition* (a traditional memory test in which the subject must discriminate 10 previously seen line drawings of common objects from 10 distracters following a delay of a few minutes), *remembering a newspaper article* (immediate and 20-minute delayed recall of a short prose passage), *face recognition* (five previously seen facial photographs must be discriminated from five distracters after a delay of a few minutes); *remembering a new route* (the tester traces out a short path between a series of specified locations in the room; subjects must retrace the same path, both immediately following demonstration and after a 10-minute delay); *delivering a message* (when the tester traces out the path, he/she leaves an envelope marked "message" at a specified location; the subject must pick it up and leave it in the right place on both immediate and delayed routes); *orientation* (to time and place); *orientation to date* (scored separately). There are four alternate forms of the RBMT, which intercorrelate between .83 to .88 (Wilson et al., 1989). Wilson et al. also demonstrated that all of the subtests significantly discriminate patients with documented brain damage (primarily head trauma and right and left unilateral stroke) from control subjects, and the RBMT subtests correlate significantly with a variety of standard memory tests, including the Recognition Memory Test (Warrington, 1984) and the Paired Associate Learning subtest from the Randt Test (Randt et al., 1983). The RBMT also correlates with rehabilitation staff ratings of memory lapses suffered by patients, and with subjective and relative-ratings of memory function (Wilson et al., 1989; interestingly, the self-rated correlations and RBMT correlations are typically higher than the correlations between self-ratings and standard memory test performance).

Additional research also supports the validity of the RBMT. Kotler-Cope (1990) reported data on RBMT performance of 34 patients with memory dysfunction (15 had AD-type dementia and most of the others had cerebrovascular disease). RBMT scores were compared to Wechsler Memory Scale-Revised (WMS-R) (Wechsler, 1987) scores, and to self- and family-rating (on the CBRS) for Depression, Higher Cognitive Deficit, Memory Disorders, and Dementia (Williams, 1987). The RBMT correlated significantly with all WMS-R Indices (values ranged from .61 for Attention/Concentration to .91 for General Memory). Self-report CBRS scores did not correlate with either the RBMT or the WMS-R. The RBMT did correlate significantly with relative-rated CBRS Higher Cognitive ($r = .43$) and Memory Disorder ($r = .38$) scales. By contrast, only the WMS-R Attention/Concentration index reflected a significant association with the relative-rated CBRS (correlation with CBRS Higher Cognitive = .43).

Finally, Wilson (1991) reported data on the utility of the RBMT in predicting long-term clinical outcome. Forty-three persons, most of whom had experienced severe closed-head injury (coma of at least six hours or a post-traumatic amnesia of at least 24 hours), were seen on 5 - 10-year follow-up. The RBMT significantly discriminated dependent from independent subjects (independence was defined as either living alone and/or in full-time education and/or in paid employment). By contrast, none of the WMS-R indices significantly discriminated dependent from independent patients.

THE EVERYDAY MEMORY INTERVIEW

West (1986b) has developed a naturalistic, everyday memory examination, the Everyday Memory Interview (EMI). The EMI assesses performance on a variety of everyday tasks in the context of a clinical interview of the subject. Tasks include incidental recall of the interviewer's name; incidental recall of the interviewer's first conversation with the subject; incidental recall of a 15-item shopping list (the items are actually generated by the subject, who is later tested on recall of the self-generated list); incidental recall of information from an informed consent form for the research study, object location recall (the subject places 10 small objects; a book, magnet, egg, rubberband, spoon, lock, ID card, coaster, penny, and bolt in 10 different locations, only half of which are in direct view of the subject); recall of a doctor's instructions (immediate and delayed recall); an imagery task requiring inspection of two photographs (one of a person and one of a building; immediate and delayed recall are evaluated for details of the two pictures); prospective memory for carrying out a task at the end of the interview (e.g., remind the examiner to make a phone call; tell the examiner about one thing the subject is going to do tomorrow); following a set of instructions to perform various activities (e.g., "place the pencil in the chair on your right side;" after the subject completes the instructions, these are reviewed once more, with the subject being made aware that recall of these instructions will be required later); recall of a prose passage on memory and habits, that the subject has read (recall is tested at a later time); and recall of a brief route within the examining office. The EMI is available in two alternate forms.

Various papers have reported on EMI performance characteristics. West and Walton (1985) reported that young adults completed more total steps in a set of instructions, as well as more steps in the correct sequence than older adults. Also, older adults recalled a lower percentage of grocery list items, as well as fewer of the doctor's instructions. Subsequently, West (1988) reported age differences on the prospective memory tasks of the EMI, with older adults performing more poorly than younger adults. West (1989) also has analyzed data demonstrating that the EMI significantly discriminated the performance of young (18-39), middle-aged (40-49), young-old (60-75), and old-old (75-90) normal volunteers. EMI scores also significantly discriminated persons whose health was rated "excellent" or "good" from those whose health was rated "poor" or "fair".

Both the RBMT and the EMI represent unique attempts to measure everyday abilities in the naturalistic setting of the clinical interview. The validity data on the RBMT are impressive, and the growing database on the EMI suggests significant potential for more widespread research and clinical applications. As West and Tomer (1989) observed, both the EMI and RBMT are lower in difficulty level, compared to simulated everyday memory tasks, such as the computerized everyday memory battery developed by Crook and colleagues (e.g., Crook & Larrabee, 1988). Larrabee and Crook (1991) observed that the lower difficulty level of the EMI and RBMT may preclude their use in clinical trials of memory-enhancing drugs in nondemented populations, because these procedures may not be as sensitive to potentially subtle treatment effects and may be subject to "ceiling" effects. In comparison, both the EMI and RBMT may be preferable in trials with demented subjects where tests such as those of Crook and Larrabee may be subject to "floor" effects.

SIMULATED EVERYDAY ASSESSMENT TECHNIQUES

In addition to measuring a subject's ability to perform everyday tasks in a naturalistic setting, others have adapted everyday task stimuli, such as grocery list items, faces and telephone numbers, to clinical testing paradigms such as supraspan list learning, signal detection, and delayed nonmatching to sample. Some of these procedures, such as the CVLT (Delis et al., 1987) are complete tests in and of themselves; others, such as the Names-Faces subtest of the Memory Assessment Scales (MAS) (Williams, 1991) are part of a more traditional battery of memory tests. Finally, there is an extensive, comprehensive set of computer-simulated everyday memory tests that comprise the Memory Assessment Clinics (MAC) computer-simulated everyday memory battery (Crook, Johnson, & Larrabee, 1990; Crook & Larrabee, 1988; Crook, Salama, & Gobert, 1986).

THE CALIFORNIA VERBAL LEARNING TEST

The CVLT was designed to evaluate multiple cognitive parameters (the process of verbal learning in addition to the amount of material retained) within the context of an everyday memory task (Delis et al., 1987). The subject is required to learn a list of 16 items (four each, in the categories of clothing, spices/herbs, tools, and fruits) over five trials, followed by a second list to serve as interference. Short delay (immediately following interference) with free and category-cued recall, long delay (20 minutes) with free and cued recall, and yes-no recognition of the original list items are assessed. Several dimensions of performance can be evaluated, including semantic and serial learning strategies, degree of vulnerability to proactive and retroactive interference, and retention of information over time. The test manual provides normative data across the age range of 17 to 80. The CVLT demonstrates good split-half reliability (.92). Test-retest values are somewhat lower (e.g., List A total recall = .59), however, the retest interval was one year. The CVLT correlates significantly with various WMS subtests, and the test manual summarizes CVLT data on a variety of clinical populations, including alcoholism, Parkinson's disease, multiple sclerosis, Huntington's disease, and Alzheimer's disease.

Additional studies further support the construct and criterion-related validity of the CVLT. Delis, Freeland, Kramer, and Kaplan (1988) reported a factor structure representing several underlying cognitive processing domains, including general verbal learning, response discrimination, proactive effect, and serial position effect, among others. Kramer, Levin, Brandt, and Delis (1989) used discriminant function analysis in demonstrating correct classification of over

76% of cases of Huntington's disease, Alzheimer's disease, and Parkinson's disease on the basis of CVLT performance. Schear and Craft (1989) reported significant correlations between CVLT, WMS, and Verbal Selective Reminding Test scores (Levin, Benton, & Grossman, 1982). Finally, Delis et al., (1991) developed an alternate, equivalent form of the CVLT.

THE NAMES-FACES SUBTEST OF THE MEMORY ASSESSMENT SCALES

The recently published MAS (Williams, 1991) contains a variety of subtests that follow traditional clinical memory test paradigms and stimuli (e.g., list learning, verbal span, visual recognition memory for geometric forms) as well as a subtest assessing memory for names and faces. In this subtest, Names-Faces, the subject is presented with 10 individual photographs, each followed by a first and last name. On the test trials, the subject must pick the correct name from three multiple choice alternatives. The procedure is repeated for two consecutive trials, followed after completion of other MAS subtests (l0-l5 minutes), by a delayed trial. The test manual reports high generalizability coefficients for both Immediate and Delayed Names-Faces scores, and both scores load on a general memory factor (in normal subjects) and verbal memory factor (in neurologically impaired subjects). Williams (1991, Table 20, p. 54) discloses that both the Immediate and Delayed Names-Faces scores are sensitive to dementia, closed head trauma, and right and left hemisphere CVA (note: the right CVAs perform at a higher level, contrasted with left CVAs, but both groups perform at a level inferior to normal subjects).

Presently, the CVLT is a well-established clinical instrument, however the MAS should see more widespread use in future clinical and research settings. One potential analysis in future investigations would be to correlate CVLT and MAS subtest performance with scores on self-rated and family-rated everyday memory skills. Demonstrations of higher correlations between behavioral ratings of everyday memory and CVLT scores than traditional clinical memory test scores would provide further support for the everyday validity of the CVLT. A similar investigation could contrast the correlations between MAS Names-Faces and everyday rated skills, with the correlations found between these everyday-rated skills and the more traditional MAS subtests.

THE MEMORY ASSESSMENT CLINICS (MAC) COMPUTER-SIMULATED EVERYDAY MEMORY BATTERY

The final everyday memory assessment procedure to be considered in this chapter is the MAC computer-simulated everyday memory battery (Crook et al., 1990; Crook & Larrabee, 1988; Crook et al., 1986). Development of the current MAC battery began in 1985, but is based on research into everyday memory functions begun in the 1970's and early 1980's by Crook and colleagues (e.g., Crook, Ferris, & McCarthy, 1979; Crook, Ferris, McCarthy, & Rae, 1980; Ferris, Crook, Clark, McCarthy, & Rae, 1980; McCarthy, Ferris, Clark, & Crook, 1981).

The MAC battery was specifically designed for research on clinical drug trials in memory disorders (Larrabee & Crook, 1991). This led to an emphasis on ecologic face validity, which is important in two respects. Cunningham (1986) called for greater face validity for clinical evaluation of psychogeriatric patients who may be threatened by the novel, unfamiliar stimuli characteristic of traditional memory tests. Second, ecologic validity is especially pertinent to clinical trials, where the goal is to develop a treatment that produces a clinically significant change in the patient's everyday life. Indeed, Leber (1986) has stated that the more clearly a test or scale is related to meaningful change in everyday behavior or performance, the more acceptable it will be as a means of documenting drug efficacy.

The MAC battery represents an attempt at simulating the reality of everyday memory tasks through the interaction of computer graphics and laser-disk technologies. Responses of subjects are either verbal or via a touchscreen and, thus, subjects are not asked to respond via keyboards, joysticks, or other manipulanda that may be alien to the daily life of some persons. This technology is combined with standard memory measurement paradigms, such as selective reminding, associate learning, signal detection, and delayed nonmatch-to-sample, to enhance the psychometric and clinical validity of the procedures. The battery incorporates several measures of everyday verbal and visual secondary memory, primary memory, reaction time, and divided attention. Name-Face learning is a task that utilizes live laser-disk recordings of persons introducing themselves and their city of residence (Crook & West, 1990). First-name recall is assessed, as well as incidental recall of the city of residence. There are two measures of everyday verbal learning: First-Last Names Paired Associate Learning and Grocery List Selective Reminding (Youngjohn, Larrabee, & Crook, 1991). Visual associative memory is assessed with the Misplaced Objects task, which requires the subject to place 20 objects in a 12-room house by touching the touchscreen. Approximately 40 minutes later, recall for object location is assessed (Crook, Youngjohn, & Larrabee, 1990a). Two facial memory tests are included in the MAC battery, one assessing facial recognition memory using a signal detection format, Recognition of Faces-Signal Detection, and one utilizing a delayed, nonmatching-to-sample format, Recognition of Faces-Delayed Nonmatch-to-Sample (Crook & Larrabee, 1992b). There is also a measure of memory for text, based on a T.V. news broadcast, The T.V. News Test, (Crook, Youngjohn, & Larrabee, 1990b). A reaction time test utilizes a simulated driving task, including traffic light, gas and brake pedals (Crook, West, & Larrabee, 1993). This test also employs a divided attention format, in which the subject must recall details of a radio broadcast played during the driving task. The Telephone Dialing test requires the subject to dial a seven or 10 digit number on a touchtone telephone, after a single visual presentation of the number. This test can be made more difficult by employing an interference condition in which the subject hears ringing or a busy signal after they have dialed the number; if the busy signal is heard, the subject must redial the number (West & Crook, 1990). Finally, there is a measure of spatial/topographic memory, the Topographic Memory test (Crook, Youngjohn, & Larrabee, 1993; Zappala, Martini, Crook, & Amaducci, 1989). This requires the subject to recall a route traced through a schema of a neighborhood map.

The MAC battery is also available, with modifications, for use in research on early stage AD. Some tests, such as Misplaced Objects and Recognition of Faces-Delayed Nonmatch-to-Sample, are not modified. Others, such as Name-Face Association and Grocery List Selective Reminding, maintain the same administration format with reduced stimuli (e.g., for Grocery List Selective Reminding, the AD Battery employs 10, rather than 15 items).

Six equivalent forms are available for Telephone Dialing, Name-Face Association, First-Last Name Memory, and Grocery List Selective Reminding, while eight equivalent forms are available for Misplaced Objects and Recognition of Faces (Crook, Youngjohn, & Larrabee, 1992). Test-retest reliabilities over a three-week follow-up were low for Recognition of Faces-Signal Detection (range .18 - .60) and Reaction Time (.44 - .68), but good for Misplaced Objects (.77) and Name-Face Association (.80 to .83; values comparable to traditional clinical memory tests) (Youngjohn, Larrabee, & Crook, 1992a). The tests are available in American English, British English, Danish, Finnish, Flemish, French, German (Austrian and German versions), Italian, Spanish, and Swedish. Current U.S. normative data average around 2,000 subjects per test, covering the age range of 17 to 90. Additional data are available on European versions, and data are also collected on over 2,000 subjects with Age-Associated Memory Impairment (AAMI) (Crook et al., 1986) and over 300 persons with Alzheimer-type dementia. Initial data show consistency of normal subjects' performance on the U.S., Belgian-French, and Italian versions of the battery (Crook, Youngjohn, Larrabee, & Salama, 1992; Crook, Zappala, Cavarzeran, Measso, Pirozzolo, & Massari, 1993).

Investigations by Crook and Larrabee (1988) and Larrabee and Crook (1989a) elucidate the factorial validity of the MAC battery, which demonstrates factors of everyday verbal and visual memory, attention-concentration, and processing speed, which are stable across the adult age range. As stated earlier, the MAC battery shows a significant association with self-rated memory in normal adults (27.9% of shared variance) (Larrabee et al., 1991). Meaningful subject performance subtypes of everyday memory function have been derived through cluster analysis (Larrabee & Crook, 1989b), and the MAC battery significantly discriminates (88.40%) between subjects with AAMI (Folstein et al., (1975) Mini-Mental State = 24 to 30) and persons with mild AD (Mini-Mental State = 20 to 23) (Youngjohn, Larrabee, & Crook, 1992b).

The MAC battery has also been utilized in several clinical trials of drugs with potential for memory enhancement in both AAMI and AD. Crook et al., (1991) demonstrated a positive treatment response of AAMI to phosphatidylserine on MAC battery scores. West and Crook (1992) demonstrated improved MAC battery performance for mature adults (the majority of whom would qualify as having AAMI) who had undergone videotape imagery-based memory training for name-face and object location recall. Conversely, McEntee et al., (1991) found no treatment response, on MAC battery scores, for AAMI subjects who had been administered guanfacine, and Crook, Wilner, Rothwell, Winterling, and McEntee (1992) reported a similar absence of treatment response in AD patients treated with guanfacine.

SUMMARY

In this chapter the authors reviewed three major methods of evaluating everyday memory function: self- and family-rated memory scales, assessment of the individual in the clinical environment, and test simulations of everyday memory skills. Although initial investigations of self-rating scales have not shown them to be powerful predictors of actual memory performance, subsequent scales, such as the MAC-S and MFQ, have shown better validity. This is particularly clear when specific everyday items are being rated (the MFQ General Frequency of Forgetting factor; MAC-S Ability factors for Remote Memory, Everyday Memory, and Semantic Memory; and MAC-S Frequency factors for Concentration and Forgetfulness).

In view of the well-established association of depression with memory complaint and the occurrence of anosognosia in neurologic disorders, self-report sales should not be employed without utilizing concurrent family ratings, and formal neuropsychological testing. Use of parallel self- and family-rating scales may be particularly useful in evaluating anosognosia, and in differentiating dementia and depressive pseudo-dementia. Scales such as the RBMT and EMI that directly assess everyday memory in the clinic have significant promise. In particular, the RBMT demonstrated ecologic validity (i.e., predicting degree of independence) in populations with severe neurologic impairment following head trauma or stroke. The EMI and RBMT may be less sensitive to more subtle changes in memory function. These subtle changes may be evaluated by psychometric simulations of everyday memory tasks such as the CVLT, the MAS Names-Faces subtests, or the MAC computer-simulated everyday memory battery. Both the CVLT and MAS have documented clinical validity across various clinical populations. However, the everyday performance dimensions covered by the CVLT and MAS Names-Faces subtests are limited. By contrast, the MAC computer-simulated memory battery developed specifically for assessment of everyday memory covers a broad range of everyday functions of memory and related abilities. Consequently, the MAC battery, which also has multiple alternative forms, has been particularly useful in clinical trials of memory-enhancing drugs in memory disorders of aging.

Ecologic validity has become an important guiding concept in clinical memory testing. It is expected that coming years will see new developments and substantial progress in this area.

REFERENCES

Banaji, M. R., & Crowder, R. G. (1989). The bankruptcy of everyday memory. *American Psychologist, 44*, 1185-1193.

Chelune, G., & Moehle, K. (1986). Neuropsychological assessment and everyday functioning. In D. Wedding, A. M. Horton, & D. Webster (Eds.) *The neuropsychology handbook*, (pp. 489-525). New York: Springer.

Crook, T. H., Bartus, R. T., Ferris, S. H., Whitehouse, P., Cohen, G. D., & Gershon, S. (1986). Age-Associated Memory Impairment: Proposed diagnostic criteria and measures of clinical change. Report of a National Institute of Mental Health work group. *Developmental Neuropsychology, 2*, 261-276.

Crook, T. H., Ferris, S. H., & McCarthy, M. (1979). The misplaced-objects task: A brief test for memory dysfunction in the aged. *Journal of the American Geriatric Society, 27*, 284-287.

Crook, T. H., Ferris, S. H., McCarthy, M., & Rae, D. (1980). The utility of digit recall tasks for assessing memory in the aged. *Journal of Consulting and Clinical Psychology, 48*, 228-233.

Crook, T. H., Johnson, B. A., & Larrabee, G. J. (1990). New methods for assessing drug effects in Alzheimer's disease and Age-Associated Memory Impairment. In O. Benkert, W. Maier,

& K. Rickels (Eds.) *Methodology of the evaluation of psychotropic drugs*, (pp. 37-55). New York: Springer.

Crook, T. H., & Larrabee, G. J. (1988). Interrelationships among everyday memory tests: Stability of factor structure with age. *Neuropsychology, 2*, 1-12.

Crook, T. H., & Larrabee, G. J. (1990). A self-rating scale for evaluating memory in everyday life. *Psychology and Aging, 5*, 48-57.

Crook, T. H., & Larrabee, G. J. (1992a). Normative data on a self rating scale for evaluating memory in everyday memory. *Archives of Clinical Neuropsychology, 7*, 41-51.

Crook, T. H., & Larrabee, G. J. (1992b). Changes in facial recognition memory across the adult life span. *Journal of Gerontology. Psychological Sciences, 47*, 138-141.

Crook, T. H., Salama, M., & Gobert, J. (1986). A computerized test battery for detecting and assessing memory disorders. In A. Bes, J. Cahn, S. Hoyer, J. P. Marc-Vergenes, & H. M. Wisniewski (Eds.), *Senile dementias: Early detection*, (pp. 79-85). London-Paris: John Libbey Eurotext.

Crook, T. H., Tinklenberg, J., Yesavage, J., Petrie, W., Nunzi, M. G., & Massari, D. C. (1991). Effects of phosphatidylserine in age-associated memory impairment. *Neurology, 41*, 644-649.

Crook, T. H., & West, R. L. (1990). Name recall performance across the adult life span. British *Journal of Psychology, 81*, 335-349.

Crook, T. H., West, R. L., & Larrabee, G. J. (1993). The Driving Reaction Time Test: Assessing age declines in dual-task performance. *Developmental Neuropsychology, 9*, 31-39.

Crook, T., Wilner, E., Rothwell, A. Winterling, D., & McEntee, W. (1992). Noradrenergic intervention in Alzheimer's disease. *Psychopharmacology Bulletin, 28*, 76-80.

Crook, T. H., Youngjohn, J. R., & Larrabee, G. J. (1990a). The Misplaced Objects Test: A measure of everyday visual memory. *Journal of Clinical and Experimental Neuropsychology, 12*, 819-833.

Crook, T. H., Youngjohn, J. R., & Larrabee, G. J. (1990b). The TV News Test: A new measure of everyday memory for prose. *Neuropsychology, 4*, 135-145.

Crook, T. H., Youngjohn, J. R., & Larrabee, G. J. (1992). Multiple equivalent test forms in a computerized everyday memory battery. *Archives of Clinical Neuropsychology, 7*, 221-232.

Crook, T. H., Youngjohn, J. R., & Larrabee, G. J. (1993). The influence of age, gender and cues on computer-simulated topographic memory. *Developmental Neuropsychology, 9*, 41-53.

Crook, T. H., Youngjohn, J. R., Larrabee, G. J., & Salama, M. (1992). Aging and everyday memory: A cross-cultural study. *Neuropsychology, 6*, 123-136.

Crook, T. H., Zappala, G., Cavarzeran, F., Measso, G., Pirozzolo, F., & Massari, D. (1993). Recalling names after introduction: Changes across the adult life span in two cultures. *Developmental Neuropsychology, 9*, 103-113.

Cunningham, W. R. (1986). Psychometric perspectives: Validity and reliability. In L. W. Poon, T. Crook, K. L. Davis, C. Eisdorfer, B. J. Gurland, A. W. Kaszniak, & L. W. Thompson (Eds.), *Handbook for clinical assessment of older adults*, (pp. 27-31). Washington, DC: American Psychological Association.

Delis, D. C., Freeland, J., Kramer, J. H., & Kaplan, E. (1988). Integrating clinical assessment with cognitive neuroscience: Construct validation of a multivariate verbal learning test. *Journal of Consulting and Clinical Psychology, 56*, 123-130.

Delis, D. C., Kramer, J. H., Kaplan, E, & Ober, B. A. (1987). *California Verbal Learning Test. Research edition. Manual.* San Antonio: The Psychological Corporation Harcourt Brace Jovanovich, Inc.

Delis, D. C., McKee, R., Massman, P. J., Kramer, J. H., Kaplan, E., & Gettman, D. (1991). Alternate form of the California Verbal Learning Test: Development and reliability. *The Clinical Neuropsychologist, 5,* 154-162.

Feher, E. P., Mahurin, R. K., Inbody, S. B., Crook, T. H., & Pirozzolo, F. J. (1991). Anosognosia in Alzheimer's disease. *Neuropsychiatry, Neuropsychology, and Behavioral Neurology, 4,* 136-146.

Ferris, S. H., Crook, T., Clark, E., McCarthy, M., & Rae, D. (1980). Facial recognition memory deficits in normal aging and senile dementia. *Journal of Gerontology, 35,* 707-714.

Folstein, M. F., Folstein, S. F., & McHugh, P. R. (1975). Mini-mental state: A practical method for grading the cognitive state of patients for the clinician. *Journal of Psychiatry Research, 12,* 189-198.

Gilewski, M. J., & Zelinski, E. M. (1986). Questionnaire assessment of memory complaints. In L. W. Poon, T. Crook, K. L. Davis, C. Eisdorfer, B. J. Gurland, A. W. Kaszniak, & L. W. Thompson (Eds.) *Handbook for clinical memory assessment of older adults* (pp. 93-107). Washington, DC: American Psychological Association.

Gilewski, M. J., Zelinski, E. M., & Schaie, K. W. (1990). The memory functioning questionnaire for assessment of memory complaints in adulthood and old age. *Psychology and Aging, 5,* 482-490.

Gruneberg, M. M., Morris, P. E., & Sykes, R. N. (1978). *Practical aspects of memory.* London: Academic Press, Inc.

Heaton, R. K., & Pendleton, M. G. (1981). Use of neuropsychological tests to predict adult patients' everyday functioning. *Journal of Consulting and Clinical Psychology, 49,* 807-821.

Hermann, D. J. (1982). Know thy memory: The use of questionnaires to assess and study memory. *Psychological Bulletin, 92,* 434-452.

Kotler-Cope, S. (1990, April). *Memory impairment in older adults: The interrelationship between objective and subjective, clinical and everyday memory measures.* Paper presented at the annual meeting of the Southern Society for Philosophy and Psychology, Louisville, Kentucky.

Kramer, J. H., Levin, B. E., Brandt, J., & Delis, D. C. (1989). Differentiation of Alzheimer's, Huntington's, and Parkinson's disease patients on the basis of verbal learning characteristics. *Neuropsychology, 3,* 111-120.

Larrabee, G. J., & Crook, T. H. (1989a). Dimensions of everyday memory in age-associated memory impairment. *Psychological Assessment: A Journal of Consulting and Clinical Psychology, 1,* 92-97.

Larrabee, G. J., & Crook, T. H. (1989b) Performance subtypes of everyday memory function. *Developmental Neuropsychology, 5,* 267-283.

Larrabee, G. J., & Crook, T. H. (1991). Computerized memory testing in clinical trials. In E. Mohr, & P. Brouwers (Eds.), *Handbook of clinical trials. The neurobehavioral approach* (pp. 293-306). Amsterdam: Swets and Zeitlinger, B. V.

Larrabee, G. J., West, R. L., & Crook, T. H. (1991). The association of memory complaint with computer-simulated everyday memory performance. *Journal of Clinical and Experimental Neuropsychology, 13,* 466-478.

Leber, P. (1986). Establishing the efficacy of drugs with psychogeriatric indications. In T. Crook, R. T. Bartus, S. Ferris, & S. Gershon (Eds.), *Treatment development strategies for Alzheimer's disease,* (pp. 1-14). Madison, CT: Mark Powley Associates, Inc.

Levin H. S., Benton, A. L., & Grossman, R. G. (1982). *Neurobehavioral consequences of closed head injury.* New York: Oxford.

Loftus, E. F. (1991). The glitter of everyday memory...and the gold. *American Psychologist. 46,* 16-18.

McCarthy, M., Ferris, S. H., Clark, E., & Crook, T. (1981). Acquisition and retention of categorized material in normal aging and senile dementia. *Experimental Aging Research, 7,* 127-135.

McEntee, W. J., Crook, T. H., Jenkyn, L. R., Petrie, W., Larrabee, G. J., & Coffey, D. J. (1991). Treatment of Age-associated memory impairment with guanfacine. *Psychopharmacology Bulletin, 27,* 41-46.

Neisser, U. (1982a). *Memory observed: Remembering in natural contexts.* San Francisco: W. H. Freeman.

Neisser, U. (1982b). Memory: What are the important questions? In U. Neisser (Ed.*), Memory observed. Remembering in natural contexts* (pp. 3-19). San Francisco: Wilt Freeman and Co.

Prigatano, G. P., & Schacter, D. L. (Eds.) (1991*). Awareness of deficit after brain injury. Clinical and theoretical issues.* New York: Oxford University Press, Inc.

Randt, C. T., Brown, E. R., & Osborne, D. P. (1983). *Randt Memory Test.* Bayport, NY: Life Science Associates.

Reisberg, B., Ferris, S. H., Borenstein, J., Sinaiko, E., de Leon, M. J., & Buttinger, C. (1986). Assessment of presenting symptoms. In L. W. Poon, T. Crook, K. L. Davis, C. Eisdorfer, B. J. Gurland, A. W. Kaszniak, & L. W. Thompson (Eds.) *Handbook clinical memory assessment of older adults.* (pp. 108-128). Washington, DC: American Psychological Association.

Schear, J. M., & Craft, R. B. (1989). Examination of the concurrent validity of the California Verbal Learning Test. *The Clinical Neuropsychologist, 3,* 162-168.

van der Cammen, T. J. M., Wright, G., Fraser, R. M., Simpson, J. M., Rai, G. S., & Exton-Smith, A. N. (1987, August). Review of the work of the memory clinic after two years. Paper presented at the Third Congress of the International Psychogeriatric Association, Chicago, Illinois.

Warrington, E. K. (1984). *Recognition Memory Test.* Windsor, Berkshire, England: NFER-Nelson Publishing Company.

Wechsler, D. A. (1945). A standardized memory scale for clinical use. *Journal of Psychology, 19,* 87-95.

Wechsler, D. (1987) *Weschler Memory Scale-Revised. Manual.* San Antonio, TX: The Psychological Corporation, Harcourt Brace Jovanovich, Inc.

West, R. L. (1985). *Memory fitness over 40.* Gainesville, FL: Triad Publishing Co.

West, R. L. (1986a). Everyday memory and aging. *Developmental Neuropsychology, 2,* 323-344.

West, R. L. (1986b). *The everyday memory interview.* Unpublished manuscript.

West, R. L. (1988). Prospective memory and aging. In P. E. Morris, & R. N. Sykes (Eds.), *Practical aspects of memory: Current research and issues* (Vol. 2) (pp. 119-125). New York: John Wiley.

West, R. L. (1989). *The everyday memory interview (EMI): Discrimination of age and health groups.* Unpublished manuscript.

West, R. L., & Crook, T. H. (1990). Age differences in everyday memory: Laboratory analogues of telephone number recall. *Psychology and Aging, 5,* 520-529.

West, R. L., & Crook, T. H. (1992). Video training of imagery for mature adults. *Applied Cognitive Psychology, 6,* 307-320.

West, R. L., & Tomer, A. (1989). Everyday memory problems of healthy older adults: Characteristics of a successful intervention. In G. C. Gilmore, P. J. Whitehouse, & M. L. Wykle (Eds.), *Memory, aging and dementia. Theory, assessment, and treatment.* (pp. 75-98). New York: Springer.

West, R. L., & Walton, M. (1985, March). Practical memory functioning in the elderly. Paper presented at the National Forum on Research in Aging, Lincoln, Nebraska.

Williams, J. M. (1987). *Cognitive behavior rating scales. Manual. Research edition.* Odessa, FL: Psychological Assessment Resources, Inc.

Williams, J. M. (1988). Everyday cognition and the ecological validity of intellectual and neuropsychological tests. In J. M. Williams, & C. J. Long (Eds.), *Cognitive approaches to neuropsychology.* (pp. 123-141). New York: Plenum.

Williams, J. M. (1991). *Memory assessment scales.* Odessa, FL: Psychological Assessment Resources, Inc.

Williams, J. M., Little, M. M., Scates, S., & Blockman, N. (1987). Memory complaints and abilities among depressed older adults. *Journal of Consulting and Clinical Psychology, 55,* 595-598.

Wilson, B. A. (1991). Long-term prognosis of patients with severe memory disorders: *Neuropsychological Rehabilitation, 1,* 117-134.

Wilson, B. A., Cockburn, J., & Baddeley, A. D. (1985). *The Rivermead Behavioral Memory Test.* Titchfield: Thames Valley Test Company.

Wilson, B. A., Cockburn, J., Baddeley, A., and Hiorns, R. (1989). The development and validation of a test battery for detecting and monitoring everyday memory problems. *Journal of Clinical and Experimental Neuropsychology, 11,* 855-870.

Winterling, D., Crook, T., Salama, M., & Gobert, J. (1986). A self-rating scale for assessing memory loss. In A. Bes, J. Cahn, S. Hoyer, J. P. Marc-Vergnes, & H. M. Wisniewski (Eds.) *Senile dementias: Early detection* (pp. 482-486). London: John Libbey Eurotext.

Yesavage, J., Brink, T., Rose, T., Lum, O., Huang, O., Adey, V., & Leirer, V. (1983). Development and validation of a geriatric depression screening scale: A preliminary report. *Journal of Psychiatric Research, 17,* 37-49.

Youngjohn, J. R., Larrabee, G. J., & Crook, T. H. (1991). First-Last Names and the Grocery List Selective Reminding Tests: Two computerized measures of everyday verbal learning. *Archives of Clinical Neuropsychology, 6,* 287-300.

Youngjohn, J. R., Larrabee, G. J., & Crook, T. H. (1992a). Test-retest reliability of computerized, everyday memory measures and traditional memory tests. *The Clinical Neuropsychologist, 6,* 276-286.

Youngjohn, J. R., Larrabee, G. J., & Crook, T. H. (1992b). Discriminating age-associated memory impairment from Alzheimer's disease. *Psychological Assessment: A Journal of Consulting and Clinical Psychology, 4,* 54-59.

Zappala, G., Martini, E., Crook, T., & Amaducci, L. (1989). Ecological memory assessment in normal aging. A preliminary report on an Italian population. In F. J. Pirozzolo (Ed.). *Clinics in geriatric medicine. New developments in neuropsychological evaluation, 5,* 583-593. Philadelphia: W. B. Saunders Company, Harcourt Brace Jovanovich, Inc.

Zelinski, E. M., Gilewski, M. J., & Anthony-Bergstone, C. R. (1990). Memory functioning questionnaire: Concurrent validity with memory performance and self-reported memory failure. *Psychology and Aging, 5,* 388-399.

12

ASSESSMENT OF SUBTLE LANGUAGE DEFICITS IN NEUROPSYCHOLOGICAL BATTERIES:
Strategies and Implications

Bruce Crosson, Ph.D.

Aphasia, of course, is a deficit in language caused by acquired brain damage. Over the last century, the term *aphasia* has become identified with syndromes evolving out of the works of Broca (1861), Wernicke (1874), and others. In general, Broca's aphasia has been identified with nonfluent language output and more subtle deficits in language comprehension. Variants of Broca's aphasia have been described. Wernicke's aphasia results in fluent jargon and comprehension difficulties. Conduction aphasia is marked by disproportionate difficulty in repetition and phonemic errors while patients with transcortical aphasias have relatively preserved repetition in the face of nonfluent output or in the face of fluent paraphasic output and comprehension difficulties (Goodglass & Kaplan, 1983). There is some evidence to suggest that conduction aphasia results from interference with a phonological transcoding system while transcortical aphasias interfere with a semantic transcoding system (e.g., McCarthy & Warrington, 1984). Although aphasias are most often considered to result from the interruption of cortical systems, aphasia has been reported with thalamic and nonthalamic subcortical lesions (see Crosson [1992] for review).

In many settings, the diagnosis of the more obvious language syndromes is accomplished by speech pathologists, especially if there are treatment implications. A more common problem for neuropsychologists is the diagnosis of subtle language disturbance when aphasic syndromes are not immediately apparent. Such diagnosis usually takes place within the context of a broader neuropsychological battery, assessing the presence or absence of cognitive impairment on a number of dimensions. Two common circumstances in which such batteries are conducted are the examination of head-injured patients and the examination of patients for progressive dementias. In the former instance, neuropsychologists may be required to evaluate what subtle effects head injury may have had on language and the implications of any such effects. In the case of suspected dementia, the presence of language impairment can act as a marker for certain degenerative dementias such as Alzheimer's disease, though not all early Alzheimer's patients have language impairment (e.g., Faber-Langendoen et al., 1988).

The diagnosis of more obvious aphasia syndromes has been covered in a number of places; however, the diagnosis and implications of more subtle language deficits has received less attention. An accurate assessment for subtle language disturbances is extremely important because the neuropsychological evaluation may be the only source of information when the more obvious clinical syndromes are not present. The purpose of this chapter is to discuss screening for more subtle language deficits in the context of a broader neuropsychological battery. The first topic discusses how to choose instruments for evaluating subtle language deficits. Then, a few instruments are briefly covered. Subsequently, the functional implications of subtle language deficits are addressed, and case examples are presented. Finally, a few conclusions are drawn.

CHOOSING AN INSTRUMENT

There are two common errors in choosing language measures for neuropsychological batteries when the diagnosis of subtle language deficits is an issue. The first is to use instruments which have been developed primarily for the purpose of discriminating amongst aphasia syndromes. The Boston Diagnostic Aphasia Examination (BDAE) (Goodglass & Kaplan, 1983) is probably the premier instrument for this purpose; it has been extensively normed on a large sample of patients with aphasia. The Western Aphasia Battery (WAB) (Kertesz, 1980) bears more than a superficial similarity to the BDAE and has become popular because classification of aphasias can be accomplished in a briefer time than with the BDAE. The Porch Index of Communicative Ability (PICA) (Porch, 1971) is often used as an index of aphasia severity in different language modalities and can be used to measure recovery.

All these instruments have common features. They are relatively lengthy and constitute batteries in themselves. Since they have been developed for use in populations with obvious aphasia, item difficulty is such that the tests discriminate language functions in the extreme range of impairment well. However, these instruments do not discriminate subtle impairment well because the relatively low item difficulty does not allow for discrimination between the normal range of language functions and subtle impairments. Further, the most extensive norms on these instruments are for an aphasic population and would not allow for this discrimination even if the item difficulty was adequate to do so.

A second error in the choice of instruments to determine subtle language deficits is to use instruments that do not have an adequate number of items to insure reliability or that are not adequately conceptualized. The Reitan-Indiana Aphasia Screening Test (Reitan, 1984) falls into this category. On this instrument, there are just a few items for naming and even less items for repetition, comprehension, and oral reading. Thus, none of these functions can be measured with any degree of reliability, and no scores can be obtained to compare different language functions (e.g., naming, repetition, auditory-verbal comprehension). The repetition items are conceptualized as measuring dysarthria, which can be assessed by listening carefully to any speech output. Oral reading is not separated from reading comprehension.

Several criteria can be applied to the selection of appropriate instruments to measure subtle language functions in the context of a neuropsychological battery[*]. These criteria are listed in Table 1. First, an adequate set of norms from a neurologically intact sample should be available. Under most circumstances, a mean and a standard deviation do not constitute an adequate set of norms. Because distributions can be skewed, it is better if a specific raw score is tied to a specific percentile in the normative sample or to a standard score. Further, since language functions can be affected by education and sometimes by age, adequate norms will take education and age into account. As a second criterion, item difficulty should be adequate to provide some level of discrimination within a normal population. Only when both of these criteria have been met can a set of norms be used to find subtle language deficits. Adequate item difficulty is necessary to address the issue of premorbidly high functioning individuals who demonstrate decreases in functioning which would otherwise be within the lower end of the normal range. If 80% or 90% of the normative sample answers all items correctly, the instrument is not likely to be useful in making discriminations for individuals with high premorbid functioning.

---

[*] The term "neuropsychological battery," as it is used here, should not be equated to a fixed battery in which the same series of tests is given to all patients regardless of the referral question. This term simply refers to a group of tests given to any individual patient and might vary widely depending upon the referral question, the patient's presenting complaints, and other factors.

TABLE 1

CRITERIA FOR SELECTING INSTRUMENTS TO MEASURE SUBTLE LANGUAGE DEFICITS

1. Adequate norms from a neurologically intact sample.
2. Adequate item difficulty to discriminate
   levels of normal functioning.
3. Assessment of multiple language functions: at least
   naming, repetition, auditory-verbal comprehension,
   and probably reading comprehension and written output as well.
4. Comparability of norms between tests to the degree possible.
5. Brevity enough to insure adequate assessment of other
   functions.

A third criterion is that the instruments used should cover a variety of language functions. In this context, some clues can be taken from routine assessments of more severe aphasias. At a minimum, naming, repetition, and auditory-verbal comprehension should be assessed. Naming is the most commonly impaired language function after brain injury (Goodglass & Kaplan, 1983). Thus, naming is likely to reveal dysfunction in cases of subtle language deficits and should be included in any assessment of language functions. Repetition is relatively intact in some cases of dominant subcortical lesion (Crosson, in press), but frequently impaired in cases of dominant perisylvian lesion, usually retrorolandic (e.g., Valdois, Joanette, Nespoulous, & Poncet, 1988). Thus, in the experience of the author, repetition tasks can be important in defining patterns of language deficits. One also should keep in mind that difficulty with repetition can also be an indicator of impaired verbal memory span (Lezak, 1995), especially if digit span is also significantly below expectations. Since every-day functioning demands understanding of others' communications, it is important to assess auditory-verbal comprehension.

In most instances, it is also desirable to assess written output and reading comprehension skills. Word fluency (e.g., giving as many words as possible beginning with a specific letter in a minute) is most frequently considered a test of frontal lobe functions, but it can be a sensitive indicator in some patients who complain of word finding difficulties but whose tested naming is otherwise unimpaired. Finally, the assessment of conversational or narrative language is also desirable.

A fourth criterion for selecting instruments to evaluate subtle language deficits is comparability of normative data between tests. It is rare in neuropsychology to have tests carefully normed on a national sample, carefully stratified across important variables. More frequently, normative data is collected in a particular locale, and normative subjects may have some peculiarities specific to the locale. Thus, one cannot assume that persons in Boston will respond the same way to test items as persons in Iowa. Since language tests meeting the above cirteria generally do not have norms from extensive national samples, it is best if individual language tests used in a neuropsychological battery have been normed on the same, or at least similar, samples. Such norms insure the best comparability between tests when attempting to establish patterns of language deficit.

A fifth criterion is the brevity to fit into a neuropsychological battery which is assessing numerous other cognitive functions at the same time. To yield maximal diagnostic efficacy, a battery has to address other functions important to the diagnosis. If too much time is spent assessing language functions, it may be at the expense of adequate assessment of other functions.

ASSESSMENT INSTRUMENTS TO EVALUATE SUBTLE LANGUAGE DEFICITS

Unfortunately, no set of instruments exists which meets all the above criteria. For this reason, one must select from available tests to best approximate the criteria. As noted above, standard aphasia batteries, such as the BDAE, the WAB, and the PICA, do not have adequate norms or item difficulty to be generally useful in evaluating subtle language deficits. However, selective subtests from the Multilingual Aphasia Examination (MAE) (Benton & Hamsher, 1989) or the Neurosensory Center Comprehensive Examination for Aphasia (NCCEA) (Spreen & Benton, 1977) do meet the criteria specified above. Both instruments have norms developed on neurologically intact samples, and item difficulty approaches adequate for measuring subtle deficits. Both instruments use age and education adjustments where appropriate and assess a variety of language functions. Norms within instruments appear to be comparable across subtests.

The author has favored the use of selective subtests the MAE because they are a little more consistent in item difficulty across subtests. The Visual Naming subtest is used to assess naming. It consists of several line drawings, and patients are required to name the drawings or parts of the pictured objects. There are 30 items; patients can score from 0 to 60 points. The maximum discrimination is the 87th percentile. The Sentence Repetition subtest is used for repetition. It consists of 14 sentences which increase in length to a maximum of 18 words. One point is given each time the sentence is correctly repeated, but since correction factors for age and education can be added to the raw score, the maximum corrected raw score used to obtain percentiles is 15. The maximum discrimination is at the 95th percentile. There are two parallel versions, but the author prefers to use Form A because its items tend to be more concrete and imageable than those of Form B. The Token Test (a version prepared for the MAE) assesses auditory-verbal comprehension. It is a 22-item test requiring patients to manipulate plastic chips (tokens) of various sizes, shapes, and colors in accordance with commands presented by the examiner. There are two parallel versions of the Token Test. The maximum raw score is 44, and the maximum discrimination is at the 82nd percentile. When necessary, Controlled Oral Word Association can be used to measure word fluency. On three separate trials, patients must generate as many words as possible that begin with a specific letter of the alphabet in a minute. There are two parallel forms of Controlled Oral Word Association. Maximum discrimination is at the 96th percentile of the normative population. Where appropriate, correction factors for age and education are applied to the raw scores of the MAE subtests.

Unfortunately, the reading subtest of the MAE does not provide as great a discrimination as the above subtests. Further, it only tests reading of words and phrases. The author elected to use Reading Comprehension of Sentences and Paragraphs from the BDAE to screen reading comprehension. Item difficulty on this particular BDAE subtest is more acceptable than that of the comparable MAE subtest, and a suggested cut off for impairment based upon the responses of a neurologically intact sample are given. However, its weakness is that it does not give specific percentiles for the various levels of performance. Screening of written output is accomplished by having the patient write a description of everything happening in the Cookie Theft picture of the BDAE. The writing can then be evaluated for paragraphic errors, other misspellings, agrammatic errors, etc. Reading and writing can be further assessed as necessary.

Because of noncomparable norms, the author sometimes shies away from use of individually developed language tests such as the Boston Naming Test (Kaplan, Goodglass, Weintraub, & Segal, 1983) or the Revised Token Test (McNeil & Prescott, 1978). Both tests are excellent measures but scores are not strictly comparable because norms have been developed on separate samples. In addition, Boston Naming Test norms are given as means and standard deviations. As noted above, normality of distribution cannot be assumed unless specifically demonstrated. Another disadvantage of the Revised Token Test is that its length can prohibit inclusion in a longer neuropsychological battery. Such disadvantages must be weighed against the assets of these instruments (e.g., adequate item difficulty) which increases the ability of these instruments to detect subtle deficits in some instances.

Normally, conversational language can be assessed during interview. The narrative language ratings from the BDAE can be used as guidelines for assessing conversational language for subtle deficits, but the examiner must keep in mind that a patient's deficits might be more subtle than in a patient with an obvious aphasia. The examiner listens for word finding difficulties, phonemic paraphasias (substitutions of one phoneme for another) or semantic paraphasias (substitutions of one word for another), circumlocutions, use of a variety of grammatical forms, awkwardness or difficulty in initiating spoken language, and any alteration in intonation patterns. Even when these are normal, patients may have difficulty switching topics of conversation when appropriate, becoming tangential, or terminating a communication at the appropriate point. These problems are common with frontal lobe injury. Some formal training in the assessment of patients with aphasia is necessary before attempting to make such judgments regarding conversational language.

Some tests have been developed to measure more complex language usage. For example, the Test of Language Competence (TLC) (Wiig & Secord, 1989) purports to measure metalinguistic abilities. The four subtests involve producing multiple meanings for ambigous sentences, recognizing inferences on the basis of incomplete information, creating sentences given three words and a context, and recognizing the meaning of figurative language. Such tests can be useful in identifying subtle problems in language usage. Unfortunately, the TLC norms only go up to older adolescence (18 years, 11 months) which limits its application to adult populations.

IMPLICATIONS OF SUBTLE LANGUAGE DEFICITS

The implications of subtle language deficits can be approached from two standpoints. First, the effects of language deficits on other functions which are dependent upon basic language functions can be examined. For example, subtle deficits in language functions might affect verbal memory. The ability to encode items into verbal memory is to some degree dependent upon a patient's ability to comprehend the items in the first place; the ability to retrieve items from verbal memory stores is to some degree dependent upon the ability to call up the name for the item. Similarly, basic language functions can affect measures of intellectual functioning. The second approach involves the effects of subtle language deficits on day-to-day functions (i.e. functional capacity). Since the ability to communicate is important to most persons on a daily basis, changes in language functions can affect functional capacity. The following paragraphs consider both approaches.

EFFECTS OF SUBTLE LANGUAGE DEFICITS ON OTHER FUNCTIONS

There is some evidence that subtle language deficits affect other related cognitive functions. The author and colleagues (Crosson, Cooper, Lincoln, Bauer, & Velozo, 1993) recently studied the relationship between four MAE subtests (Visual Naming, Sentence Repetition, Token Test, Controlled Oral Word Association) and verbal memory in 75 chronic blunt-head-injury patients. There were few patients with obvious aphasias in this population, but a larger number of patients with subtle language deficits were tested. Several verbal memory measures from the California Verbal Learning Test (CVLT) (Delis, Kramer, Kaplan, & Ober, 1987) were used in this analysis.

Results indicated several interesting relationships. First, the absolute number of items recalled during learning trials, immediately after an interference list, and after a 20-minute delay were all highly related to Visual Naming scores. This relationship existed for both free- and cued-recall trials. However, when recognition memory was tested after a 20-minute delay, language measures demonstrated a smaller correlation than for recall trials, and this smaller correlation was with Token Test scores as opposed to Visual Naming scores. This pattern of results indicates that the ability to retrieve information from verbal memory on recall trials is dependent upon a patient's ability to retrieve lexical items from long-term stores. In fact, when delayed recall scores are equated for the number of items recalled during learning trials, the relationship with Visual Naming becomes significantly smaller. The minor relationship between Token Test scores and correct recognitions on the CVLT recognition trial indicates the role that auditory-verbal comprehension plays in encoding verbal memories. Finally, intrusion errors during recall (learning trials or delayed recall trials) and the number of false recognitions on the recognition trial also showed a strong relationship to Visual Naming scores. One might conjecture that a retrieval difficulty secondary to a naming deficit results in retrieving non-list items during recall trials, but the relationship between false recognitions and Visual Naming scores is more difficult to explain.

The relationship between these MAE subtests and measures of intellectual functions was also explored (Lincoln, Crosson, Bauer, Cooper, & Velozo, 1994). Subtests of the Wechsler Adult Intelligence Scale-Revised (WAIS-R) (Wechsler, 1981) constituted the intellectual measures. With the exception of Arithmetic and Digit Span, Verbal subtests showed the strongest relationship with Visual

Naming. Arithmetic and Digit Span both demonstrated stronger relationships with Sentence Repetition than other MAE subtests. Controlled Oral Word Association scores also contributed significant variance to five of six Verbal subtests. The variance in WAIS-R Verbal subtests accounted for by language measures was substantial, with multiple R^2s ranging from .317 to .516. The strength of these relationships most likely reflects the dependence of verbal intellectual measures on more basic language skills.

WAIS-R Performance subtests showed smaller but significant relationships with MAE measures. The relationship between Visual Naming and Picture Completion reflects the naming component on this WAIS-R subtest. The other Performance subtests were correlated with Controlled Oral Word Association and Token Test scores. The relationship of Performance subtests with Controlled Oral Word Association may reflect the dependence of both on frontal lobe capacities.

Thus, in this head-injured sample, there is evidence of the relationship between language abilities, on the one hand, and verbal memory and verbal intellectual functions, on the other. It does not seem to be too much of a leap to deduce that verbal memory and intellectual capacities are to some degree dependent upon more basic language skills to support them. In other words, one implication of subtle language impairments is deficits in other abilities dependent upon the language system. To some degree, this interdependence is reflected in relationships between psychometric indicators such as those discussed above. However, it is more important from a practical viewpoint to consider the functional implications of subtle language impairments.

FUNCTIONAL IMPLICATIONS OF SUBTLE LANGUAGE IMPAIRMENTS

Many neuropsychologists who spend most of their time in diagnosis and assessment will not have the opportunity to experience the functional implications of patients' subtle language impairments on a first-hand basis. However, those who participate in rehabilitation planning and treatment may see directly how less obvious language impairments affect daily functioning. In some ways, the effects can be more devastating than more obvious language deficits if not recognized. Others in the environment will expect communication difficulties from patients with easily identifiable aphasic syndromes, but unless informed of subtle language deficits, others may miss the implications for communication.

Patients with subtle deficits in verbal expression may have difficulty conveying their thoughts and needs to others. They may be misunderstood by persons who do not take the time to understand their communications. Less obvious deficits in verbal expression are evident from impaired scores on naming or word fluency tasks, or from the evaluation of conversational output by a trained observer. Implications can be managed in a number of ways. First, the patient and persons interacting regularly with the patient can be educated about difficulties in expression and their cause. Second, others can be taught the ways therapists have found most effective in communicating with the patient. Third, patients can be taught strategies to facilitate word-finding or substituting equivalent words.

Subtle auditory-verbal comprehension deficits can cause patients not to understand others' verbal requests and communications. If the language deficit is not identified in such cases, patients can be mistaken as having problems with memory, motivation, problem solving, or other functions. There are effective ways for managing subtle comprehension problems. Often times, patients will understand a communication if they hear it a second time; therefore, such patients can be taught to request repetition from others. A slower pace of communication will facilitate understanding with many patients; thus, these patients can be taught to ask others to slow the pace of their communications, or therapists can teach other persons regularly interacting with the patients to slow their communication. The degree of grammatical complexity of communications may also affect the ability to comprehend. Minimizing potential distractors may also be beneficial, as is supplementing verbal communications with actual demonstrations of requests or other visual supplementation when appropriate.

In dealing with functional implications, one should understand that standardized test scores are only a point of departure. Deficits are most easily addressed by clinicians when they have access to extensive observations in a rehabilitation environment. Careful observation of patients' communication within functional contexts will allow clinicians to further refine observations gleaned from standardized test scores. The patient can be involved in activities which will help to determine their functional communication capacity. A number of techniques to improve functional communication can be tried so that the most effective methods for a particular patient can be found. This type of extended functional evaluation and treatment of subtle language deficits is best carried out in the context of an interdisciplinary team where a professional with extensive training in communication, such as a Speech/Language Pathologist, can participate. The role of assessment in this process is to identify accurately the nature and degree of subtle language deficits so that further functional assessment and treatment can be accomplished.

The issue of functional evaluation and intervention is somewhat more complicated when neuropsychological findings are not being used directly for rehabilitation purposes. In such instances, test results can be used as a springboard for discussing the patient's communication patterns in greater depth with relatives or significant others. Frequently in such instances, relatives or significant others can be educated regarding language problems and how to handle them.

CASE EXAMPLES

The assessment of subtle language deficits is illustrated in the following two case examples. In particular, the relationship between this type of language dysfunction and functional communication capacity will be illustrated. In the first case, language deficit was obvious only after formal testing, yet its impairment had an impact on the patient's functioning. In the second case, a mild anomic aphasia was evident when his verbal output was carefully analyzed, but his tested deficit was much worse than that level of output normally would indicate. Both cases demonstrate some of the reasons for assessing subtle language problems, as well as some of the problems in doing so.

Case 1 was a 24-year-old man enrolled in an intensive rehabilitation program. He experienced a head injury with a depressed skull fracture in a fall during an industrial accident. He had obtained 14 years of education, and he was first tested five and one-half months after his accident. His period of coma was determined to be 16 days, but his post-traumatic amnesia lasted approximately 75 days. When the patient developed a right hemiplegia from herniation of the left cerebral peduncle against the tentorium cerebelli, a partial right temporal lobectomy was performed to relieve pressure. A tracheostomy had also been performed acutely. Acute CT scans were not available, but reports indicated contusion and edema of the right temporal lobe, as well as edema in the left temporal, parietal, and occipital lobes. At the time of evaluation, the patient was taking seizure medication. Later during his rehabilitation, he demonstrated seizures which were preceded by sensory changes in the right arm and during which he became aphasic.

Partial results of the initial evaluation are presented in Table 2. Although language deficit could not be detected by carefully listening to conversational language, MAE subtests demonstrated significant impairment in naming, repetition, auditory-verbal comprehension, and word fluency. Comprehension may have been somewhat less impaired than other language functions. Written language functions were also impaired. The effects of these deficits on cognition can be seen in the uniformly decreased performance on the WAIS-R, and in the impaired performance on the CVLT. Problem solving demonstrated some impairment as well.

TABLE 2
CASE 1: SELECTED TEST RESULTS

MAE Subtests	WAIS-R
Visual Naming - 0 %ile	Information - 5
COWA - 1st %ile	Digit Span - 5
Sentence Repetition - 0 %ile	Vocabulary - 7
Token Test - 5th %ile	Arithmetic - 4
	Comprehen. - 6

BDAE Subtests	Similarities- 5
Reading Sentences and	Picture Com.- 9
Paragraphs - 5/10 (impaired)	Picture Arr.- 11
Narrative Writing - 2.5/5	Block Design- 7
(impaired)	Obj. Assem. - 7
	Digit Symbol- 4

CVLT	
Trial 1 - 3/16	VIQ - 75
Trial 2 - 5/16	PIQ - 81
Trial 3 - 7/16	
Trial 4 - 7/16	
Trial 5 - 6/16	Wisconsin Card Sort
Short Delay	
Free Recall - 6/16	Categories - 3
Cued Recall - 5/16	Persev. Errors - 39
Long Delay	
Free Recall - 6/16	
Cued Recall - 5/16	
Recognition	
Correct Recognitions - 15	
False Positives - 3	

Through observation and interaction with the patient during rehabilitation, it was noted that his subtle language deficits affected his ability to communicate with others as well as his ability to understand others. Some attempts were made to educate the patient and his family about these deficits. Therapists worked with him on word-finding strategies, and he was receptive to others' attempts to assist him in conveying an idea. Regarding comprehension, it was found that repetition increased his understanding, and he was encouraged to ask others to repeat themselves.

It is of some interest that the patient showed excellent awareness of his deficits. For example, he was not only able to learn about a right visual neglect, but he was also able to develop compensations for it. This phenomenon would not have been predicted from his tested language, verbal memory, verbal intellectual, or problem-solving skills, but it was a definite asset in his rehabilitation. Although this case example indicates the importance of formal evaluation for subtle language deficits, it also indicates that observation of functional communication skills is needed to best understand this patient's capacities.

Case 2 was a 46-year-old man who was injured when an automobile struck his bicycle. He had 20 years of education and taught college level courses. He was unconscious for only a few minutes; his acute language disturbance prevented accurate assessment of post-traumatic amnesia. The chronic T2 weighted magnetic resonance scan (see Fig. 1) demonstrated rather severe damage primarily to the left temporal lobe as follows: There was cerebral spinal fluid collection in the anterior left temporal lobe secondary to encephalomalacia. The left temporal horn of the lateral ventricle was markedly enlarged, secondary to volume loss in the left temporal lobe. Areas of reduced signal intensity consistent with hemosiderin deposition (remaining from acute hemorrhagic lesions) were seen in the left temporal lobe and in the left frontal-parietal region. (The frontal lesion is not shown in Fig. 1.) The patient was offered language therapy for his deficit, but he and his family refused this treatment.

Neuropsychological evaluation was first done about seven weeks post-injury. The patient presented as mildly anomic with circumlocutions during interview. Some of the formal testing results are presented in Table 3. Although the patient's word-fluency, repetition, and auditory-verbal comprehension were basically intact, the patient had a severe deficit in naming, beyond what might have been predicted from his conversational language. The effects of the lesion also can be seen in verbal memory (CVLT) and verbal intellectual assessment.

Ordinarily, we would have discouraged this patient from trying to re-enter the college classroom, since teaching at that level is quite demanding and since naming and memory deficits as well as decreased Verbal IQ could negatively impact teaching. However, the patient was insistent that he return to teaching. He was able to tap his colleagues for help in preparation, and he had adequate time to do so. He had a reduced load upon re-entry. In anticipation of potential failure, close follow-up was conducted. However, in spite of continuing naming and verbal memory deficits, the patient made an adequate re-entry into college level teaching. This case example points out the limitations of formal testing in predicting ultimate outcome. In retrospect, the greater impairment of tested naming than conversational language and somewhat circumscribed deficits may have been predictors of successful re-entry in this case.

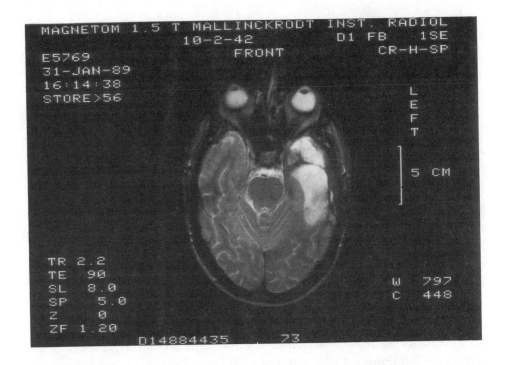

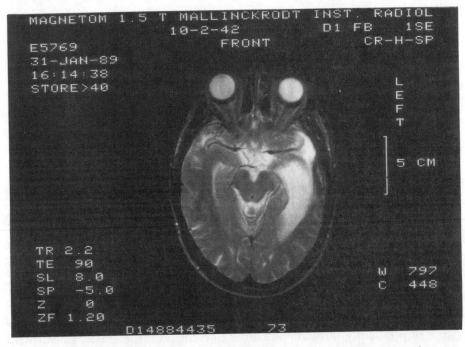

Figure 1. Magnetic resonance scan for Case 2. These two slices show severe damage to the left temporal lobe. See text for greater detail.

TABLE 3
CASE 2: SELECTED TEST RESULTS

MAE Subtests	WAIS-R
Visual Naming - 0 %ile	Information - 9
COWA - 75th %ile	Digit Span - 8
Sentence Repetition - 43rd %ile	Vocabulary - 12
Token Test - 82nd %ile	Arithmetic - 13
	Comprehen. - 11
CVLT	Similarities- 8
Trial 1 - 3	
Trial 2 - 7	Picture Com.- 11
Trial 3 - 4	Picture Arr.- 11
Trial 4 - 4	Block Design- 8
Trial 5 - 7	Obj. Assemb.- 8
Short Delay	Digit Symbol- 12
Free Recall - 2	
Cued Recall - 2	VIQ - 102
Long Delay	PIQ - 111
Free Recall - 1	
Cued Recall - 3	
Recognition	
Correct Recognitions - 12	
False Positives - 9	

CONCLUSIONS

Case 1 illustrated the importance of evaluating patients for subtle language deficits from a functional standpoint; however, both case examples have pointed out the limitations of formal testing in predicting functional outcome. There are at least two reasons why standardized tests might underestimate functional capacity. The first is that standardized instruments attempt to isolate particular functions, but in doing so, they prevent compensations which might be available to patients under more natural circumstances. The second reason is that standardized tests attempt to put all patients on an equal footing by using tasks with which they have limited familiarity. This facet of standardized tests may obscure individual strengths and knowledge which can be applied to their various life tasks.

In comparison, it is also possible to overestimate functional capacity from standardized test results. This problem often occurs because standardized testing attempts to optimize performance by providing a high degree of structure in an environment free from distraction. The actual environment in which most of us operate is less structured and filled with distractions which detract from performance.

Thus, even with attempts to develop more functional test instruments, accurate prediction of functional outcomes from limited test data will continue to be inexact at best. It is essential for neuropsychologists and other professionals to know the limitations of their test instruments in this regard. In an intensive rehabilitation environment, test scores act as a starting point for intervention and continuing evaluation of functional skills. Even in a nonrehabilitation environment, the sensitive clinician can use interviewing during feedback to help establish the relevance of test findings and assist patients and families in adjusting to deficits.

REFERENCES

Benton, A. L., & Hamsher, K. deS. (1989). *Multilingual aphasia examination* (2nd ed.). Iowa City, IA: AJA Associates, Inc.

Broca, P. (1861). Perte de la parole. Ramollissement chronique et destruction partielle du lobe anterieur gauche du cerveau. *Bulletin de la Societe d'anthropologie*, II, 235-238.

Crosson, B. (1992). *Subcortical functions in cognition: Language and memory*. New York: Guilford Press.

Crosson, B., Cooper, P. V., Lincoln, R. K., Bauer, R. M., & Velozo, C. A., (1993). Relationship between verbal memory and language after blunt head injury. *The Clinical Neuropsychologist, 7*, 250-267.

Delis, D. C., Kramer, J. H., Kaplan, E., & Ober, B. A. (1987). *California verbal learning test*. San Antonio, TX: The Psychological Corporation.

Faber-Langendoen, K., Morris, J. C., Knesevich, J. W., LaBarge, E., Miller, J. P., & Berg, L. (1988). Aphasia in senile dementia of the Alzheimer type. *Annals of Neurology, 23*, 365-370.

Goodglass, H., & Kaplan, E. (1983). *The assessment of aphasia and related disorders* (2nd ed.). Philadelphia: Lea & Febiger.

Kaplan, E., Goodglass, H., Weintraub, S., & Segal, O. (1983). *Boston naming test*. Philadelphia: Lea & Febiger.

Kertesz, A. (1980). *Western Aphasia Battery*. London, ON: The University of Western Ontario.

Lezak, M. D. (1983). *Neuropsychological assessment* (3rd. ed.). New York: Oxford University Press.

Lincoln, R. K., Crosson, B., Bauer, R. M., Cooper, P. V., & Velozo, C. A. (1994). Relationship between WAIS-R subtests and language measures after blunt head injury. *The Clinical Neuropsychologist, 8*, 140-152.

McCarthy, R. & Warrington, E. K. (1984). A two-route model of speech production: Evidence from aphasia. *Brain, 107*, 463-486.

McNeil, M. R., & Prescott, T. E. (1978). Revised Token Test. Austin, TX: Pro-Ed.

Porch, B. E. (1971). *Porch index of communicative ability.* Palo Alto, CA: Consulting Psychologists Press.

Reitan, R. M. (1984). *Aphasia and sensory-perceptual deficits in adults.* Tuscon, AR: Reitan Neuropsychology Laboratories, Inc.

Spreen, O., & Benton, A. L. (1977). *Neurosensory Center Comprehensive Examination for Aphasia (NCCEA).* Victoria, BC: Neuropsychology Laboratory, Department of Psychology, University of Victoria.

Valdois, S., Joanette, Y., Nespoulous, J-L, & Poncet, M. (1988). Afferent motor aphasia and conduction aphasia. In H. A. Whitaker (Ed.), *Phonological Processes and Brain Mechanisms.* New York: Springer-Verlag.

Wechsler, D. (1981). *Wechsler Adult Intelligence Scale-Revised.* San Antonio, TX: The Psychological Corporation.

Wernicke, C. (1874). *Der Aphasische Symptomencomplex.* Breslau: Cohen & Weigert.

Wiig, E. H. & Secord, W. (1989). *Test of Language Competence-Expanded Edition.* San Antonio, TX: The Psychological Corporation.

13

PRACTICAL APPROACHES TO ECOLOGICAL VALIDITY OF NEUROPSYCHOLOGICAL MEASURES IN THE ELDERLY

Linas A. Bieliauskas, Ph.D., A.B.P.P.

INTRODUCTION

Neuropsychological test data provide measures of general cognitive abilities among the following: Orientation, Attention/Concentration, Memory, Language, Motor Coordination, and Intentional Use of Objects, Judgment and Reasoning, General Intellectual Ability, and Affective Functioning. Neuropsychological measures can categorize a patient's abilities in these broad areas of cognitive functioning and indicate how they compare with those of same-aged and similarly educated peers, whether abilities can be classified as "impaired" based on similar normative data, and whether the pattern of preserved and impaired abilities is consistent with particular traumatic, disease, or toxic/metabolic processes affecting the brain.

Among the elderly, neuropsychological measures are often concerned with a patient's presentation of cognitive strengths and weaknesses as they relate to diseases associated with aging. These include degenerative dementias, vascular dementias, medication side-effects, and changes in cognition associated with normal aging as areas of most common concern. However, while the pattern of cognitive change as measured by neuropsychological tests is of diagnostic and research interest, the practical implications of test scores have received less attention in the literature. This chapter takes a practically relevant look at performance on tests of cognitive functioning in the elderly and how it translates into everyday behavior. This topic is approached by bifurcating it into sections dealing with how tests in various cognitive domains best relate to behaviors of interest and how various more complex behaviors can be predicted by neuropsychological test performance. Obviously, not all available tests will be covered; rather, fairly commonly used tests are presented as examples of how various cognitive functions can be measured. Only very brief descriptions of those tests are given here, with the reader referred to either source documents for the various tests cited or to Lezak (1995) for a compendium and annotated description of these tests and more which might be of interest. The reader is also referred to earlier reviews of general relationships between neuropsychological tests and functional behavior (Heaton & Pendleton, 1981; Tupper & Cicerone, 1990).

ORIENTATION

MEASURES

Broadly speaking, orientation is simply the ability to locate oneself in time and space. The standard medical mental status examination generally assesses what is called "orientation to time, place, and person." Typically, the patient is asked to indicate the current date, month, year, day of the week, and possibly season (time), the name of the present city, county, state, building, and possibly floor of building (place), and their own age, birthdate, and name (person). Orientation is an important facet of examination as its impairment is a primary presenting symptom of delirium which is often seen in more acute (reversible) medical conditions, though it is also present in the later stages of degenerative dementias (Francis, 1992; Lipowski, 1989).

Necessarily, to the extent that disorientation reflects delirium-like states, it will affect performance on most other neuropsychological tests. Tests of orientation, generally encompassing specific questions as noted above are part of most general mental status screening exams, including the Mini-Mental State (MMSE) (Folstein, Folstein, & McHugh, 1975), the Neurobehavioral Cognitive Status Examination (NCSE) (Kiernan, Mueller, Langston, & Van Dyke, 1987), the Wechsler Memory Scale (Wechsler, 1945); and its revised version (Wechsler, 1987). A more extensive measure, The Temporal Orientation Test (Benton, Hamsher, Varney, & Spreen, 1983) can be utilized if a more reliable test score specific to orientation is desired.

PRACTICAL IMPLICATIONS

As mentioned above, measures of orientation will relate directly to an individual's ability to locate themselves in time and space in such a way as to meaningfully guide behavior in context. When patients do not know where they are or when they are there, behaviors can be generally disorganized, as in the case of delirium-like states, or inappropriate to the surroundings. Delirium can be described as "confusion with an overlay of excitement" (p. 1177, Walton, 1977). In this case, disorientation is manifest primarily as behavior in general disarray, with the patient seemingly unable to follow through to or even identify meaningful purposes for their actions. The author restates that delirium-like behaviors are suspicious for more acute medical etiologies such as drug side effects, acute illness, etc., with the elderly being "uniquely prone to delirium as a consequence of almost any physical illness or intoxication..." (p. 578, Lipowsky, 1989). Poorly oriented behavior which appears less overtly confused but is yet inappropriate to surroundings is more characteristic of moderate to late stages of degenerative dementia. From the author's experience, this ranges from a patient who is arguing with his reflection in the mirror to the case of an elderly woman with diagnosed Alzheimer's disease whose husband noticed her leaving their home with a packed suitcase because she was tired of visiting and wanted to go home (the couple had lived there for 15 years).

Unfortunately, to this author's knowledge, there is nothing which can practically be done to directly affect poor orientation. The identification and reversal of acute causes for disorientation, is, of course, most desirable. However, without an acute cause being found, there is little that can be done to modify inappropriate behaviors. Treatment approaches such as "Reality Orientation Therapy" (Folson, 1968) have not shown any evidence of efficacy (Goldstein & Ruthven, 1983). Some approaches to less overt disorientation (or mild confusion) are described in the section entitled *Abstract Reasoning and Analytical Thinking* later in this chapter. The major practical impact of disorientation is the need for the patient to be generally monitored in a way which assures safety and attention to basic needs.

ATTENTION/CONCENTRATION

MEASURES

When we describe "attention/concentration" abilities, to what we are referring? *Attention* can be defined as "the capacity for selective perception" and *concentration* as "an effortful, usually deliberate, and heightened state of attention in which irrelevant stimuli are selectively excluded from conscious awareness..." (p. 34, Lezak, 1983). In other words, when we *attend*, we perceive some aspect of our environment to the exclusion of other aspects, and we *concentrate* when we sustain that attention, usually on purpose, while actively ignoring other competing stimuli. Noting a mathematics book and finding a section on algebra demonstrates attention processes while solving an algebra problem which has been located demonstrates concentration processes.

The Digit Span and Arithmetic subtests of the Wechsler Adult Intelligence Scale - Revised (WAIS-R) (Wechsler, 1981) comprise a derived factor named "Freedom from Distractibility" (Parker, 1983) which can be calculated in relation to other WAIS-R factors (e.g., a verbal and a visuospatial factor). In addition, there are various subtests of larger instruments specifically designed for measuring attention/concentration abilities. An attention/concentration index is also calculated from the WMS-R, with normative scores provided through age 74. The Mental Control and Digits subtests of the old Wechsler Memory Scale provide similar information (Wechsler, 1945). The Digit Span, Arithmetic, and Digit Symbol subtests of the WAIS-R, in and of themselves, give an idea of how well an individual can repeat strings of digits, perform mathematical calculations, and engage in visuomotor tracking in comparison to aged norms. The WAIS-R provides percentile ranks for subtest performance up to the age of 74. Separate tests designed to measure relatively similar areas of attention/concentration include the Trails test (Reitan & Wolfson, 1985), another timed visuomotor tracking task with available norms through age 64 (Fromm-Auch & Yeudall, 1983), Serial Digit Learning (Benton, Hamsher, & Varney, 1983), a supraspan digits forward repetition/learning task with norms through age 64, and the Symbol Digit Modalities Test (Smith, 1968), a timed symbol-number matching task, similar to the Digit Symbol test from the WAIS-R, with norms provided through age 75.

Finally, it is often of interest to measure simple and complex reaction times (Wasserman & Kong, 1979) as at least a general indicator of speed of information processing and response. Some norms for older age groups (through 75 years of age) are available (Era, Jokela, & Heikkinen, 1986), and reaction time has been demonstrated to be a potent predictor of safe driving in younger head-injured subjects (Stokx & Gaillard, 1986).

PRACTICAL IMPLICATIONS

The ability to accurately attend to surrounding stimuli and to sustain that attention sufficiently to perform mental operations will affect all other areas of cognitive functioning. If one cannot listen and perceive, then obviously one will not remember, not carry out more complex instructions, and cannot adequately make judgments or reason through problems. Conditions affecting the elderly which can disproportionately affect attention/ concentration abilities include more acute etiologies, such as head trauma, toxic reaction (including side effects of medications), metabolic disturbances (such as can occur with acute illness), and cerebrovascular dementing conditions (such as small multiple infarcts). In a proportion of these cases, etiologies are reversible and disproportionate attention/concentration difficulties should always be viewed as suspicious in this regard. From a practical standpoint, however, patients with such difficulties need to have instructions concretely repeated to them and stimuli clearly exposed. It is the responsibility of the individual interacting with a patient with such difficulties to make sure that information is understood (i.e., received; if the comprehension of information is insured, it is possible, in a number of instances, for the patient to act on the information in an informed manner.

MEMORY

MEASURES

The ability to remember what has happened can be broken down into a number of practical components, most of which should be considered in assessing memory functions. These would include memory for verbal vs. memory for visuospatial stimuli, recall vs. recognition, and recent vs. remote memory. There are, of course, more sophisticated distinctions in the appreciation of memory processes (Squire, 1987), but those are generally of more interest to the researcher studying the components of memory processes in normal and abnormal aging. An extensive annotation of memory testing in the elderly can also be found in Poon (1986).

As a start, the Wechsler Memory Scale (WMS) (Wechsler, 1945) and Wechsler Memory Scale-Revised (WMS-R) (Wechsler, 1987) are probably the most popularly used memory tests in clinical practice. The WMS provides a global scored called the Memory Quotient (MQ) which is designed to be similar to a Wechsler scale Intelligence Quotient (IQ); that is, the score is supposed to represent an average performance score for age of 100 with a standard deviation of 15, just as for an IQ derived from the Wechsler Adult Intelligence Scale (Wechsler, 1955). For a number of years, it was common practice to equate the two quotients, MQ and IQ and thus assess for relative slippage of memory functions versus more general intellectual abilities. However, there are criticisms raised about such interpretations and it appears that such comparisons are increasingly questionable when one compares the MQ and IQ from the

Wechsler Adult Intelligence Scale-Revised (Larrabee, 1987). Keep in mind, however, that the MQ is not a pure measure of memory functions; in addition to verbal and figural short-term recall, this composite score includes measures of orientation and attention/concentration.

The WMS-R provides IQ-like indices for various cleaner memory functions, again with a standard score reference of an average performance being 100 with a standard deviation of 15. In addition to a General Memory index, which is subject to the same general caveats as the MQ mentioned above, there are age-normed indices for Verbal Memory, Visual Memory, and Delayed Recall.

For verbal memory, there are also various measures of learning word lists which are commonly employed. These include the Rey Auditory Verbal Learning Test (Rey, 1964), the Selective Reminding Test (Buschke, 1973), the California Verbal Learning Test (Delis, Kramer, Kaplan, & Ober, 1986), and the Hopkins Verbal Learning Test (Brandt, 1991). All give measures of ability to recall words after repeated presentations with the Hopkins Verbal Learning Test being developed specifically for elderly populations and providing measures of cued recall and recognition in addition to simple recall. The Hopkins also has the advantage of having six parallel forms available for situations where repeated testing over time is necessary. Of course, the MMSE and the NCSE also have abbreviated screening measures of verbal memory. An easily administered test of simple recognition memory for words, the Recognition Memory Test (Warrington, 1984) can be used with more difficult-to-test patients and this test also provides a parallel test of simple recognition memory for faces for testing nonverbal memory as well.

Finally, a commonly used individual test of nonverbal memory should be mentioned. The Rey-Osterrieth Complex Figure (Rey, 1941; Osterrieth, 1944) is a measure of ability to recall and reconstruct a complex visual figure. Norms for the use of this test with elderly patients have been published by Boone, Lesser, Hill-Gutierrez, Berman, and D'Elia (1993).

PRACTICAL IMPLICATIONS

The implications of an inability to recall what has recently taken place ranges in implication from a simple loss of experiences (e.g., forgetting a recent visit, trip) to the inability to maintain enough constancy of ongoing events to keep an intelligible conversation. The practicality of memory for experiences also includes a range from inconvenience and embarrassment (e.g., forgetting experiences with friends or family) to major difficulty with carrying out daily living activities. The employment of tests of memory such as those mentioned above provide an estimate of the degree and, hopefully, type of memory deficit.

In terms of practical breakdown of memory components, decreased memory for verbal materials will affect primarily conversational and read materials while decreased memory for visuospatial stimuli will affect abilities to locate where objects have been placed, to recall pictorial events (e.g., motion pictures, photographs), and to navigate in space. A particularly important distinction between memory components is that of recall vs. recognition. Recall is the ability to freely remember past stimuli or events. Many conditions, such as delirium-related illness, will particularly affect recall. Under those conditions, elderly patients can frequently remember prior events if they are cued, (i.e., given reminders (cued recall). And, with more acute conditions, elderly patients can perform even better if given a choice of previously occurring or non-occurring stimuli or events (recognition). Cued recall and recognition are important indicators that the ability to register memories is still intact even if the ability to access them may be impaired. From a practical standpoint, preserved recognition memory indicates that an individual is capable of operating on the basis of past information if they are steadily reminded. This is important in terms of informed decision making and management of personal affairs if effective support is available. In primary degenerative dementing conditions, the actual ability to register memories is deficient and measurement of recognition memory reflects as much impairment as does measurement of recall.

Finally, the distinction between recent and remote memory has utilitarian implications for the ability to place current events in a historical context. In general, memories for recent events appear to be among the earliest indicators for dementing conditions in the elderly and these are the most sensitively measured by the memory tests mentioned above. Frequently, elderly patients with dementia appear to have difficulty with recent memories while memories from the distant past appear to be well-preserved. However, this is more a misconception on the part of relatives than an actual fact. Wilson, Kaszniak and Fox (1981) demonstrated that patients with Alzheimer's disease had similar memory deficits for recent and remote events. From this author's viewpoint, what relatives likely see in their relatives with dementia is some relatively greater ability to access long-term, probably frequently repeated memory segments from the past vs. ability to access more recent, probably single events. However, if the general quantity and quality of these memories from long ago is objectively evaluated, the impairments in recent and remote memory will be found to be similar. Deficits in remote memory for extremely familiar materials, such as one's home address or phone number, generally do not occur until a dementing condition is fairly advanced and can cause particular problems if an individual loses their way from home.

LANGUAGE

MEASURES

In very simplistic terms, the assessment of language in elderly patients concerns itself primarily with expressive ability, the ability to say what one wants to say, and receptive ability, the ability to comprehend what is said. While there are certainly many subtle distinctions in language which can be measured when classifying aphasia (loss of specific functions of speech), this section concentrates more on measurement of practical communication difficulties. The reader is referred to the classic book by Benson (1979) for a sophisticated exposition of neurological language disorders.

Expressive language in the elderly is generally measured in terms of ability to name objects, ability to spontaneously produce words, ability to correctly use grammar, and ability to write legibly. A commonly used general test of language abilities which quickly screens such expressive as well as receptive language functions is the Reitan-Indiana Aphasia Screening Test (Reitan, 1984). Other commonly used expressive language tests in the elderly include the Controlled Oral Word Association Test, a test of verbal fluency, and the Visual Naming test, a measure of ability to provide names for pictured objects (Benton & Hamsher, 1976). The latter test has particular utility for minority populations as appropriate norms have been developed (Roberts & Hamsher, 1984). An additional commonly used naming task for the elderly is the Boston Naming Test (Kaplan, Goodglass, & Weintraub, 1978); it's 60 items provide for a wide range of responses though the norms are based on rather small samples. Again, the MMSE and NCSE provide brief measures of naming as well and also short samples of sentence repetition.

Receptive language, or the ability to understand, is generally measured in two ways: understanding of words and understanding of the meaning of sentence constructions. Perhaps one of the best measures of the level of single word understanding (especially in patients who are minimally fluent) is the Peabody Picture Vocabulary Test (Dunn, 1965) or the Peabody Picture Vocabulary Test-Revised (Dunn & Dunn, 1981). Age equivalent vocabulary comprehension levels can be obtained, providing an estimate of the overall level of vocabulary which the patient has at his or her command. Understanding the meaning of sentence constructions is usually done by having the patient follow sequential commands. Of course, the patient may be able to understand what is said but not be able to carry out a command, thus confounding the interpretation of such a test. Nevertheless, from a functional point of view, tests of understanding do indicate the degree to which a patient can functionally respond to their language environment. Again, the MMSE and NCSE provide brief, multi-stage screens of language comprehension. One of the more popular tests in this domain is the Token Test (De Renzi & Vignolo, 1962) which has the patient carry out more and more complex commands with a variety of differently sized, shaped, and colored tokens; a shortened version, which may be especially appropriate for older subjects, has also been normed by education (De Renzi & Faglioni, 1978).

PRACTICAL IMPLICATIONS

The inability to communicate one's wishes or intentions may be a particularly frustrating aspect of dementing conditions. The types of neuropsychological tests described above give some idea as to what degree of communication the patient is capable. They may, for example, indicate the need to speak with a person in very concrete, low age-level terms. Alternatively, they may also indicate that though a patient has a fairly well-preserved vocabulary, putting words together in meaningful sentences may be difficult; in more complex cases of language deficit, a patient may appear to have fairly intact vocabulary comprehension but inconsistent follow commands, indicating a disruption in the ability to understand syntax. Finally, the expressive language tests often reveal the presence of paraphasias (misuse of spoken words) which is often symptomatic of local brain dysfunction, such as is seen with strokes, or a degenerative dementing process, including the occasional progressive aphasia syndrome (Mesulam, 1981; Green, Morris, Sandson, McKeel, & Miller, 1990).

In the case of patients who suffer fairly abrupt loss in language function, likely due to cerebrovascular complication, some recovery can be expected and it is prudent to engage the patient in language-stimulating exercises, especially shortly after the onset of deficit. Alternatively, in slowly progressive language deterioration or if further recovery of language functions is not reasonable to expect, methods for compensation need to be explored. Occasionally, patients may be able to express themselves by writing or better understand written than spoken communication. All too often, written communication is equally or even preferentially impaired in elderly persons, especially in degenerative dementing conditions (Faber-Langendoen et al., 1988). In general, compensatory strategies for the absent language abilities need to be created, some of which will necessarily be quite creative (e.g., Hooper & Dunkle, 1985). In any event, repeated neuropsychological language tests can provide an ongoing indication of the level of a person's ability to communicate.

MOTOR COORDINATION AND INTENTIONAL USE OF OBJECTS

MEASURES

Motor function can grossly be classified into the ability to execute certain muscle movements and the ability to coordinate groups of muscle movements to achieve an intended goal. With increasing age, motor coordination generally becomes less efficient though older persons can generally still accomplish the actions for which they set out. Some diseases of the elderly, especially Parkinson's disease, primarily affect motor control while often sparing higher level coordination of intention and action; peripheral physical diseases, such as arthritis in its various forms, may also significantly limit motility while not affecting higher cognitive functions. For such unfortunate individuals, this is an extremely frustrating situation wherein they know what they want to do but can't effectively control the muscle movements to do it. Therefore, psychological depression is not uncommon with motor dysfunction disease in the elderly (Bieliauskas & Glantz, 1989).

Measures of fine motor control include the Finger Oscillation Test (Reitan & Wolfson, 1985) which counts finger tapping speed for each hand, and the Grooved Pegboard Test (Matthews & Kløve, 1964) which measures the speed of manipulating small pegs in a series of exact-fitting holes. More general visuomotor coordination is measured by the Trail Making Test (Reitan & Wolfson, 1985) where simple numerical, and more complex alternating numerical and alphabetic symbols are connected in sequence as fast as a subject is able. Strength is often measured using a hand dynamometer (Grip Strength) (Reitan & Wolfson, 1985). Older age norms through age 69 (Bornstein, 1985) and 80 (Heaton, Grant, & Matthews, 1991) are available for these tests.

The loss of ability to perform intentional movements is generally termed "dyspraxia" and, in the elderly, can either be the result of more focalized parietal or frontal cortical dysfunction, such as is seen with cerebrovascular insult, or a late manifestation of degenerative dementia. "Praxis," or the ability to perform such intentional movements is often formally measured less formally by having the patient demonstrate intentional use of real or imagined objects. The Reitan-Indiana Apasia Screening Test (Reitan, 1984) contains several specific praxis-measuring items.

PRACTICAL IMPLICATIONS

Primary motor impairment (i.e., decreased fine or more gross motor coordination and decreased strength) results in significant impediment to a patient's ability to accomplish what they wish, even to the end of performing simple, everyday activities. A loss of independence frequently ensues with an understandable accompanying sense of frustration, if not more serious despair. Such afflicted elderly individuals generally require supportive assistance and emotionally need to make an adjustment to an altered lifestyle. While neuropsychological tests can help identify the degree of such motor impairment, they offer little in the way of remedy. It is at least some help to elderly motor-impaired patients to assist them in adapting to a "different," not necessarily "worse," manner of living. For example, rather than pursuing athletically related activities, individuals may learn to enjoy more aesthetic pursuits. Nevertheless, as mentioned above, psychological depression and a sense of despair are not uncommon for such persons and treatment for depression should always be considered as a possible adjunct to other supportive care.

The loss of ability to form intentioned movements is generally serious in the elderly and reflective of various advanced dementing processes. Neuropsychological tests of praxis can help explain why the elderly patient cannot perform what appear to be relatively simple tasks, assistance for which will generally need to be provided by someone else. For persons with advanced degenerative dementias, even basic tasks such as dressing or toileting may need to be assisted.

JUDGMENT AND REASONING

MEASURES

With judgment and reasoning we enter an area of measurement which has very frequent practical import— the assessment of competence to manage one's own affairs or to make informed decisions. Tests used to assess judgment generally present the patient with verbal or pictorial situations which require the patient to identify inappropriate contexts or to prescribe appropriate actions. In other words, to provide some simulation of the kinds of decisions we make in everyday life. Tests used to assess reasoning are more attuned to measure the ability to follow logical process in assessing evidence and reaching a decision.

The Comprehension subtest of the WAIS-R is one common measure of judgment and, like other WAIS-R subtests, provides an age-related percentile estimate of performance on this task. The NCSE also provides a brief screen of judgment abilities. The Picture Absurdities subtest of the Stanford-Binet Intelligence Scale, Form L-M (Terman & Merrill, 1973) and the Stanford-Binet Intelligence Scale (Thorndike, Hagen, & Sattler, 1986) are also two of the most straightforward measures of the ability to extract unusual or bizarre features of absurdly depicted social situations. A potential drawback of the Picture Absurdities test is that it is normed only through the ages of early adulthood, though if one assumes that judgment should not naturally decline with age, Picture Absurdities still provides a general estimate capability for judgment.

Reasoning is often measured with the Similarities subtest of the WAIS-R which gives the patient pairs of words and has them identify what is common to both (i.e., under which larger rubric could they be grouped). The NCSE has a similar screening subtest. More complex reasoning tasks include the Categories test (Reitan & Wolfson, 1985) and the Wisconsin Card Sorting Test (Heaton, 1981) which, using different formats, require the identification of rules for proper responding based on grouping of the features of presented stimuli. These tests also change the rules at different times with the patient being required to identify the change.

PRACTICAL IMPLICATIONS

The level of judgment measured by neuropsychological tests gives an idea where the patient fits in with their respective age peers in terms of being able to correctly identify proper responses in different situations. For example, an older person scoring at the 25th percentile on a test of judgment would be expected to have 75% of his or her peers make better decisions when faced with social situations. This provides an estimate on how easily the patient in question may be taken advantage of by others, how well the patient will react when faced with making a stressing decision, and how effective they will be in interpersonal situations.

Measures of reasoning more directly approaches one's ability to make informed decisions. Basically, if one is faced with various bits of information and a problem, how well can one put facts together in a logical way to arrive at an efficient solution? Individuals who score low on these tests have difficulty making decisions about things like sales of property, transfer of assets, and even the desirability of medical procedures.

However, tests of judgment and reasoning also reflect more subtle and complicated aspects of behavior in the elderly. Perhaps a terse but effective term for individuals whose reasoning is impaired is to describe them as wearing "blinders." Fundamentally, each one of us has a perceptual hierarchy about what we experience. For example, if a person is sitting in a doctor's office and does not see their car, they know that the car is in a garage which requires them to leave the office, cross the street, and take an elevator to a given floor. When a patient's reasoning is impaired (i.e., when a patient has on "blinders," he or she may reason if the car isn't there, it's gone. Measures of reasoning give an idea of how complexly an idea can be conceived. With "blinders," what you see is what you get.

Similarly, this notion of complexity of information processing frequently affects elderly who perseverate with various notions. For example, it is not uncommon for families of older patients to complain that the patient has called the police many times to report their house being broken into. The family is frustrated because no amount of argument will convince the patient otherwise. If we consider the concept of "blinders," we realize that the perceptual hierarchy which distinguishes silly from effective thinking for all of us is no longer working. We all have silly thoughts at one time or another, but we tell ourselves these thoughts are silly. Imagine what would happen if one operated on every thought that came up as if it were genuine. That is what happens with "blinders" and from clinical experience, it is suggested that the notion of being robbed must be in the back of many people's minds. If one understands that the patient is operating as if the thought is real, one can much more effectively tell the patient that the FBI has been called and that they are watching the house. In that way, the patient's pressing concern is addressed, even if it isn't logical.

Finally, the perceptual hierarchy which reasoning tasks measure also governs the dimension of time. It is not uncommon for a distressed patient's family to report that the patient was told a relative was coming to visit in a week and that the patient has asked about the visit every 10 minutes since. In dementing conditions it is clear that memory is not 100% lost and that emotionally charged stimuli may be remembered, even if in an inappropriate context. The call from a cherished relative might be one such stimulus— the anticipation of the relative visiting is recalled, but no other context to the visit. With "blinders," the call promising a visit is all that is perceived, not how far away the visit might be or where it might take place. If such a collapse of response hierarchy is taken into account when dealing with a patient with impaired reasoning, one would readily see that visits or other emotional activities should not be promised or announced in advance but rather told to the patient just as they are about to happen.

These examples give some insight as to the layers of thought that go into judgment and reasoning, layers which are often negated in dementing conditions. Advice to families of patients whose reasoning is shown to be deficient on testing generally includes a suggestion to "go with the flow," i.e., to deal directly with a patient's perception or thought rather than argue that it is wrong or inappropriate.

GENERAL INTELLECTUAL ABILITY

MEASURES

Perhaps the easiest way to conceptualize what we mean by intelligence is as "the tendency for each organism to process all kinds of information at a similar level of efficiency" (Lezak, 1976, p. 15). In other words, general intellectual ability refers to an overall level of capability to process information. Even though some question the validity of such general summary indices as an "Intelligence Quotient" (Lezak, 1988), there is, nevertheless, value in knowing the general capacity of an individual in terms of tailoring expectations of behavior and understanding for health care purposes (Bieliauskas, 1983). Such an index gives us some idea of how a patient perceives their symptoms, how he or she can process information about appropriate health care, and how effectively the patient can engage health-promoting behaviors.

The Wechsler Adult Intelligence Scale-Revised (WAIS-R), already mentioned for the utility of its various subtests for assessment of attention/concentration and judgment and reasoning, is one of the most frequently used measures for general intelligence. It consists of a variety of subtests designed to give an overall idea of the patient's level of cognitive processing. It is normed through age 75, and additional norms have been published for patients who are older (Ryan, Paolo, & Brungardt, 1990). A drawback to the WAIS-R is its fairly lengthy administration time, usually over an hour, leading to the possibility of fatigue effects or frustration on the part of elderly patients. For this reason, more brief summary measures which estimate general IQ are often given, most of them taking only 5 to 15 minutes. Brief intellectual screening tests include the Peabody Picture Vocabulary Test-Revised (Dunn & Dunn, 1981), normed through age 23 but with performance tending to hold through old age in our clinical experience, even in the face of functional cognitive deterioration; the New Adult Reading Test (Nelson, 1982), recently shown to closely match WAIS-R IQ scores in elderly patients (Ryan & Paolo, 1992); and The Shipley Institute of Living Scale (Zachary, 1986), a self-administered test which also approximates the age range of WAIS-R IQ scores if the patient is capable of taking the test by themselves. In addition, there is a method for attempting to estimate an individual's potential performance on intellectual tests based solely on demographic factors (Barona, Reynolds, & Chastain, 1984).

PRACTICAL IMPLICATIONS

The upper ranges of IQ measurement are generally not difficult to interpret; they indicate that the patient at least has (or has had) the potential to process information at fairly high levels. If IQ levels are measured as relatively high in comparison to other functional measures, such as in the areas of memory or attention, one can surmise that while the patient was highly functional at one time, their current cognitive difficulties represent a decline from their previous capabilities. Lower ranges of measured intellectual abilities, if outside of what would be expected based on the patient's educational and occupational background, likely represent general deterioration in the sense of the patient now no longer processing information efficiently. Depending on the test used, lowered intellectual measures can also indicate more specific dysfunction; for example, scores on the Peabody Picture Vocabulary Test Revised would be adversely affected by left hemisphere dysfunction which would affect language abilities. The clinician also needs to be careful when using an estimate of general intellectual ability since it might be precisely the limited functions to which the test is tied that are uniquely impaired and underestimates of general intellectual potential may result.

From a day-to-day standpoint, general intellectual abilities indicate a patient's ability to understand more complex communications, especially those related to health maintenance behaviors as stated above. These measures may also suggest how far an individual has deteriorated from their previous levels of complex behaviors. Such information, when transmitted to a patient's family, may serve to realistically realign their expectations of what the patient can and cannot do. Finally, measures of intellectual function may serve to indicate a potential for improvement through rehabilitation or retraining. It is a general rule-of-thumb that the more resources an individual has before an event which might cause deterioration, the more chance that individual has of recovering to a noticeable degree. This is of particular relevance for those patients whose cognitive impairments are due to acute insult (e.g., from a cerebrovascular incident), where some recovery is usually expected.

Measures of general intellectual function do have fairly strong relationships with other cognitive measures and certain ranges of performance on many cognitive measures are quite related to scores such as IQ. Thus, there are realistic expectations of how a patient should perform on other neuropsychological tests if their IQ level represents their potential prior to cognitive decline (Heaton et al., 1991; Warner, Ernst, Townes, Peel, & Preston, 1987). Intellectual measures are also of value in determining the validity of certain measures of psychopathology, such as the *MMPI* (Hathaway & McKinley, 1951), and its more recent version, the *MMPI-2* (Butcher, Dahlstrom, Graham, Tellegen, & Kaemmer, 1989) which generally require the patient to have an IQ of 80 to be considered valid.

AFFECTIVE FUNCTIONING

MEASURES

For the elderly with dementing conditions, estimates of prevalence rates for various forms of psychopathology range from 16 to 50% (Bieliauskas, 1993a); summarizing various studies, estimates of rates of depression can range from 20 to 35% in medically ill elderly, 50 to 68% in patients with CVA's, around 30% in patients with Alzheimer disease, and from 39 to 90% of patients with Parkinson's disease (Bieliauskas, 1993c). The identification of clinically significant psychopathological symptoms is of considerable interest within neuropsychological assessment of the elderly.

As with younger individuals, the *MMPI* (Hathaway & McKinley, 1951) and *MMPI-2* (Butcher et al., 1989) are among the most popular measures of a wide range of psychological and psychiatric symptoms. These tests are generally considered valid for most populations, including the elderly, though the MMPI has separate norms specific to populations aged 70 and over (Dahlstrom, Welsh, & Dahlstrom, 1972). A drawback to these tests, however, is their length—566 true/false items on a self-administered test. In our experience, many elderly patients do not have the patience or perseverance to complete such lengthy tests, particularly if they are required to do it on their own. However, many shorter indicators of psychopathological change in the elderly are readily available. There are a number of brief screening measures for depression including the Geriatric Depression Scale (Yesavage, Brink, Rose, & Adey, 1983), the Symptom Checklist for Major Depressive Disorders (Kashani, McKnew, & Cytryn, 1985) which follows DSM-III diagnostic criteria for depression, the MMPI Mini-Mult (Kincannon, 1968) depression scale which has been shown to be quite valid in elderly neurological populations (Bieliauskas, 1987), and the Beck Depression Inventory (Beck, Ward, Mendelson, Mock, & Erbaugh, 1961). For more general psychiatric disturbance, the Langner Psychiatric Status Index (Langner, 1962) is quite useful as a screening measure with particular relevance for acute psychiatric exacerbation such as the hallucinatory phenomena associated with treatment for Parkinson's disease (Glantz, Bieliauskas, & Paleologos, 1986).

PRACTICAL IMPLICATIONS

The identification of psychiatric conditions, depression, in particular, in elderly patients is crucial in terms of assuring appropriate care from a quality-of-life perspective. Depression, or depressive symptoms, are especially amenable to treatment and afford us one venue where we can reasonably expect to improve life situations in the elderly. When using tests of depression, however, care must be taken not to overdiagnose primary depression or to readily assume that a patient's cognitive decline is due primarily to its influence. In fact, many health-related changes in the elderly have depressive-like features associated with them and simple test scores, while perhaps reflecting misery or illness-associated vegetative changes, cannot be immediately interpreted as indicating the presence of clinically significant depression. Some guidelines for evaluating the nature of depressive symptoms, including test scores indicating depression, are provided in Bieliauskas (1993b).

The primary emphasis on use of tests of affective and other psychiatric symptoms in the elderly is to alert the clinician that appropriate psychiatric or psychological care is warranted, regardless of the actual etiology of the symptoms. Both the patient's quality-of-life and the patient's family will benefit by straightforward and effective treatment.

DIRECT ASSESSMENT OF DAILY LIVING ACTIVITIES

MEASURES

The advantage of using neuropsychological instruments in assessing cognitive functions, as described above, is that they provide an estimate of a patient's general capabilities in given areas and thus afford a fair degree of predictability to more general living situations (Dunn, Searight, Grisso, Margolis, & Gibbons, 1990; McSweeny, Grant, Heaton, Prigatano, & Adams, 1985). This permits maximizing the effectiveness of the planning of patient care (Alessi, 1991; Naugle & Chelune, 1990).

Nevertheless, there are direct measures of specific behavioral functions (e.g., using a telephone, addressing a letter, tuning a television). Such measures will provide direct indications of the patient's ability to perform a specific task though there will not be direct inference to superordinate cognitive abilities. In that sense, such instruments are more related to the role of occupational therapy than to psychology. Direct measures of patients' behaviors include the Adult Functional Adaptive Behavior Scale (Pierce, 1989; Spirrison & Pierce, 1992), Direct Assessment of Functional Status (Loewenstein et al, 1989), and the Blessed Dementia Rating Scale (Blessed, Tomlinson, & Roth, 1968) among others. A general review of measures relating to everyday life functioning can be found in McSweeney (1990).

PRACTICAL IMPLICATIONS

Direct measures of individual patient behaviors are of obvious value in that they give a straightforward indication of how well a person can perform that behavior. If there are questions such as "Can this patient live alone?" a measure of whether or not the person can make a telephone call will let one know whether or not the person can contact help if he or she is faced with an emergency. Similarly, a measure of making change will let one know whether or not the person can be expected to effectively do their grocery shopping. Obviously, the importance of the individual behaviors measured depends on the living situation of the person. Assessment of whether or not an individual can cook, for example, will be far more important to a person living alone than for a person in an assisted living situation. These kinds of measures offer some additional information when performing neuropsychological assessment with the elderly, though more extensive evaluation of daily living activities seem to fall more under the purview of occupational therapists.

GENERAL CONSIDERATIONS

Taking a practical approach to the ecological validity of neuropsychological tests is always in the patient's interest. All too frequently, neuropsychologists write reports which list test scores and perhaps address various functional domains, but fail to delineate the significance of test performance for the patient's daily life. When instructing students in report writing, the author always stresses that once they have formulated their conceptions of the case, they need to answer the question "So what?" It is of little help to a referring physician or to the patient, for example, if when a patient is referred for evaluation of their aphasia, the neuropsychological test report confirms that the patient has a problem with language.

Obviously, continued research in establishing the criterion validity of neuropsychological tests is desirable and encouraged. Nevertheless, a combination of common sense, an understanding of the domains of cognitive functions, and attention to studies which have examined the relationship between daily activities and test performance serve us well in patient care. If the goal of establishing the impact of cognitive dysfunction on quality of life remains with us throughout our assessments as a bottom line, neuropsychological tests will generally provide the consistent and predictive documentation necessary for optimal support of our elderly patients.

REFERENCES

Alessi, C. A. (1991). Managing the behavioral problems of dementia in the home. *Clinics in Geriatric Medicine, 7*, 787-801.

Barona, A., Reynolds, C. R., & Chastain, R. (1984). A demographically based index of premorbid intelligence for the WAIS-R. *Journal of Consulting and Clinical Psychology, 25*, 885-887.

Beck, A., Ward, C. H., Mendelson, M., Mock, J., & Erbaugh, J. K. (1961). An inventory for measuring depression. *Archives of General Psychiatry, 4*, 561-571.

Benson, D. G. (1979). Aphasia, alexia, and agraphia. New York: Churchill Livingston.

Benton, A. L., & Hamsher, K. DeS. (1976). *Multilingual Aphasia Examination.* Iowa City: University of Iowa.

Benton, A. L., Hamsher, K. deS., Varney, N. R., & Spreen, O. (1983). *Contributions to neuropsychological assessment.* New York: Oxford.

Bieliauskas, L. A. (1993a). Cognitive and psychopathological change in degenerative disease in the elderly. *Journal of Clinical and Experimental Neuropsychology, 15*, 421-438.

Bieliauskas, L. A. (1993b). Depressed or not depressed? That is the question. *Journal of Clinical and Experimental Neuropsychology, 15*, 119-134.

Bieliauskas, L. A. (1993c). Psychological depression in the elderly in medical/rehabilitation/ nursing care settings. *Neurorehabilitation, 3,* 42-50.

Bieliauskas, L. A. (1987). Use of the Mini-Mult D scale in patients with Parkinson's Disease. *Journal of Consulting and Clinical Psychology, 55*, 437-438

Bieliauskas, L. A. (1983). *The influence of individual differences in health and illness.* Boulder, CO: Westview Press..

Bieliauskas, L. A., & Glantz, R.H. (1989). Depression type in Parkinson disease. *Journal of Clinical and Experimental Neuropsychology, 11*, 597-604.

Blessed, G., Tomlinson, B. E., & Roth, M. (1968). Association between quantitative measures of dementing and senile change in the cerebral grey matter of elderly subjects. *British Journal of Psychiatry, 114*, 797-811.

Boone, K. B., Lesser, I. M., Hill-Gutierrez, E., Berman, N. G., & D'Elia, L. F. (1993). Rey-Osterrieth Complex Figure performance in healthy, older adults: Relationship to age, education, sex, and IQ. *The Clinical Neuropsychologist, 7*, 22-28.

Bornstein, R. A. (1985). Normative data on selected neuropsychological measures from a nonclinical sample. *Journal of Clinical Psychology, 41*, 651-659.

Brandt, J. (1991). The Hopkins Verbal Learning Test: Development of a new memory test with six equivalent forms. The Clinical Neuropsychologist, 5, 125-142.

Buschke, H. (1973). Selective reminding for the analysis of memory and learning. *Journal of Verbal Learning and Verbal Behavior, 12,* 543-550.

Butcher, J. N., Dahlstrom, W. G., Graham, J. R., Tellegen, A., & Kaemmer, B. (1989). Minnesota Multiphasic Personality Inventory (MMPI-2). *Manual for administration and scoring.* Minneapolis: University of Minnesota Press.

Dahlstrom, W. G., Welsh, G. S., Dahlstrom, L. E. (1972). *An MMPI Handbook. Minneapolis:* University of Minnesota Press.

Delis, D. C., Kramer, J. H., Kaplan, E., & Ober, B. A. (1986). *California Verbal Learning Test.* New York: The Psychological Corporation.

De Renzi, E., & Faglioni, P. (1978). Normative data and screening power of a shortened version of the Token Test. *Cortex, 14,* 41-49.

De Renzi, E., & Vignolo, L. A. (1962). The Token Test: A sensitive test to detect disturbances in aphasics. *Brain, 85,* 665-678.

Dunn, L. M., & Dunn, L. M. (1981). *Peabody Picture Vocabulary Test-Revised manual.* Circle Pines, MN: American Guidance Service.

Dunn, E. J., Searight, H. R., Grisso, T., Margolis, R. B., & Gibbons, J. L. (1990). The relation of the Halstead-Reitan neuropsychological battery to functional daily living skills in geriatric patients. *Archives of Clinical Neuropsychology, 5,* 103-117.

Era, P., Jokela, J., & Heikkinen, E. (1986). Reaction and movement times in men of different ages: A population study. *Perceptual and Motor Skills, 63,* 111-130.

Faber-Langendoen, K., Morris, J. C., Knesevich, J. W., LaBarge, E., Miller, J. P., & Berg, L. (1988). Aphasia in senile dementia of the Alzheimer type. *Annals of Neurology, 23,* 365-370.

Folson, J. C. (1968). Reality orientation for the elderly mental patient. *Journal of Geriatric Psychiatry, 1,* 291-307.

Folstein M. F., Folstein, S. E., & McHugh, P. R. (1975). Mini-mental state. *Journal of Psychiatric Research, 12,* 189-198.

Francis, J. (1992). Delirium in older patients. *Journal of the American Geriatrics Society, 40,* 829-838.

Fromm-Auch, D., & Yeudall, L.T. (1983). Normative data for the Halstead-Reitan neuropsychological tests. *Journal of Clinical and Experimental Neuropsychology, 5,* 221-238.

Glantz, R. H., Bieliauskas, L. A., & Paleologos, N. (1986). Behavioral indicators of hallucinosis in Levodopa-treated Parkinson's disease. In M. D. Yahr & K. J. Bergmann (Eds.), *Advances in Neurology, 45,* 417-420.

Goldstein, G., & Ruthven, L. (1983). *Rehabilitation of the brain-damaged adult.* New York: Plenum.

Green, J., Morris, J. C., Sandson, J., McKeel, D. W., and Miller, J. W. (1990). Progressive aphasia: A precursor of global dementia? *Neurology, 40,* 423-429.

Hathaway, S., & McKinley, J. (1951). *The Minnesota Multiphasic Personality Inventory manual.* Minneapolis: University of Minnesota Press.

Heaton, R. K. (1981). *A manual for the Wisconsin Card Sorting Test.* Odessa, FL: Psychological Assessment Services.

Heaton, R. K., Grant, I., & Matthews, C. G. (1991). *Comprehensive norms for an expanded Halstead-Reitan battery.* Odessa, FL: Psychological Assessment Resources.

Heaton, R. K., & Pendleton, M. G. (1981). Use of neuropsychological tests to predict adult patients' everyday functioning. *Journal of Consulting and Clinical Psychology, 49,* 807-821.

Hooper, C. R., & Dunkle, R. E. (1985). *The older aphasic person.* Rockville, MD: Aspen.

Kaplan, E. F., Goodglass, H., & Weintraub, S. (1983). *The Boston Naming Test.* Philadelphia: Lea & Febiger.

Kashani, J., McKnew, D., & Cytryn, L. (1985). Symptom checklist for major depressive disorders. *Psychopharmacology Bulletin, 21,* 957-958.

Kiernan, R. J., Mueller, J., Langston, J. W., & Van Dyke, C. (1987). The neurobehavioral cognitive status examination: A brief but differentiated approach to cognitive assessment. *Annals of Internal Medicine, 2107*, 481-485.

Kincannon, J. C. (1968). Prediction of the standard MMPI scale scores from 71 items: The Mini-Mult. *Journal of Consulting and Clinical Psychology, 32*, 319-325.

Langner, T. S. (1962). A twenty-two item screening score of psychiatric symptoms indicating impairment. *Journal of Health and Human Behavior, 3*, 269-276.

Larrabee, G. J. (1987). Further cautions in interpretation of comparisons between the WAIS-R and the Wechsler Memory Scale. *Journal of Clinical and Experimental Neuropsychology, 9*, 456-460.

Lezak, M. D. (1976). *Neuropsychological Assessment.* New York: Oxford.

Lezak, M. D. (1988). IQ: RIP. *Journal of Clinical and Experimental Neuropsychology, 10*, 351-361.

Lezak, M. D. (1995). *Neuropsychological Assessment* (3rd ed.). New York: Oxford.

Lipowski, Z. J. (1989). Delirium in the elderly patient. *The New England Journal of Medicine, 320*, 578-582.

Loewenstein, D. A., Amigo, E., Duara, R., Guterman, A., Hurwitz, D., Berkowitz, N., Wilkie, F., Weinberg, G., Black, B., Gittelman, B., & Eisdorfer, C. (1989). A new scale for the assessment of functional status in Alzheimer's disease and related disorders. *Journal of Gerontology: Psychological Sciences, 44*, 114-121.

Matthews, C. G. & Kløve, H. (1964). *Instruction manual for the Adult Neuropsychology Test Battery.* Madison, WI: University of Wisconsin Medical School.

McSweeny, A. J. (1990). Qualify-of-life assessment in neuropsychology. In Tupper, D. E. & Cicerone, K. D. (Eds.), *The neuropsychology of everyday life: Assessment and basic competencies* (pp. 185-217). Boston: Kluwer Academic Publishers.

McSweeny, A. J., Grant, I., Heaton, R. K., Prigatano, G. P., & Adams, K. M. (1985). Relationship of neuropsychological status to everyday functioning in healthy and chronically ill persons. *Journal of Clinical and Experimental Neuropsychology, 7*, 281-291.

Mesulam, M. (1981). Slowly progressive aphasia without generalized dementia. *Annals of Neurology, 11*, 592-598.

Naugle, R. I., & Chelune, G. J. (1990). Integrating neuropsychological and real-life data: A neuropsychological model for assessing everyday functioning. In Tupper, D. E. & Cicerone, K. D. (Eds.), *The neuropsychology of everyday life: Assessment and basic competencies* (57-73). Boston: Kluwer Academic Publishers.

Nelson, H. E. (1982). *National Adult Reading Test (NART) Test Manual.* Windsor, Berkshire, England: NFER-Nelson.

Osterrieth, P. A. (1944). Le test de copie d'une figure complex: Contribution à létude de la perception et de la mémoire. *Archives de Psychologie, 30*, 206-353.

Parker, K. (1983). Factor analysis of the WAIS-R at nine age levels between 17 and 74 years. *Journal of Consulting and Clinical Psychology, 51*, 302-308.

Pierce, P. S. (1989). *Adult Functional Adaptive Behavior Scale: Manual of directions.* (Available from the author, VA Medical Center, Togus, ME)

Poon, L. W. (Ed.) (1986). *Clinical memory assessment of older adults.* Washington, DC: American Psychological Association.

Reitan, R. M. (1984). *Aphasia and sensory-perceptual deficits in adults.* Tucson, AZ: Neuropsychology Press.

Reitan, R., & Wolfson, D. (1985). *The Halstead-Reitan Neuropsychological Test Battery.* Tucson, AZ: Neuropsychology Press.

Rey, A. (1941). L'examen psychologique dans les cas d'encéphalopathie traumatique. *Archives de Psychologie, 28,* 286-340.

Rey, A. (1964). *L'examen clinique en psychologie.* Paris: Presses Universitaires de France.

Roberts, R. J., & Hamsher, K. DeS. (1984*). Effects of minority status on facial recognition and naming performance.*

Ryan, J., & Paolo, A. (1992). A screening procedure for estimating premorbid intelligence in the elderly. *The Clinical Neuropsychologist, 6,* 53-62.

Ryan, J. J., Paolo, A. M., & Brungardt, T. M. (1990). Standardization of the Wechsler Adult Intelligence Scale-Revised for persons 75 years and older. *Psychological Assessment, 2,* 404-411.

Smith, A. (1968). The Symbol-Digit Modalities Test: A neuropsychologic test for economic screening of learning and other cerebral disorders. *Learning Disorders, 3,* 83-91.

Spirrison, C. L., & Pierce, P. S. (1992). Psychometric characteristics of the adult functional adaptive behavior scale (AFABS). *The Gerontologist, 32,* 234-239.

Squire, L. R. (1987). *Memory and brain.* New York: Oxford.

Stokx, L. C., & Gaillard, A. W. K. (1986). Task and driving performance of patients with a severe concussion of the brain. *Journal of Clinical and Experimental Neuropsychology, 8,* 421-436.

Terman, L. M., & Merril, M. A. (1973). *Stanford-Binet Intelligence Scale, Form L-M.* Boston, MA: Houghton Mifflin.

Thorndike, R. L., Hagen, E. P., & Sattler, J. M. (1986). *Stanford-Binet Intelligence Scale.* Chicago: Riverside.

Tupper, D. E., & Cicerone, K. D. (1990). *The neuropsychology of everyday life: Assessment and basic competencies.* Boston, MA: Kluwer Academic Publishers.

Tupper, D. E., & Cicerone, K. D. (1991). *The neuropsychology of everyday life: Issues in development and rehabilitation.* Boston, MA: Kluwer Academic Publishers.

Walton, J. N. (1977). *Brain's diseases of the nervous system.* New York: Oxford.

Warner, M. H., Ernst, J., Townes, B. D., Peel, J., & Preston, M. (1987). Relationships between IQ and neuropsychological measures in neuropsychiatric populations: Within-laboratory and cross-cultural replications using WAIS and WAIS-R. *Journal of Clinical and Experimental Neuropsychology, 9,* 545-562.

Warrington, E. K. (1984). *Recognition memory test.* Windsor, Berkshire, England: NFER-NELSON.

Wasserman, G. S., & Kong, K. L. (1979). Absolute timing of mental activities. *Behavioral and Brain Sciences, 2,* 243-304.

Wechsler, D. (1945). A standardized memory scale for clinical use. *Journal of Psychology, 19,* 87-95.

Wechsler, D. (1955). *Wechsler Adult Intelligence Scale manual.* New York: Psychological Corporation.

Wechsler, D. (1981). *WAIS-R manual.* New York: Psychological Corporation.

Wechsler, D. A. (1987). *Wechsler Memory Scale-Revised.* New York: The Psychological Corporation.

Wilson, R. S., Kaszniak, A. W., & Fox, J. H. (1981). Remote memory in senile dementia. *Cortex, 17,* 41-48.

Yesavage, J. A., Brink, T. L., Rose, T. L., & Adey, M. (1983). The geriatric depression scale: Comparison with other self-report and psychiatric rating scales. In T. Crook, S. Ferris, & R. Bartus (Eds.), *Geriatric Psychopharmacology* (pp. 153-167). New Canaan, CT: Mark Powley Associates, Inc.

Zachary, R. A. (1986). *The Shipley Institute of Living Scale.* Los Angeles: Western Psychological Services.

14

NEUROPSYCHOLOGICAL ASSESSMENT OF ETHNIC-MINORITIES:
The Case of Assessing Hispanics Living in North America

Patricia Perez-Arce, Ph.D.
Antonio E. Puente, Ph.D.

In mental testing, society's preconceptions and presumptions especially resist reformulation because of the widespread use of professional authority to establish the reference groups and standards by which to categorize individual performance.

John Garcia (1984, p. 44)

INTRODUCTION

The reality of a polyethnic, polycultural, and polyglot American society is ineluctably imposing itself upon the field of neuropsychology. However, investigators do not have a conceptual framework nor appropriate methodology to guide their research, while clinicians lack not only adequate testing tools but also a comprehensive understanding of how ethnic/cultural variables may impinge on brain function and neuropsychological test performance. Consequently, neuropsychologists working with people from nonmajority groups find themselves improvising, adapting, translating, and/or adjusting existing neuropsychological measures and norms to provide a critically needed service. Concurrently, those that are asked to evaluate individuals from unfamiliar cultures, who may speak a different language, may use untrained interpreters, invalid tests, and unrepresentative norms that severely misrepresent the actual abilities and/or competencies of the referred individual. Such approaches not only reflect poor science but are highly suggestive of unethical, even illegal practice. For example, Public Law 94-142 requires the use of "nondiscriminiatory" testing and the American Psychological Association Ethical Guidelines (APA, 1992) require cultural sensitivity in assessment situations.

This chapter seeks to address some critical issues and problems frequently encountered by neuropsychologists who assess people from outside the majority group. The authors take, as an example, the specific case of working with Hispanics. Hispanics represent the fastest growing and second largest ethnic minority group in the United States. Further, Hispanics share many common characteristics with other ethnic-minorities such as a high proportion of low socioeconomic status, limited and/or poor education, few economic resources, poor health care, unskilled jobs, provenance from foreign, developing countries, discrimination, English as a second language, unique cultural values, rural life experiences, and low acculturation level. These myriad variables complicate the already difficult demands of a neuropsychological evaluation.

Puente and McCaffrey (1992) have suggested that our previous approach to neuropsychological assessment has been traditionally based on the assumption that the neuropsychologist must fully appreciate both the limits and possibilities of test instruments and brain function. Nevertheless, they argue that this approach still leaves much to be desired. Puente and McCaffrey suggest that neuropsychological assessment must be based on placing an understanding not only of tests and brain function, but must also be based on the patient within a biopsychosocial context. That is, the patient must be understood not only in terms of tests and what is commonly known about brain function, but they must be understood within the context of the life they live. This approach increases what is currently being considered ecological validity and is reflective in the theme of this book. The concept of ecological validity of neuropsychological testing emphasizes the effect that socioeconomic, cultural, language, and related factors have on the way information is processed and on the manner of response to situational demands.

The psychological testing literature has raised psychologists' awareness of ecological validity with the caveat, "By far the most important considerations in the testing of culturally diverse groups...pertains to the interpretation of test scores," (Anastasi, 1976). Cauce and Jacobson (1980) cogently argued both implicit and incorrect assumptions concerning the assessment of the Hispanic in the United States. Besides the problem of overt prejudice, the authors outlined several problems involving biased assumptions. They included bilinguality, homogeneity in English language proficiency, equivalence of literal translations, population homogeneity, language uniformity, and culture-free testing. Olmedo (1981) further emphasized the problems of bilingualism, acculturation, and the generalizability of cognitive constructs from linguistic majorities to linguistic minorities.

Unfortunately, clinical neuropsychology lags sorely behind other forms of clinical psychology, especially school psychology. One has to look no further than the most seminal book in neuropsychological assessment to understand this lag. In Lezak's (1983) book, Neuropsychological Assessment, there is a prevalent belief that "given reasonably normal conditions of physical and mental development, there is one intellectual performance level that best represents each person's intellectual abilities generally," (Lezak, 1983). Lezak's assumption does not take into account the relative nature of what is a normal condition for development.

In Lezak's (1983) chapter delineating history-taking, no mention is made of the need to assess the patient's dominant language, preferential mode of processing information or of cultural context (e.g., definitions, beliefs, values, and attitudes regarding achievement, school, and work, and the potential impact of these variables on testing performance). Moreover, Lezak clusters the term *cultural deprivation*, with brain injury, poor work habits, and anxiety as variables that "can only depress intellectual functioning." There is no elucidation of what cultural deprivation means in this context. Does it allude to low socioeconomic level, to cultures dissimilar to that of European Americans? Clearly there is a serious gap between neuropsychological knowledge and culturally relevant cognitive assessments.

Given the present state of affairs, it is not surprising that many psychologists in the field have continued to believe that the plea for programmatic reforms that take into account cognitive differentiation and linguistic diversity have gone unanswered by the testing industry (Garcia, 1984). Some propose that this unresponsiveness by those in the testing industry has been partly due to the lack of understanding of the effect that cultural values and perceptions, as well as the structure of language, have on cognition (Ardila, 1983; LeVine, 1988; Manuel-Dupont, Ardila, Rosselli, & Puente, 1992). Others have suggested that empirical evidence is so limited as to have little impact on practical knowledge. Kaufman (1979), for example, suggests that our understanding of brain-behavior relationships is too recent to have had an impact on the structure and format of intelligence type of tests. Kaufman and others (Ardila, Roselli, & Puente, 1994; Kaufman, 1979; Ornstein, 1973) do acknowledge that diverse cultural groups may emphasize different modes of processing information and that current cognitive tests may penalize specific cultural/ethnic populations.

The chapter focuses on two main issues. In the first part, three major variables which affect neuropsychological assessment of minority group cultures are discussed. Next, the effects of these variables on neuropsychological assessment are addressed. Specific focus is placed on intellectual assessment since recent practice surveys (e.g., Putnam & De Luca, 1991) indicate that this is the most common type of neuropsychological test and its implications for both neuropsychological and related fields (e.g., education) are most critical.

DEFINING SOCIOCULTURAL VARIABLES

Race has been defined primarily as an anatomical differentiation between groups of people. Kechnie (1983) wrote, "Any of the major biological divisions of mankind, are distinguished by color and texture of hair, color of skin and eyes, stature, bodily proportions, etc. Many ethnologists now consider that there are only three primary divisions, the Caucasian..., Negroid..., and Mongoloid..., each with various subdivision." In contrast, ethnicity is more behaviorally oriented and may be defined as "designating any of the basic divisions or groups mankind, as distinguished by customs, characteristics, language, etc." (Kechnie, 1983). One example of ethnicity is that of the Hispanic. Culture is a broader behavioral concept and has been defined as designating "a cognitive system, that is, a set of 'propositions,' both descriptive... and normative..., about nature, man, and society that are more or less embedded in interlocking higher-order networks and configurations," (Spiro, 1988). An additional corollary of culture is that it is not the sole determinant of behavior; behavior results from cultural, situational, ecological, motivational, economic, political, biological, emotional, and other factors (Kagan, 1984; Spiro, 1988).

These definitions clarify the confusion that many people exhibit in the inappropriate use of "racial group" when ethnic/cultural groups is meant. In other words, race is often confused with ethnicity and vice versa. Even though most Hispanics are primarily Caucasian, Hispanics can be from any of the three basic races. There are Hispanics who are born of European descendants on both sides of the family, others of Latin American Indians, still others are of African ancestry bilaterally, and many others have ancestors of mixed races. Hispanics share over-arching cultural values, dominant language, and norms. However, depending on their country of origin, they have unique vocabulary, religious traditions, music, and communication styles. This same pattern applies to African Americans, Native Americans, Asian Americans, and European Americans. Research in education, sociology, and psycholinguistics, among others, must be considered to understand the deeper influence of culture on cognition and its manifestations. The topic of race is not be considered in any detail in this chapter because of the lack of adequate empirical information on the topic coupled with the variables' strong affective and political connotations.

CULTURE

The significant impact of culturally specific values and norms on a cognitive variable (e.g., academic achievement) is epitomized by the scholastic performance demonstrated by immigrant children from different cultures. Caplan, Chow, and Whitmore (1992) studied a sample of 536 school-age children of refugee nuclear families (i.e. "boat people") from Indochina, most of whom attended low-income, inner-city American schools. In the California sample, their mean overall score on the California Achievement Test was in the 54th percentile and only 4% had a GPA below a C grade. The factors most related to achievement were a large family, daily parental involvement with homework tasks, particularly reading aloud regularly to their children. Further, it was found that the parents' values were deeply rooted in Confucian and Buddhist traditions.

In contradistinction, Hispanic children's school drop out rate is extremely high. For them, large family is associated with poorer school performance. In addition, there is little evidence that Latino parents are highly involved in their children's homework tasks. One characteristic of many Mexican-Americans is that they are migrant field workers with very little formal education. Their children tend to help the family in the fields and, unless they are settled, usually can escape the government's demand for school attendance. The parents, if originally educated in rural areas, have only a rudimentary knowledge of reading, writing, and the demands of a formal education. The value of a scholastic education is not particularly salient for a successful life.

Mexican-American children and young adults show a high degree of cooperative behaviors and significantly less competitive motivation across situations, regions, and socioeconomic levels when compared to their European-American peers (Kagan, 1984; Madsen & Kagan, 1973; Knight & Kagan, 1982). Yet, regardless of their cultural norms they must conform to classroom learning environments that emphasize individual achievement and advancement through time- and norm-referenced competition. In fact, Kagan (1980, 1983) writes of the "structural bias hypothesis" of the classroom where children from nonmajority group cultures are required to fit into the more culturally syntonic cooperative teamwork process. Competitive motives and behaviors are learned in the United States through socialization provided by institutions such as school, as well as organized sports, video games, and the media. This is not the case with Chicano children where socialization is maintained under the control of the family, rather through the influence of peers and institutional forces (Avellar & Kagan, 1976; Kagan, 1984).

Acculturation must be considered in interpreting performance on cognitive tasks. In a large study of social motives the modal response of Anglo-American children was rivalry/superiority, the modal response of second generation Mexican-American children was equality, closely followed by altruism, while third-generation Mexican-American children showed equal preference for equality and rivalry/superiority (Knight & Kagan, 1977).

Apparent achievement deficits found in first generation and/or unacculturated people with low or no education, may be related to differences in motivation, practice, and lack of perceived need (Bruner, Oliver, & Greenfield, 1966; Garcia, 1984; Greenfield, 1966; Shweder, 1988), as well as to learned social motives such as cooperation and competition (Kagan, 1984). In his extensive research in child development, Kagan (1984) found that both social (cultural) values and cognitive processes determine how children will behave in relation to competitive games. If a child is yet unable to conceptualize alternative solutions to problems, he or she will respond at the most self-referent, concrete level. Once greater cognitive complexity is attained, social values will determine the quality of the response choice.

EDUCATION/COGNITIVE DEVELOPMENT

Educational experience and level are frequently confounded with cultural and ethnic factors in the study of people from nonmajority group cultures. In a common syllogistic analysis, the assumption is made that people who hold unskilled occupations are less intelligent than the general population, and, since a sizable majority of Hispanics and African-Americans work in unskilled jobs, they, as an ethnic/cultural group, must be less intelligent than European-Americans. This false premise can be traced to the early work of Terman (1914) and others.

It is rare for a neuropsychologist to encounter adult patients who have not achieved a minimum of six years of education. However, for those patients who have emigrated from rural areas of Latin American countries or even from the inner cities of the United States a low level of education is the norm. Many of these adults never mastered basic literacy skills such as reading and writing in their indigenous language, and, consequently, even if they speak English, they do not read or write English. Nevertheless, they emigrated under high-risk conditions, found jobs, brought their families to the United States, and even managed to buy a house. In essence, they never had the opportunity to learn the relationship between the spoken word and its abstract representation through linguistic symbols. Their conceptual abilities may be immaturely developed, and they may be constricted in their ability to comprehend higher-order abstractions. In addition, their appreciation for and experience with standardized testing tends to be highly limited. Most frequently, testing is a "foreign" experience which is typically used for detrimental outcomes (e.g., special education placement). However, despite their poor educational background they have survived and thrived admirably in a foreign and sometimes unwelcoming culture. Their intelligence and cognitive capacity clearly cannot be measured with tests that are highly correlated with school and culture-based achievement.

Anecdotal observations indicate that little educational experience coupled with early rural upbringing in Latin America is frequently associated with impaired performance on a range of neuropsychological measures, including tests that are not language-based and often considered to be higher-order in nature (e.g., Category Test). The interpretation of neuropsychological test results of these patients necessitates a different type of analysis because, besides the presenting problem related to possible brain trauma, one must take into account the possible mitigating effects of language dominance, culturally determined perceptual interpretations, the variability of educational experience related to having gone to school in rural Latin American pueblos and pueblitos, the usual lack of access to medical care, poor nutrition, a social environment that does not appreciate nor has the opportunity support the pragmatic value of school education, and/or an occupational work history that has precluded cognitive stimulation and practice.

A number of perspectives allow for an understanding as to why individuals with little education and living in an environment that does not require literacy skills for successful living may present with deficient neuropsychological scores. In educational psychology the concept of maturation of functional scholastic behaviors includes a stage of "readiness to learn," (i.e., readiness to acquire literacy skills). This is a concept that has been integrated into the purpose of Head Start programs, stimulating the thinking processes of preschool children to prepare them to understand and manipulate information at school. Immigrant children raised in illiterate environments, who may be transient in their living situations as many farm workers' families are, may be severely handicapped when and if they are enrolled in American public schools in second, third, or higher grades without any school readiness skills necessary to analyze multiple levels of meaning. Further, these students may also be very unfamiliar with school type of tasks as are found in neuropsychological tests.

In Piaget's (1978) cognitive developmental theory, the progression to increasingly complex systematic mental activity requires the need to communicate with others, "only by means of friction against other minds, by means of exchange and opposition does thought come to be conscious of its own aims and tendencies." (Piaget, 1928). Within his theory, the social environment provides the opportunity for stimulation, practice, and learning through different kinds of activities, concepts, and relationships (e.g., cooperation and competition, respect, values). While these ideas support current ethnographic theories and educational research, that social context is intimately related to cognitive functioning in general, Piaget's theory is flawed by the presumption of the homogeneity of all children regardless of their environment. To illustrate, Piaget and his Geneva group maintained that conservation is achieved "naturally" regardless of environmental variables such as schooling. However, the predicted orderliness in the development of the concept of conservation appears to apply mostly to Western (i.e., European-based) cultures (de Lemos, 1965). His methods, like most methods evaluating cognitive abilities (Kaufman, 1979), rely heavily on verbal input and output, and, therefore, penalize children who are from less verbal cultures and environments.

These assumptions of homogeneity in cognitive development were challenged by studies comparing unschooled rural Senegalese children with French-style educated urban Senegalese children (Bruner, Oliver, & Greenfield, 1966; Greenfield, 1966). It was demonstrated that the unschooled children, after ages 8 or 9, failed to progress in their comprehension of quantity conservation, and, instead, persisted with perceptual rather than conceptual explanations for a much longer time. Moreover, with proper instruction, some of the unschooled children acquired conservation easily. The results of these studies support the tenet that cultural factors influence cognitive processes and they help us to understand the close association between Western education and Western modes of thought.

These findings are presented because of their potential implications in regards to testing performance. A number of factors are involved in demonstrating motivation to do well on academic types of tests. These include speed of response under timed conditions and applying oneself to the task without needing support from the examiner, both very North American and European concepts. The structural and process components of cognitive tests are consistent with culturally reinforced individualistic and competitive American behavior, and for those who are unacculturated to American values and behaviors or are recent immigrants from non-European countries, measuring these types of behaviors might be meaningless. At most, such an approach would reflect level of neuropsychological acculturation, but not necessarily neuropsychological deficiency.

INTELLIGENCE TESTING

Intellectual assessment of nonmajority people is important yet difficult not only because the most developed body of literature exploring the relationship between ethnicity and cognition is in the assessment of "intelligence," but also because interpretation of neuropsychological results must have as its basis, an estimate of the individual's previous and current general cognitive capacity. This interpretation would include the ability to attend, perceive, analyze, problem solve, communicate, and understand various levels of symbolic meaning (Lezak, 1983). Ironically, determining the intellectual capacity of nonmajority people in the United States poses a dilemma and a paradox. A brief overview of this research will be presented as it elucidates the failures in the current neuropsychological framework and highlights how essential it is to consider the effects of sociocultural variables on test performance.

"Intelligence" has been placed in quotation marks because it is a construct defined by a set of test scores that are heavily correlated with American educators-defined measures of scholastic success. Garcia (1984) writes that "IQ tests postulated a model [child/adult] whose intelligence was congruent with the socioeconomic status and political power of its parents." His point is that those in any society that are in positions of power and who control resources, whether economic or intellectual, are the determinants of what is "normal" and desirable in the "average" individual, the average being one's own kind. Given these natural inclinations, it is not surprising that, in the United States, the field of psychology and neuropsychology has been and continues to be defined and led predominantly by researchers and clinicians of European-American descent. Surprisingly, a review of the literature over the last 25 years on intelligence assessment of Hispanics reveals that the vast majority of researchers do not have an Hispanic surname. Further, most research on nonmajority group cultures have focused on African-Americans and Hispanics have typically been another variable when studying "minority" issues.

Finally, when Hispanics are considered, most studies tend to ignore the heterogeneity of Hispanics. For example, Hispanics from the European "Peninsula" are quite different than those from the "Americas," Mexican-Americans, are quite different from Cubans, and so on. Further, the majority of studies involve Mexican-Americans which, although comprise a large segment of Hispanics, by no means represent the only segment of this ethnic group.

However, the reality of our heterogenous population and its diverse needs is inexorable. American society is beginning to wake up from the dream that Americans, and even minorities, are a homogenous group in which any individual's cognitive capacities can be measured in the same way and compared to the "norm." It is important to remember that it has not been very long since Little Rock, Arkansas's historical victory of 1953 (Brown vs. Board of Education, see Dreger, 1985) giving equal access to educational opportunities to Blacks and opening the door for people of color to enter diverse professional fields. Furthermore, it has been only in the last 20 years that the number of ethnic minorities have increased to the point where in California, as a group, they will constitute the majority by the year 2000 (U.S. Bureau of Census, 1994).

The literature on the intellectual assessment of children and adults shows thus far that traditional measures of intelligence such as Wechsler Intelligence scales and the Stanford Binet test may not be interpreted in the standardized manner when administered to people from developing countries (Smith, 1974), as well as to African-Americans (Jensen, 1980; Reynolds, Chastain, Kaufman, & McLean, 1987), Hispanics (Kaufman, 1979; Whitworth & Gibbons, 1986; McCollough, Walker, & Diessner, 1985; McShane & Plas, 1984; Teeter, Moore and Petersen, 1982).

One of the primary findings of intelligence testing research in the United States is that Hispanic and Native American children score substantially higher on the Wechsler Performance subscales than on the Verbal ones, and that this discrepancy is maintained through adulthood although it decreases with increasing age on both the WAIS and the WAIS-R (Kaufman, 1990; Whitworth & Gibbons, 1986). Taylor and Richards (1991) reported that when IQ is held constant, Hispanic children tend to perform better on visuospatial tasks. Additionally, Sandoval, Zimmerman, and Woo-Sam (1983) suggested that careful analysis of WISC-R Verbal subtests identified only a small number of items differentially difficult for one group of minority children or another. The WAIS-R (Picture Arrangement) subtest appears to be an "excellent" measure of general intelligence while the Vocabulary and Block Design subtests are considered only "fair" measures of this variable (Kaiser, see Kaufman, 1990). For European-Americans, comparatively, the latter two subtests are considered the most solid measures of crystallized and fluid intelligence, respectively (Kaufman, 1990; Lezak, 1983).

When examining the issue of adult intelligence with the WAIS and WAIS-R, interesting patterns have been reported by Whitworth and Gibbons (1986). Anglo-Saxons scored higher than Mexican-Americans and Blacks. The differences previously reported with the WAIS were once more found and such differences carried over into the revised version of the test. Verbal subtest scores on the WAIS and WAIS-R were similar and lower for both ethnic groups. However, as reported earlier, Hispanics perform better on the Performance Subtests.

Commentary on the difference between the WAIS and the Escala de Intelligencia Weschler Para Adultos (EIWA) is also warranted. Lopez and Romero (1988) reported that most significant differences between the two tests was the conversion of raw scores to scaled scores. In some cases, the scores were "very different." Considering the standardization sample, the age of the test and other related variables, extreme caution is suggested by Lopez and Romero. A more recent and detailed analysis by Melendez (1994) suggested that the two forms are not comparable. Indeed, the overestimation of IQs and the poor standardization sample led Melendez to suggest that the EIWA should be used only under unusual circumstances.

Explanations for the disparity between the performance on intellectual measures between Hispanics and people of color and their European-American counterparts include differences in intellectual abilities due to genetic factors (Jensen, 1980), linguistic factors (Padilla & Lindholm, 1984), cross-cultural cognitive styles (Duran, 1984; Gonzales & Roll, 1985), the cultural specificity of psychometric measures and norms (Adler, 1970; Palmer, Olivarez, Wilson, & Fordyce, 1989; Smith, 1974; Valencia, Henderson, & Rankin, 1985), socioeconomic level (Laosa, 1984; Padilla & Lindholm, 1984), language spoken at home (Laosa, 1984), and/or to verbal ability and reading proficiency (Duran, 1984; Kaufman & Kaufman, 1983). Unfortunately, there is a glaring lack of well-controlled studies that would help determine which of these factors make the greatest contribution to the above-mentioned pattern of differential performance. Inadequate methodology confounds most studies relating cognitive abilities and ethnicity in that they usually do not control for environmentally related variables (e.g., cultural norms, language, socioeconomic level, prenatal and postnatal medical care, nutrition, environmental stimulation, occupational health hazards, substance abuse history, level of stress due to lower status in society). (Amante, VanHouten, Grieve, Bader, & Margules, 1977; Caplan, Choy, & Whitmore, 1992; Padilla & Lindholm, 1984).

Some investigators have postulated that if health and medical variables affecting test performance were parceled out, there would be no significant differences on cognitive testing between children of diverse ethnic/cultural groups. For example, Amante et al. (1977) found that when perceptually normal Black children were compared with perceptually normal Anglo-American children of similar socioeconomic level, there were no significant differences in IQ scores between the two groups. However, when perceptual neurological intactness was not controlled, 28% of the black children, as compared to 3% of the Anglo-

Americans, obtained an IQ score lower than 85 on the Culture Fair Test even though these children were matched by socioeconomic level and residence.

While critical questions regarding the validity and applicability of current intelligence tests for ethnic-minorities are being actively explored, the importance of taking into account specific cultural and linguistic differences continues to be ignored in much of the neuropsychological literature. Most formula estimates of premorbid intelligence give weights to race based on whether a person is "white," "black," or "other," (Barona, Reynolds, & Chastain, 1984). Race is collapsed into generic categories that give no consideration to ethnicity-specific and/or language factors. The advantage of utilizing demographic methods to estimate premorbid intelligence is touched on in Spreen & *Strauss's Compendium of Neuropsychological Tests: Administration, Norms, and Commentary* (1991). However, no mention is made of the inadvisability of using with ethnic-minorities "the best indicators of premorbid intelligence," the Vocabulary and Information subtests of the WAIS-R. Furthermore, no recommendations are made as to how to evaluate intellectual level, premorbid intelligence, and/or neuropsychological functioning of ethnic-minority patients.

A related issue is how IQ scores relate to academic achievement and ecological factors play a role here as well. In the numerous studies that have explored this relationship, there is a consensus that IQ scores and school achievement are highly correlated (Matarazzo, 1972). However, the overall correlation of .50 still leaves 75% of the variance in school performance unaccounted (Kaufman, 1990). Neuropsychologists are best equipped through their knowledge of brain-behavior relationships to parse out the contribution of demographic variables to performance on cognitive testing. For example, Matarazzo and Herman (1984) have suggested that one way to estimate premorbid IQ is to equate years of schooling. However, other disciplines (e.g., ethnography) may provide possible explanations to understand this accounting gap.

Within the ethnographic field there is a growing recognition that one must comprehend social context to understand cognitive functioning (Shweder, 1988). Ethnographic research related to the symbols-and-meanings conception of culture suggests that "meaning, a subjective conventional fact, totally overrides, and alters our reaction to its [a symbol, an object] objective...properties" (Shweder, 1988). In fact, there appears to be strong evidence that sociocultural factors, such as family values and school experience, more so than linguistic factors, may influence scholastic motivation and achievement level and may have the power to override the impact of disruptive demographic factors such as childhood traumas (Bruner et al., 1966; Caplan et al., 1992; Greenfield, 1966).

A growing awareness and concern about the effects of environmental circumstances on cognition has been partly impelled by the intelligence testing literature. A number of articles and books have been published that explore the relationship between intellectual abilities and performance on a variety of neuropsychological tests (Dodrill, 1981; Reitan 1985) and on the influence of subject variables, such as education, culture, gender, and race, on the interpretation of conventional cut-off scores of neuropsychological measures (Ardila et. al, 1993; Karzmark, Heaton, Grant, & Matthews, 1985; Thompson, Heaton, Matthews, & Grant, 1987).

Nevertheless, the knowledge base is scarce when answering questions such as, "Do current neuropsychological tests measure what they are supposed to measure when administered to ethnic-minorities?" and "May one use the common interpretation paradigm of level-of-performance, pattern of results, pathognomonic signs, and lateralizing indicators with sociocultural groups that may speak a different language, have a unique learning style, and employ distinct communication, educational, and socialization practices (Martinez & Mendoza, 1984)?" These and related questions raised by neuropsychologists working in the field with people from minority group cultures need to be answered for a number of reasons. Foremost is the accuracy of neuropsychological test results when applied to people outside the mainstream culture, as inaccurate results lead to faulty conclusions as well as misguided diagnosis and prognosis.

OTHER NEUROCOGNITIVE FUNCTIONS

Unfortunately, this section remains largely unwritten. Despite the importance of examining the effects of biopsychosocial variables in neuropsychological performance, the literature is very weak. To help illustrate this situation, the variable of language is briefly considered. Communication with the patient is assumed intact in all but the "language" sections of a neuropsychological evaluation. It is often assumed that literal translations are acceptable. However, the structures of the English and Spanish languages are not equal. Phonological and grammatical concerns would warrant most literal translations as totally unacceptable. Back translations of tests and the use of literal translation would render most tests as useless.

The work on Hispanics by Ardila and colleagues (e.g., Ardila, Rosselli, & Rosas, 1989) buttresses and extends the issues raised here. For example, Rosselli and Rosas (1989) reported that Hispanic illiterates differed from matched controls in standard language assessment including phonological discrimination.

What was unexpected was that illiterates further differed from controls on tests of naming, praxis, coordinated movements, and cancellation. This line of research points to the importance of understanding the role of education and related sociocultural variables in neuropsychological assessment (see Ardila, Rosselli, & Ostroky-Solis, 1992).

CONCLUSIONS

There are numerous dilemmas encountered in understanding and assessing the neurocognitive capabilities of non-English-speaking children and adults who are unschooled in the European-based educational system that includes literacy skills. Clinically, when a patient with these characteristics is referred for a neuropsychological evaluation, a trained interpreter who has mastered the art of writing verbatim, has been trained to discern subtle alterations in expressive and receptive language, understands the critical importance of verbal and non-verbal communication, and can communicate and translate back to the examiner these myriad observations must be employed. All things being equal, it should go without saying that translators with psychological training would be the second best alternative. If possible, clients should be evaluated by someone trained in both the sociocultural and neuropsychological issues.

It is hoped that neuropsychology will profit from the experience in the field of psychological testing and that greater strides will be achieved in integrating cultural diversity and all that it entails into the methodology of neuropsychological assessment. Sanchez (1928) emphasized the importance of understanding bilingualism in mental measurement. The question of whether such a concern has been transferred to clinical neuropsychology is at issue here. Unfortunately, the literature does not appear to support a positive prognosis for this situation. For example, Santos de Barona (1993) reported that a "significant decline" in the number of articles containing ethnic minorities issues occurred between 1970 and 1989. Clearly, knowledge of the relationship between cognition and culture can only come about through investigations that focus specifically on the effects of non-European cultural variables and of non-Anglo-Saxon languages on performance on the currently used neuropsychological tests. These efforts must include appropriate and culturally relevant, measures of concurrent validity, (e.g., achievement, adaptability and survival). It may be that new neuropsychological measures must be developed for specific ethnic groups. Current measures might apply to various non-European-American cultural groups, but more appropriate norms would be required.

A final comment should be made with regards to the concept of "neuropsychological acculturation." If the question involves the appreciation of a person's ability to integrate into a particular society as measured by such variables as problems solving or memory tasks, then the issue of culturally sensitive measures is at best academic. One might argue like Clarizio did in 1982 that "if the goal of achieving a desegregated society is still as worth pursuing (a value judgment), then the minority child should be compared against a national reference group, for this is the group with which the minority child must compete." Even this statement, however, might be pursued as culturally biased in that the final criterion is competition and not understanding. Clearly, both the question of cultural sensitivity and understanding coupled with the ultimate criterion for testing remains open to scrutiny.

REFERENCES

Adler, S. (1970). Auditory retention ability in five year old lower and middle class children: A pilot study. *Journal of Communication Disorders, 3*, 133-139.

Amante, D., VanHouten, V. W., Grieve, J. H., Bader, C. A., & Margules, P. H. (1977). Neuropsychological deficit, ethnicity, and socioeconomic status. *Journal of Consulting and Clinical Psychology, 45*, 524-535.

American Psychological Association (1992). Ethical principles of psychologists and code of conduct. *American Psychologist, 47*, 1597-1611.

Anastasi, A. (1976). *Psychological testing,* 4th. Ed.. New York: MacMillan Publishing Co.

Ardila, A. (1983). *Psicologia del lenguaje.* Mexico: Editorial Trillas.

Ardila, A., Rosselli, M., & Ostrosky-Solis, F. (1992). Socioeducational. In A. E. Puente, & R. J. McCaffrey, III, (Eds.), *Handbook of neuropsychological assessment: A biopsychosocial perspective. Critical issues in neuropsychology* (pp. 181-192). New York, NY: Plenum Press.

Ardila, A., Rosselli, M., & Puente, A. E. (1993). *Neuropsychological evaluation of the spanish speaker.* New York: Plenum.

Ardila, A., Rosselli, M., & Rosas, P. (1989). Neuropsychological assessment in illiterates: Visuospatial and memory abilities. *Brain and Cognition, 11*(2), 147-166.

Avellar, J., & Kagan, S. (1976). Development of competitive behaviors in Anglo-American and Mexican-American children. *Psychological Reports, 39*(1), 191-198.

Barona, A., Reynolds, C. R., & Chastain, R. (1984). A demographically based index of premorbid intelligence for the WAIS-R. *Journal of Consulting and Clinical Psychology, 52*, 885-887.

Bruner, J. S., Oliver, R. R., & Greenfield, P. M. (1966). *Studies in cognitive growth.* New York: Wiley.

Caplan, N., Choy, M.H., & Whitmore, J. (1992). Indochinese refugee families and academic achievement. *Scientific American, 266*, 36-45.

Cauce, A. M. & Jacobson, L. I. (1980). Implicit and incorrect assumptions concerning the assessment of the Latino in the United States. *American Journal of Community Psychology, 8*,(5), 571-585.

Clarizio, H. (1982). Intellectual assessment of Hispanic children. *Psychology in the Schools, 19*, 61-70.

de Lemos, M. M. (1965). The development of conservation in aboriginal children. *International Journal of Psychology, 4*, 2155-269.

Dodrill, C. B. (1981). An economical method for the evaluation of general intelligence in adults. *Journal of Consulting and Clinical Psychology, 49*(5), 668-673.

Dreger, R. M. (1985). School desegragation. American Psychologist, 40, 124-125.

Duran, R. P. (1984). Assessment and instruction of at-risk Hispanic students. *Exceptional Children, 56,* 154-158.

Figueroa, R. A. (1966). Test bias and Hispanic children. *The Journal of Special Education, 17*, 431-440.

Garcia, J. (1984). The logic and limits of mental aptitude testing. In J. L. Martinez & R. H. Mendoza (Eds.), *Chicano psychology* (pp. 41-58). Orlando: Academic Press.

Gonzales, R., & Roll, S. (1985). Relationship between acculturation, cognitive style and intelligence: A cross-sectional study. *Journal of Cross-Cultural Psychology, 16*, 190-205.

Greenfield, P. M. (1966). On culture and conservation. In J. S. Bruner, R. R. Oliver, & P. M. Greenfield (Eds.), *Studies in cognitive growth* (pp. 334-335). New York: Wiley.

Jensen, A.R. (1980). *Bias in mental testing.* New York: The Free Press.

Kagan, J. (1983). The emergence of self. *Journal of Annual Progress in Child Psychiatry and Child Development*, 5-28.

Kagan, J. (1980). Family experience and the child's development. *Journal of Annual Progress in Child Psychiatry and Child Development*, 23-30.

Kagan, S. (1984). Interpreting Chicano cooperativeness: Methodological and theoretical considerations. In J. L. Martinez & R. H. Mendoza (Eds.), *Chicano psychology*, pp. 289-334. Orlando, FL: Academic Press.

Karzmark, P., Heaton, R. K., & Grant, I., Matthews, G. (1985). Use of demographic variables to predict full scale IQ: A replication and extension. *Journal of Clinical and Experimental Neuropsychology, 7*(4), 412-420.

Kaufman, A. S. (1990). *Assessing adolescent and adult intelligence.* Needham, MA.: Allyn & Bacon.

Kaufman, A. S. (1979). WISC-R research: Implications for interpretation. *Journal of School and Psychology Review, 8*(1), 5-27.

Kaufman, A. S., & Kaufman, N. L. (1983). *K-ABC Kaufman Assessment Battery for Children: Interpretive Manual.* Circle Pines, MN: American Guidance Service.

Kechnie, J. L., (1983). *Webster's new universal unabridged dictionary.* Cleveland, OH: Dorset & Baber.

Knight, G. P., & Kagan, S. (1982). Siblings, birth order, and cooperative-competitive social behavior: A comparison of Anglo-American and Mexican-American children. *Journal of Cross-Cultural Psychology, 13*(2), 239-249.

Knight, G. P., & Kagan, S. (1977). Acculturation of prosocial and competitive behaviors among second- and third-generation Mexican-American children. *Journal of Cross-Cultural Psychology, 8*, 273-284.

Laosa, L. M. (1984). Ethnic, socioeconomic, and home language influences upon early performance on measures of abilities. *Journal of Educational Psychology, 76*(6), 1178-1198.

LeVine, R. A. (1988). Properties of culture: An ethnographic view. In R. A. Shweder & R. A. LeVine (Eds.), *Culture theory: Essays on mind, self, and emotion.* Cambridge: Cambridge University Press.

Lezak, M. (1983). *Neuropsychological assessment*. New York: Oxford University Press.

Lopez, S. & Romero, A. (1988). Assessing the intellectual functioning of Spanish-speaking adults: Comparison of the EIWA and the WAIS. *Journal of Professional Psychology: Research and Practice, 19*(3), 263-270.

Madsen, M. C., & Kagan, S. (1973). Mother-directed achievement of children in two cultures. *Journal of Cross Cultural Psychology, 4*(2), 221-228.

Manuel-Dupont, S., Ardila, A., Rosselli, M., & Puente, A. E. (1992). Bilingualism. In A. E. Puente, R. J. McCaffrey, III, (Eds.), *Handbook of neuropsychological assessment: A biopsychosocial perspective. Critical issues in neuropsychology* (pp. 193-210). New York, NY: Plenum Press.

Martinez, J. L., & Mendoza, R. H. (Eds.) (1984). *Chicano psychology*. Orlando, FL: Academic Press.

Matarazzo, J. D. (1972). *Wechsler's measurement and appraisal of adult intellegence* (5th ed.). New York: Oxford Press.

Matarazzo, J. D., & Herman, D. O. (1984). Relationship of education and IQ in the WAIS-R standardization sample. *Journal of Consulting and Clinical Psychology, 52*(4), 631-634.

McCullough, C. S., Walker, J. L., & Diessnea, R. (1985). The use of the Wechsler Scales in the assessment of Native Americans of the Columbia River Basin. *Psychology in the Schools, 22*, 23-28.

McShane, D. A., & Plas, J. M. (1984). The cognitive functioning of American Indian children: Moving from the WISC to the WISC-R. *Journal of School Psychology Review, 13*(1), 61-73.

Melendez, F. (1994). The use of the EIWA in neuropsychological assessment of Hispanics. *The Clinical Neuropsychologist, 6*, 38-44.

Olmedo, E. (1981). Testing linguistic minorities. *American Psychologist. 36*, 1078-1085.

Ornstein, R. (1973). *The nature of human consciousness*. San Francisco, CA.: Freeman.

Padilla, A. M. & Lindholm, K. J. (1984). Child bilingualism: The same old issues revisited. In J. L. Martinez Jr. & R. H. Mendoza (eds.), *Chicano psychology*, (pp. 369-408). Orlando, FL.: Academic Press.

Palmer, D. J,. Olivarez, A. Jr., Wilson, V. L., & Fordyce, T. (1989). Ethnicity and language dominance–Influence on the prediction of achievement based on intelligence test scores in nonreferred and referred samples. *Learning Disability Quarterly, 12*, 261-274.

Piaget, J. (1928). *Judgment and reasoning in the child*. Trans. M. Worden. New York: Harcourt, Brace & World.

Puente, A. E., & McCaffrey, R. J., III. (1992). *Handbook of neuropsychological assessment: A biopsychosocial perspective*. New York, NY: Plenum Press.

Putnam, S. H., & DeLuca, J. W. (1991). The TCN professional practice survey: II. An analysis of the fees of neuropsychologists by practice demographics. *Clinical Neuropsychologist, 5*(2), 103-124.

Reynolds, C. R., Chastain, R. L., Kaufman, A. S., & McLean, J. E. (1987). Demographic characteristics and IQ among adults: Analysis of the WAIS-R standardization sample as a function of the stratification variables. *Journal of School Psychology, 25*(4), 323-342.

Rosselli, M., Ardila, A., & Rosas, P. (1990). Neuropsychological assessment in illiterates: II. Language and praxic abilities. *Brain and Cognition, 12*(2), 281-296.

Rosselli, M., & Rosas, P. (1989). Neuropsychological assessment in illiterates: Visuospatial and memory abilities. *Brain and Cognition, 11*(2), 147-166.

Sandoval, J.,Zimmerman, I. L., Woo-Sam, J. M. (1983). Cultural differences on WISC-R verbal items. *Journal of School Psychology, 21*(1), 49-55.

Shweder, R. A. (1988). Preview: A colloquy of culture theorists. In R. A. Shweder & R. A. LeVine (Eds.), *Culture theory: Essays on mind, self, and emotion*. Cambridge: Cambridge

University Press.

Smith, M. W. (1974). Alfred Binet's remarkable questions: A cross-national and cross-temporal analysis of the cultural biases built into the Stanford-Binet Intelligence Scale and other Binet test. *Genetic Psychology Monographs, 80*, 307-334.

Spiro, M. E. (1988). Is the Oedipus complex universal? In G. H. Pollock, & J. M. Ross, (Eds.), *The Oedipus papes. Classics in psychoanlaysis mongraph 6.*, pp. 435-473.

Spreen, O., & Strauss, E. (1991). *A compendium of neuropsychological tests: Administration, norms, and commentary.* New York, NY: Oxford University Press.

Taylor, R. L. & Richards, S. B. (1991). Patterns of intellectual differences of black, Hispanic and white children. *Psychology in the Schools, 28*, 5-8.

Teeter, A., Moore, C. L., & Petersen, J. D. (1982). WISC-R Verbal and Performance abilities of Native American students referred for school learning problems. *Psychology in the Schools, 19*, 39-44.

Thompson, L. L., Heaton, R. K., Grant, I., & Matthews, C. G. (1987). Comparison of preferred and nonpreferred hand performance on four neuropsychologifal motor tasks. *Journal of Clinical Neuropsychology, 1*(4), 324-334.

U.S. Bureau of the Census. *Statistical Abstract of the United States, 1994* (14th ed.). Washington, DC.

Valencia, R. R., Henderson, R. W., & Rankin, R. J. (1985). Family status, family constellations, and home environmental variables as predictors of cognitive performance of Mexican American. *Journal of Educational Psychology, 77*, 321-331.

Whitworth, R. H. & Gibbons, R. T. (1986). Cross-racial comparison of the WAIS and the WAIS-R. *Educational and Psychological Measurement, 46*, 1041-1049.

15

ECOLOGICAL ISSUES AND CHILD NEUROPSYCHOLOGICAL ASSESSMENT

Lawrence C. Hartlage, Ph.D.
Donald I. Templer, Ph.D.

Ecological validity considerations involving childhood neuropsychological assessment require attention to two special features. One feature involves the developmental diversity of child neuropsychological functions. As opposed to adults, for whom age groupings may span age ranges of 8 to 10 years or more, a matter of even a few years can be related to important differences in neuropsychological organization. The other feature involves the relative imprecision of measurements usually applied to children. School performance, for example, is apparently a meaningful criterion, and is further a criterion which appears to contain some sort of inherent objective measurement with at least ordinal scaling characteristics. School performance, in typical practice, may in fact be neither meaningful nor objective, at least insofar as a criterion measure against which neuropsychological assessment can be validated. Before exploring empirical data concerning ecological validity of neuropsychological assessment with children, it is important to review these developmental and criterion features to provide an appropriate conceptual context from which to evaluate such data.

The nature of what neuropsychological functions are available and accessible to measurement in children of differing ages has clear implications for what is to be assessed. In the first year of life, for example, while there may be differential verbal vs. nonverbal functions available to the child, such functions are not accessible to very sophisticated measurement. By around age two, rudimentary precursors of eventual language vs. nonlanguage abilities are accessible to the point of permitting the assessment of relative developmental levels for each, and procedures appropriate to such assessment are available (Hartlage & Lucas, 1973; Hartlage & Telzrow, 1981). By beginning school age, precursors of discrete academic skills; measures of constructional praxis; receptive and expressive language skills; and other specific neuropsychological functions are present in sufficient degree as to permit more definitive profile mapping (Hartlage, 1974; Hartlage & Lucas, 1972). For some time, it has been known that by early primary grades there is a shift from proximoceptive (somatosensory) to teloreceptive (visual) prepotency, with changing correlations of these types of central processing functions with criterion measures such as reading (Hartlage, 1975a, 1975b; Kaufman, Belmont, Birch, & Zach, 1973; Lawton & Seim, 1973). Progressively, the frontal lobes exert influence over functions of given neuropsychological systems, especially around the age of puberty (Golden, 1981; Hynd & Hartlage, 1982; Luria, 1969), so that relationships between a functional neuropsychological system and a criterion variable at one age may not be presumed to have the same relationship with the same criterion variable at a subsequent age. Reference to a traditional IQ test may help emphasize this point: The Stanford Binet (Terman & Merrill, 1960) test at mental age six has none of the items used at mental age three, although presumably the criterion measure—Stanford Binet IQ—is the same.

From a clinical perspective, perhaps the most useful and readily available criterion variables against which childhood neuropsychological assessment can be validated relate to school performance. Unfortunately, school performance, although putatively dependent to considerable degree on neuropsychological function, is influenced by a host of other factors whose interactive effect with neuropsychological phenomena is difficult to determine. Global intellectual level, to the extent it can be separated from neuropsychological function, represents one such factor. A child with intact neuropsychological function but low IQ may do poorly in school, while a neuropsychologically impaired child with residual high IQ may not appear to experience academic problems. Similarly, the context of school expectancy can be an important factor in school success, somewhat independent of neuropsychological status. A reasonably bright youngster with mild neuropsychological impairment may meet academic expectations of performance in an inner city school, but be identified as experiencing academic difficulty in a high-achieving college preparatory private school. Type of neuropsychological deficit also may be expected to interact with school performance differentially at given grade levels. The child with neuropsychological impairments involving left hemisphere functioning may experience somewhat more academic difficulty, especially in higher grades; while the child with right hemisphere neuropsychological impairment may experience early school problems but appear to outgrow them in later grades (Hartlage, & Telzrow,

1986). In later school grades, such factors as course of study may relate differentially to given neuropsychological impairments, depending on whether or not the subject matter at hand typically addresses the child's neuropsychological impairments (Hartlage, 1982). Thus, school success, a ubiquitous criterion measure for validation of child neuropsychological assessment, has a number of limitations which can combine to obviate its use as a meaningful and valid criterion.

What remains in terms of determining the ecological validity of neuropsychological assessment of children is a body of literature in which neuropsychological assessment data, either from batteries or individual tests, are correlated with discrete psychometric measures. While such measures (e.g., estimates of reading ability based on standardized tests of reading) may be considered to be only indirect or metameasures of ecological validity, they offer the advantage of (typically) interval scaling, demonstrated reliability, and demonstrated validity for predicting the criterion measure at issue. A look at some of these data may help suggest the relevance of the given neuropsychological assessment to the ecological validity criterion measures involved.

EMPIRICAL VALIDATION

HALSTEAD-REITAN BATTERY

One important research focus of the Halstead-Reitan Neuropsychological Battery for Children (HRNB-C) with implications for ecological validity has involved studies involving learning-disabled children, using school performance measures or tests of same as criterion variables. Prominent among research in this area has been that of Dean and his coworkers (e.g., D'Amato, Gray, & Dean, 1988; Rattan, Rattan, Dean, & Gray, 1989; Strom, Gray, Dean, & Fischer, 1987). Strom et al. demonstrated a substantial increase (from 16 to 30%) in the variability accounted for in school achievement with the addition of the HRNB tests to information obtained from the WISC-R. Using regression equations from each Wide Range Achievement Subtest, each WISC-R and each HRNB scale, they demonstrated individual beta weights, and subsequently reported canonical weights (> $\pm$ .30) for WISC-R, WRAT, and HRNB subtests to illustrate unique contributions of each HRNB scale to the prediction of each of the three WRAT measures (Reading, Spelling, and Arithmetic).

More specific relationships with discrete verbal comprehension factors were reported in the D'Amato et al. (1987) paper, which found highest loadings for school achievement on two HRNB tests (Speech Sounds Perception and TMT-B) and one WISC-R subtest (Arithmetic) again suggesting that HRNB measures may address school achievement criterion measures as well as or better than strictly intellective (e.g., WISC-R) measures. The work of Rattan et al. (1989) and Rattan, Rattan, Gray, & Dean (1987) assessed the commonality of HRNB and WISC-R factors with learning-disabled children, and found that Speech Perception best predicted Similarities, Information, and Vocabulary subtests, with Tactual Performance Test total time the best predictor of Comprehension, Picture Completion and Picture Arrangement. Rhythm Test predicted Digit Span and Arithmetic, while Category Test accounted for the greatest amount of variability in the Block Design subtest. TPT-Memory best predicted Object Assembly, and TMT-B accounted for the greatest portion of variability in the Digit Symbol subtest. While these Rattan studies address HRNB correlates of WISC-R scales rather than specifically ecological measures, the elucidation of HRNB correlates involving these familiar WISC-R scales may help cast some light on the neuropsychological substrates of performance on these (WISC-R) scales, and thus provide some guidelines concerning specific HRNB substrates of given ecological measures.

In an early series of factor analyses of neuropsychological tests, Klonoff and his associates (e.g., Crockett, Klonoff, & Bjerring, 1969; Klonoff, 1971; Klonoff, Robinson, & Thompson, 1969) had identified approximately 14 factors independent of psychometric measures of intelligence. These factors interdependent with WISC performance variables, one factor interdependent with WISC verbal variable and one factor derived from WISC verbal variables. This early research was intended to provide clinical investigators with data which could be used to produce accurate estimates of the cognitive dimensions, through use of regression weights used to compute factor scales. These studies, especially Klonoff (1971) provide a fairly comprehensive overview of how discrete neuropsychological measures contribute to such ecological constructs as verbal fluency, motor speed, manipulative dexterity, form reproduction accuracy, and auditory recognition.

Other investigators have looked more closely at age and sex correlates of the HRNB, including both psychometric and behavioral measures. Klesges (1983) and Klesges and Fisher (1981) reported a number of behavioral checklist (CACD) correlates with Halstead-Reitan tests, as well as some age and sex covariates, and proposed that better age and sex correlated norms may be needed to optimally evaluate performance on HRNB measurements with children. Perhaps the greatest interest in HRNB correlates has involved common variance with intellective measures, and a number of investigators have emphasized the importance of considering IQ level in the interpretation of HRNB children's performance (e.g., Seidenberg, Giordani, Berent, & Boll, 1983), although some researchers have addressed more ecologically relevant issues such as the relationship of given HRNB Children's Test items with measures like nonverbal cognitive ability or reasoning (e.g., Telzrow & Harr, 1987); or finger recognition skills with reading achievement (e.g., Fletcher, Taylor, Morris, & Satz, 1982). In general, most studies have not combined to contribute a great deal of specific information concerning the ecological validity of the specific HRNB scales, insofar as factors such as IQ, age, and sex have not been systematically controlled. In large sample studies where some attempt has been made to partial out or covary one or more of these variables, however (e.g., Strom et al., 1987), HRNB scales have demonstrated impressive relationships with such validity criteria as academic skill levels.

LURIA NEBRASKA NEUROPSYCHOLOGICAL BATTERY FOR CHILDREN

Although of fairly recent origin, the Luria-Nebraska Neuropsychological Battery-Children's Revision (LNNB-C) (Golden, 1981; Plaisted, Gustavson, Wilkening, & Golden, 1983) has been the subject of a fair amount of research with implications for ecological validity. Sweet and associates (e.g., Carr, Sweet, & Rossini, 1985; Sweet, Carr, Rossini, & Kaspar, 1986) found that the LNNB-C and WISC-R contained relatively unique information for psychiatric and control groups, but not for neurologically impaired patients: that is, correlations between WISC-R and LNNB-C approached significance mainly with the neurologically impaired children. Using the Kaufman WISC-R factors, Sweet et al. (1986) found that earlier studies showing relationships between LNNB-C and WISC-R factors had this apparent relationship spuriously elevated by the inclusion of brain-injured children, and that with a non-neurologic population the LNNB-C and WISC-R, in fact, had few correlations. This is a potentially important distinction, as it suggests that, at least with non-neurologically impaired samples, correlations of LNNB scales with external criterion measures of ecological validity there would be no need to partial out or covary mental ability

As a demonstration of how this might have implications in an applied setting, Hale and Foltz (1982) found that the addition of the LNNB-C Pathognomonic scale not only increased the predictability of adolescent academic achievement, but the amount of variance shared between achievement and the 34 items composing the modified Pathognomonic scale was greater than that shared between the intelligence and achievement measures. Further, the modified Luria Pathognomonic scores by themselves were viable predictors of academic achievement. Specifically, regression procedures for reading, spelling, and arithmetic produced R^2 values significant at p .0001, .0002, and .0001, respectively using Pathognomonic scale as the predictor.

In a study comparing K-ABC and LNNB-C, Kruszecki (1987) found essentially comparable-sized relationships between LNNB-C and SRA reading, language, and math scores as occurred between LNNB-C and K-ABC subtest scales, suggesting somewhat greater overlap among LNNB-C and these (K-ABC) psychometric measures than those prevailing between LNNB-C and WISC-R scales. Viewed from a somewhat different perspective, low correlations were found between the LNNB-C and the Minnesota PerceptoDiagnostic Test (Snow, Hartlage, Hynd, & Grant, 1983), although the MPD correlated with all nine subscales of the California Achievement Test (Fuller & Wallbrown, 1983). Research with the LNNB-c suggests that the individual factor scores may have potential for prediction to ecological validity criteria, independent of overlap with psychometric intellective factors, to an extent considerably greater than that of the HRNB-C (e.g., Snow, Hynd, & Hartlage, 1983).

OTHER MEASURES

Although there is no doubt that the Wechsler Intelligence Scale for Children (WISC-R) has potential for some level of neuropsychological assessment, and in fact is typically included in neuropsychological assessment batteries (e.g., Hartlage & Telzrow, 1980; Seretny, Dean, Gray, & Hartlage, 1986), there is little support for its use as an independent measure of neuropsychological status. There are data suggesting relationships between given subtests and discrete achievement measures (e.g., Kaufman, 1975), with perhaps greatest coherence between the verbal comprehension factor and all achievement measures; the perceptual organization factor and reading and spelling measures; and the freedom from distractibility factor and arithmetic measures (e.g., Stedman, Lawlis, Cortner, & Achterberg, 1978). In general, the nature of these correlations is well described by White (1979), who reports that information yielded by the Peabody Individual Achievement Test may be obtained through WISC-R results.

In a fashion somewhat similar to that which prevails for the WISC-R, the Bender Visual Motor Gestalt Test, while often used in neuropsychological assessment, cannot be defended as a single item test for neuropsychological assessment. Unlike the WISC-R, however, the Bender-Gestalt is heavily weighted by maturational factors which do not have the same type of age factors inherent in the Wechsler scales. As a result, the Bender Gestalt may assess somewhat different factors at differing developmental stages, with its potential for predicting academic success greater at younger age levels (Keough & Smith, 1967). Although the magnitudes of correlations between Bender Gestalt scores and academic achievement tend to be sufficient to reach statistical significance in early school grades, this instrument is not considered to represent a neuropsychological assessment procedure which offers a unique contribution to the prediction of academic achievement or other ecological relevant criteria (Chang & Chang, 1967; Wright & DeMers, 1982). Other instruments, scales, or procedures commonly used in neuropsychological assessment of children tend to be of such a specialized or narrow focus that their predictive validity to a range of ecological criterion measures is not supported, except insofar as has been demonstrated by individual validation studies. The Beery Test of Visual Motor Integration, for example, has a number of studies relating performance to some ecological criterion referents (Beery, 1982), but is not an independent neuropsychological scale and has many of the same ecological relationship features as the Bender Gestalt.

In an attempt to determine whether some neurologic phenomena typically assessed in the child neurological examination relate to classroom success, Hartlage and Hartlage (1973) compared neurological examination findings with teacher ratings of children. Subsequent work involving a larger sample of presumably normal third graders with an expanded list of classroom behaviors named by teachers as important to school success correlated these items with 19 measures from neurologic examination (quantified to ordinal scaling, using essentially the same format as LNNB-C scaling). Results are listed in Table 1. As can be seen, teacher ratings of attention (paying attention) and attention span tended to produce significant correlations, ranging as high as .82 for left hand symbol recognition with attention span .78 with paying attention. WRAT reading and arithmetic rank in class also tended to approach significance with a number of neurologic examination items, such as correlations of .84 and .77 between fact dominance and WRAT reading and arithmetic rank, respectively. Behavioral phenomena tended to be less related to neurologic examination items, with one classroom behavior considered by teachers to be important for classroom success (frequently volunteers) not related to any of the 19 neurologic examination items. While these neurological examination items are not typically included in neuropsychological examinations of children, the overlap of some items (e.g., finger tip symbol writing, tapping speed, dominance) from both examination procedures to suggest a degree of ecological relevance to at least some classroom behaviors considered important for school success by teachers. Perhaps of more consequence are the collected data relating neurologic substrates to a variety of external criterion measures, since these help suggest possible relationships potentially involved in comparable neuropsychological test items with these ecological measures.

TABLE 1
CORRELATIONS BETWEEN NEUROLOGICAL MEASURES AND VARIOUS COGNITIVE AND BEHAVIORAL VARIABLES

Neurological Measure	Arithmetic Rank	WRAT Reading	D-A-P S.S.	"Attention"	"Sits Still"	"Attention Span"	"Follows Directions"
Finger Tip Symbol Writing (Rt. Hand)	*** .559	*** .621	-.121	*** .720	.205	*** .742	*** .739
Finger Tip Symbol Writing (Lt. Hand)	*** .522	*** .588	-.183	*** .780	** .293	*** .826	*** .820
Seconds Balancing on One Foot	*** .357	*** .393	*** .497	*** .535	** .304	*** .617	*** .580
Tapping Speed/10 Seconds (Right Hand)	.231	.242	*** .440	*** .446	.174	*** .462	*** .449
Tapping Speed/10 Seconds (Left Hand)	.085	.097	*** .347	** .297	.164	*** .370	** .308
Tapping Speed/10 Seconds (Right Foot)	.181	.126	*** .415	*** .404	.142	*** .393	*** .342
Tapping Speed/10 Seconds (Left Foot)	.121	.154	*** 339	*** .548	.185	*** .492	*** .463
Hand Tremor, Eyes Closed (Right Hand)	*** .377	*** .464	-.221	*** .695	* .245	*** .666	*** .732
Hand Tremor, Eyes Closed (Left Hand)	* .264	.205	-.198	*** .457	.222	*** .503	*** .569
Hand Tremor, Eyes Closed (Both Hands)	.225	*** .442	-.100	*** .422	* .272	*** .338	*** .384
Hand Dominance	*** .662	*** .717	*** .338	*** .679	** .296	*** .695	*** .719
Foot Dominance	*** .773	*** .841	** .291	*** .670	.231	*** .644	*** .704
Eye Dominance	*** .468	*** .368	* .278	-.006	.063	-.002	.042
Right-Left Orientation (Single)	*** .424	*** .429	.113	.279	.108	.302	* .282
Right-Left Orientation (Complex)	*** .394	*** .430	.192	.219	.197	.196	** .297
Right-Left Orientation (Very Complex)	*** .511	*** .526	.035	.184	.203	.185	* .243
Mirror Movements (Right Hand)	*** .453	*** .585	.089	*** .586	.276	*** .601	*** .587
Mirror Movements (Left Hand)	*** .501	*** .647	-.037	*** .593	** .307	*** .617	*** .636
Tongue Dysdiadochokinesis	*** .618	*** .598	*** .368	*** .341	.100	*** .391	*** .447

(Continued on next page)

TABLE 1
CORRELATIONS BETWEEN NEUROLOGICAL MEASURES AND VARIOUS COGNITIVE AND BEHAVIORAL VARIABLES

Neurological Measure	Easy to Control	Even Tempered	Neatly Written Work	Works Hard for Approval	Frequently Volunteers	Cooperative	Well-liked	Friendly
Finger Tip Symbol Writing (Rt. Hand)	.045	.004	.167	.056	-.177	.128	-.020	-.093
Finger Tip Symbol Writing (Lt. Hand)	.149	.065	.089	.034	-.221	.120	.001	-.025
Seconds Balancing on One Foot	-.189	-.076	.065	-.129	.103	-.209	-.064	-.192
Tapping Speed/10 Seconds (Right Hand)	.110	.119	-.067	-.214	-.205	-.189	-.189	.111
Tapping Speed/10 Seconds (Left Hand)	.035	.074	.073	-.204	-.231	-.108	-.218	.161
Tapping Speed/10 Seconds (Right Foot)	-.014	.076	.106	-.321**	-.028	-.225	-.084	.072
Tapping Speed/10 Seconds (Left Foot)	.024	.026	-.053	-.138	-.024	-.075	-.114	.212
Hand Tremor, Eyes Closed (Right Hand)	.145	.038	-.011	.182	-.126	.251*	-.100	-.191
Hand Tremor, Eyes Closed (Left Hand)	.268*	.096	.041	.257*	-.107	.324**	.055	-.108
Hand Tremor, Eyes Closed (Both Hands)	.431***	.349***	.080	.239	.005	.262*	.070	.141
Hand Dominance	-.186	-.230	.136	-.083	.129	-.273*	.093	-.123
Foot Dominance	-.194	-.342***	.158	.114	.242	.005	.004	-.018
Eye Dominance	-.166	-.232	.134	-.106	-.189	-.350***	-.213	-.131**
Right-Left Orientation (Single)	-.018	-.039	-.030	-.260*	-.119	-.108	-.120	.294
Right-Left Orientation (Complex)	-.139	-.184	-.145	-.246*	-.042	-.115	-.153	.076
Right-Left Orientation (Very Complex)	.320**	.233	-.093	-.203	-.154	.015	-.266*	.249
Mirror Movements (Right Hand)	-.178	-.115	-.048	-.004	.065	-.052	-.201	-.278*
Mirror Movements (Left Hand)	.001	.024	.096	.097	.215	.166	-.122**	-.002
Tongue Dysdiadochokinesis	-.060	-.139	-.286*	-.162	.157	-.066	-.308**	-.205

***p<.001   **p<.01   *p<.05

So what is the status of ecological validity of neuropsychological assessment with children? As has been mentioned, the relative fluidity and amorphous nature of such criterion measures as school grades suggests that more objective but indirect criterion measures (e.g., achievement test scores) may offer the most defensible measures of relevant ecological validity. Using that criterion, the venerable and well-researched Halstead-Reitan Neuropsychological Battery for Children offers correlations of rather consistently impressive magnitude, although the overlap of intellectual factors tends to obscure the nature of the actual relationships. By contrast, the Luria-Nebraska Neuropsychological Battery-Children's Revision appears to assess—at least in normal and psychiatrically impaired children—discrete abilities which do not have a major intellectual component. Certainly the comparatively discrete and crystallized nature of abilities sampled by the given LNNB-C scales lends itself to multivariate correlations with given ecological validity criterion measures, and research has in fact shown that the LNNB-C is a powerful predictor of academic achievement, both superseding predictive validity of the WISC-R and combining with the WISC-R to increase its predictive validity (e.g., Hale & Foltz, 1982). As with any relatively new neuropsychological procedure, the early research has necessarily tended to address validity for accurate neuropsychological diagnosis, with secondary emphasis on consideration with existing neuropsychological test batteries. Now that the LNNB-C has addressed these two requirements, it can move to the new arena, that of ecological validity. It is hoped that the attention to this issue, addressed by this volume and especially in this brief overview, will be enhanced and accelerated by this attention, and that a review of the topic at the conclusion of this decade of the brain will be able to cite a broader and more comprehensive range of ecological validity criterion measures than now grace the literature in this exciting and promising arena.

REFERENCES

Beery, K. E. (1982). *Revised administration scoring and teaching manual for the developmental test of visual-motor interpretation.* New York: Follett Publishing Co.

Carr, M. A., Sweet, J. J., & Rossini, E. (1985). Diagnostic validity of the Luria-Nebraska Neuropsychological Battery-Children's Revision. *Journal of Clinical and Consulting Psychology, 54,* 354-358.

Chang, T. M., & Chang, V. A. (1967). Relation of visual-motor skills and reading achievement in primary-grade pupils of superior ability. *Perceptual and Motor Skills, 24,* 51-53.

Crockett, D., Klonoff, H., & Bjerring, J. (1969). Factor analysis of neuropsychological tests. *Perceptual and Motor Skills, 29,* 791-802.

D'Amato, R. C., Gray, J. W., & Dean, R. S. (1988). Construct validity of the PPVT with neuropsychological, intellectual, and achievement measures. *Journal of Clinical Psychology, 44(6),* 934-935.

Fletcher, J. M., Taylor, H. G., Morris, R., & Satz, P. (1982). Finger recognition skills and reading achievement: A developmental neuropsychological analysis. *Developmental Psychology, 18(1),* 124-132.

Fuller, G. B., & Wallbrown, F. H. (1983). Comparison of the Minnesota Percepto-Diagnostic test and Bender-Gestalt: Relationship with achievement criteria. *Journal of Clinical Psychology, 39(6),* 985-988.

Golden, C. J. (1981). The Luria-Nebraska children's battery: Theory and formulation. In G. W. Hynd & J. E. Obrzut (Eds.), *Neuropsychological assessment and the school-age child: Issues and procedures.* New York: Grune & Stratton.

Hartlage, L. C. (1974). Pre-reading screening to determine optimum reading instructional approaches. *Reading Improvement, 11(1),* 7-9.

Hartlage, L. C. (1975a). Differential age correlates of reading ability. *Perceptual and Motor Skills, 41,* 968-970.

Hartlage, L. C. (1975b). Neuropsychological approaches to predicting outcome of remedial educational strategies for learning disabled children. *Pediatric Psychology, 7(3),* 23.

Hartlage, L. C. (1979). *Management of common clinical problems: Learning disabilities. School Related Health Care* (pp. 28-37). (Ross Laboratories, Monograph #9)

Hartlage, L. C. (1982). Overview of neuropsychological evaluation of learning disabilities. In *Vocational rehabilitation of persons with learning disabilities: Evaluation eligibility. Planning and placement.* Washington, DC: George Washington University RIUI.

Hartlage, L. C., & Hartlage, P. L. (1973). *Relative contributions of neurology and neuropsychology in the diagnosis of learning disabilities.* International Neuropsychological Society, New Orleans (Feb.).

Hartlage, L. C., & Lucas, D. G. (1973). Predicting reading ability in first grade children. *Perceptual and Motor Skills, 34,* 447-450.

Hartlage, L. C., & Telzrow, C. F. (1980). The practice of clinical neuropsychology in the U.S. *Clinical Neuropsychology,* (3), 200-202. 17

Hartlage, L. C., & Telzrow, C. F. (1981). *Neuropsychological assessment and intervention with children and adolescents.* Sarasota, FL: Professional Resource Exchange.

Hartlage, L. C., & Telzrow, C. F. (1986). *Neuropsychological assessment and intervention with children.* Sarasota, FL: Professional Resource Exchange.

Hynd, G. W., & Hartlage, L. C. (1982). Brain-behavior relationships in children: Neuropsychological assessment in the schools. In G. W. Hynd (Ed.), *The school psychologist: An introduction.* Syracuse: Syracuse University Press.

Kaufman, A. S. (1975). Factor analysis of the WISC-R at 11 age levels between 6 1/2 and 16 1/2 years. *Journal of Consulting and Clinical Psychology, 43,* 135-147.

Kaufman, J., Belmont, I., Birch, H., & Zach, L. (1973). Tactile and visual sense system interactions: A developmental study using reaction time models. *Developmental Psychobiology, 6(2),* 165-176.

Keough, B. H., & Smith, C. E. (1967). Visuo-motor ability for school prediction: A seven year study. *Perceptual and Motor Skills, 25,* 101-110.

Klesges, R. L. (1983). The relationship between neuropsychological, cognitive, and behavioral assessments of brain functioning in children. *Clinical Neuropsychology, 5(1),* 28-37.

Klesges, R. L., & Fisher, L. P. (1981). A multiple criterion approach to the assessment of brain damage in children. *Clinical Neuropsychology, 3,* 6-11.

Klonoff, H. (1971). Factor analysis of a neuropsychological battery for children aged 9 to 14. *Perceptual and Motor Skills, 32,* 603-616.

Klonoff, H., Robinson, G., & Thompson, G. (1969). Acute and chronic brain syndromes in children. *Developmental Medicine and Child Neurology, 2,* 198-213.

Kruszecki, L. S. (1987). *The relationship between the Kaufman Assessment Battery for Children and the Luria-Nebraska Neuropsychological Battery-Children's Revision in a sample of black low academic achievers.* Dissertation submitted to California School of Professional Psychology-Berkley.

Lawton, M. S., & Seim, R. D. (1973). Developmental investigation of tactual-visual integration with reading achievement. *Perceptual and Motor Skills, 36,* 375-382.

Luria, A. R. (1969). Frontal lobe symptoms. In P. J. Vicken & G. W. Bruyn (Eds.), *Handbook of clinical neurology* (Vol. II). Amsterdam: North Holland Publishing Company.

Plaistedn, J. R., Gustavson, J. L., Wilkening, G. N., & Golden, C. J. (1983). The Luria-Nebraska Neuropsychological Battery-Children's Revision: Theory and current research findings. *Journal of Clinical Child Psychology, 12,* 13-21.

Rattan, A. I., Rattan, G., Dean, R. S., & Gray, J. W. (1989). Assessing the commonality of the WISC-R and the Halstead-Reitan Neuropsychological Test Battery with learning disordered children. *Journal of Psychoeducational Assessment, 7,* 296-303.

Rattan, A. I., Rattan, G., Gray, J. W., & Dean, R. S. (1987, March). *Defining neuropsychological constructs of the WISC-R with learning disabled children.* Paper presented at 19th Annual National Association of School Psychologists' Convention, New Orleans, LA.

Seidenberg, M., Giordani, B., Berent, S. A., & Boll, T. (1983). IQ level and performance on the Halstead-Reitan Neuropsychological Test Battery for older children. *Journal of Consulting and Clinical Psychology, 51(3),* 406-413.

Seretny, M., Dean, R., Gray, J., & Hartlage, L. (1986). The practice of clinical neuropsychology in the United States. *Archives of Clinical Neuropsychology, 1(1),* 5-12.

Snow, J. H., Hartlage, L. C., Hynd, G. W., & Grant, D. H. (1983). The relationship between the Luria-Nebraska Neuropsychological Battery-Children's Revision and the Minnesota Percepto-Diagnostic Test with learning disabled students. *Psychology in the Schools, 20,* 415-419.

Snow, J. H., Hynd, G. W., & Hartlage, L. C. (1983). Differences between mildly and more severely learning-disabled children on the Luria-Nebraska Neuropsychological Battery-Children's Revision. *Journal of Psychoeducational Assessment, 2(1),* 23-28.

Stedman, J. M., Lawlis, G. F., Cortner, R. H., & Achterberg, G. (1978). Relationship between WISC-R factors, wide range achievement test scores, and visual-motor maturation in children referred for psychological evaluation. *Journal of Consulting and Clinical Psychology, 46(5),* 859-872.

Strom, D. A., Gray, J. W., Dean, R. S., & Fischer, W. E. (1987). The incremental validity of the Halstead-Reitan Neuropsychological Battery in children. *Journal of Psychoeducational Assessment, 2,* 157-165.

Sweet, J. J., Carr, M. A., Rossini, E., & Kaspar, C. (1986). Relationship between the Luria-Nebraska Neuropsychological Battery-Children's Revision and the WISC-R: Further examination using Kaufman's factors. *Clinical Neuropsychology, 8(4),* 177-180.

Telzrow, C. F., & Harr, G. A. (1987). Common variance among three measures of nonverbal cognitive ability: WISC-R performance scale, WJPB-TCA reasoning cluster, and Halstead category test. *Journal of School Psychology, 25,* 93-95.

Terman, L. M., & Merrill, M. A. (1960). *Stanford-Binet Intelligence Scale manual for the third revision, form L-M.* Boston: Houghton-Mifflin Co.

White, T. W. (1979). Correlations among the WISC-R, PIAT and DAM. *Psychology in the Schools, 16(4),* 497-500.

Wright, D., & DeMers, S. T. (1982). Comparison of the relationship between two measures of visual-motor coordination and academic achievement. *Psychology in the Schools, 19,* 473-477.

16

PERSONALITY TESTS

Tedd Judd, Ph.D., A.B.P.P., A.B.C.N.
David Fordyce, Ph.D.

ABSTRACT

Ecologically valid assessment of personality and emotions following brain injury requires innovations beyond psychology's traditional self-report personality inventories and psychiatry's criterion-based diagnostic classifications. New techniques are specific to neuropsychological phenomena, use informants to circumvent anosognosia, and attempt to distinguish pre- from post-injury personality. Many include behavioral observations, and accommodate to cognitive limitations. Still lacking are adequate theories of post-brain injury personality, generalization of validity to various specific contexts (e.g., home, school, work, community, different cultures), adequate techniques for assessing pre-injury personality and distinguishing adjustment reactions from organic changes, and integrated assessment of personality and cognition.

INTRODUCTION

One night a drunk was searching the ground under a street lamp. A passerby asked, "What are you looking for?"
"My keys."
"Where did you drop them?"
"Over there."
"Then why are you looking for them here?"
"Because the light is better."

Clinical neuropsychology has sometimes been accused of acting like that drunk. Lavish attention has been given to measuring the changes in cognition resulting from brain injury because this can be done relatively easily, that is, the light is better, while the changes in emotions and personality, though perhaps the most disabling of the changes which follow brain injury, are harder to measure and often get neglected.

In recent years, the changes of personality and emotions following brain injury have begun to receive the attention they deserve, largely due to the increasing realization that they are often the changes which have the greatest impact on the quality of life after brain injury (Ponsford, 1990). The importance of these changes has been recognized largely through the experiences of post-acute head trauma rehabilitation facilities and confirmed through surveys of persons with brain injury and their families. Catalogs of these changes are common in the proliferation of books and journals on head trauma rehabilitation (e.g., Corey, 1987; Pepping & Roueche, 1991; Prigatano, 1992; Sohlberg & Mateer, 1989; Williams & Long, 1987; Ylvisaker & Gobble, 1987). But many difficulties with our science are also being recognized. How can we best conceptualize, evaluate, predict, and treat the changes in personality resulting from brain injury? How can we relate those changes to pre-brain-injury personality? How can we make sure the measures used are ecologically valid? These are all still unanswered questions in a rapidly developing field.

This chapter attempts to address some of these nascent issues. The authors review the nature of personality and emotions in the person with brain injury as it is currently understood. There is a description of the implications of this understanding for the accurate neuropsychological assessment of personality and emotions, with particular emphasis on desirable features of tests. Then these implications are compared with currently available and prevalent tests and practices, and followed by a discussion on prudent approaches to neuropsychological personality assessment with currently available techniques. Finally, directions for future research are outlined.

APPROACHES TO PERSONALITY ASSESSMENT

The general purpose of clinical personality assessment is to evaluate individual differences in order to assist in the prediction of human behavior. Thus, any personality assessment tool or program has as its goal to achieve high predictive validity for the person's behavior in some specific setting (American Psychological Association, 1954; Cronbach & Meehl, 1955). For example, the Minnesota Multiphasic Personality Inventory (MMPI) has been shown to be a good clinical predictor of an individual's personality behavior which may later be seen in the workplace (Heaton, Chelune, & Lehman, 1978; Newman, Heaton, & Lehman, 1978; Prigatano et al., 1984).

In general, neuropsychology has focused on diagnosis and description rather than prediction of behavior. Historically, the most-emphasized purpose of clinical neuropsychological evaluation has been to determine the presence or absence of brain injury (at least in the U.S.). In addition, traditional neuropsychology has attempted to elucidate and describe clinical syndromes and formulate knowledge of brain-behavior relationships. While of great interest, these activities are not, in and of themselves, related to either the theory or practice of behavioral prediction. Certain studies compared performance on neuropsychological tests to other measures of psycho-social function (for review see Acker, 1986; Chelune, 1985; Heaton & Pendelton, 1981). These post hoc analyses gratifyingly yielded significant correlations, albeit modest in scope. Currently there is an increasing appreciation of a need to change orientation towards the "ecological validity" of neuropsychological assessment, that is, relating the consequences of brain injury to behaviors of importance in daily life. Hopefully this change in orientation will prevail and not be impeded by our diagnostic-descriptive heritage.

While this chapter focuses on tests of personality and emotional behavior, it should be understood that this is for the sake of organization only. Any attempt to understand the personality and emotional functioning of a brain-injured person also requires an assessment of cognitive functioning. Furthermore, distinctions between cognitive and emotional variables are unclear. The following discussion of the multiple factors which contribute to personality and emotional behavior highlights the importance of not imposing artificial categorizations on human behavior. The validity issues discussed apply to both cognitive and personality tests.

Neuropsychologists should have a working knowledge of the psychology of individual differences in personality traits; of the means by which the environment may modify behavioral and emotional dispositions; of whether test or behavioral measures reflect "signs" or "samples" of behavior; and of the implications of all these factors and others on issues of reliability, validity, and generalizability of test behaviors (e.g., Wiggins, 1973). However, traditional personality theory and assessment practice is heterogenous in nature and differing opinions and strategies exist. These differences have important implications for more refined assessment of emotional variables following brain injury. A good text on personality assessment should occupy a primary place in the neuropsychologist's library and be reviewed frequently, especially when considering the merits of a new psychological tool, whether it measures personality or cognitive skills. In reality, the evaluation of personality and emotions after brain injury is usually based on a mixture of theory and methods from behavioral neurology, traditional psychiatry, psychometric testing, and neuropsychology.

BEHAVIORAL NEUROLOGY APPROACH

The primary approach of behavioral neurology to the evaluation of personality and emotions after brain injury has been the qualitative evaluation of behavior primarily through interviews and direct observation during the neurological examination and the mental status examination. These techniques are an indispensable part of the neuropsychologist's repertoire, especially when testing proves impossible or inadequate. Behavioral rating scales have sometimes been used to supplement and standardize these techniques.

PSYCHIATRIC MODEL

The psychiatric model seeks to classify the disorders of personality and emotions. Some diagnostic categories are based on known or suspected brain injury. The most recent and authoritative example of this model is the Diagnostic and Statistical Manual IV (DSM-IV) (American Psychiatric Association, 1994). This system employs a criterion-based approach to classifying psychiatric disorders by the presence or absence of certain combinations of signs and symptoms at specified times. While more objective than past psychiatric diagnostic methods, the determination of the presence or absence of these criteria is usually based on clinical judgment, often drawing on unspecified or unstandardized procedures.

The DSM-IV psychiatric classification system reasonably attempts to distinguish long-term personality disorders from more acute emotional disorders. It also allows for a rough assessment of general medical condition, level of recent stress, and general level of recent adaptive functioning as part of a multiaxial evaluation format. Some diagnostic categories relate directly to the presence of brain injury (e.g., Delirium, Mental Disorders due to a General Medical Condition, Dementia, Amnestic Disorder, various conditions related to substance abuse) though their applicability and utility varies (Grant & Alves, 1987).

The DSM-IV system is somewhat helpful in separating persons with disorders of personality and behavior not due to brain injury from those where brain injury is a factor. It is an improvement over its predecessor, DSM-III-R, (American Psychiatric Association, 1987), in that it more clearly recognizes that changes in personality may result directly from brain injury and that they may be distinct from mental disorders not resulting from brain injury. It is also useful for certain health care administrative functions. DSM-IV can typically be used with some accuracy by many mental health workers. It is not adequate, however, for the more detailed distinctions that are typically elaborated in a competent neuropsychological assessment. For example, the system provides only minimal methods for describing personality qualities that fall short of a formal personality disorder, cultural factors are given only superficial treatment, and several important diagnostic entities are considered provisional (e.g., post-concussional disorder, mild neurocognitive disorder).

In spite of considerable advantages, this particular category-criteria system has significant limitations for neuropsychology. The person equipped with only this system is much like the person whose only tool is a hammer, and who therefore sees screws, hooks, bolts, and other hardware as nails. Much of the research on emotional problems following brain injury presupposes that the categories and criteria of emotional difficulties represented in DSM-IV and especially its predecessors also apply to people with brain injury. Typical research might ask questions such as, "What is the incidence of depression following right- as contrasted with left-hemisphere stroke?" It is less common that such research will ask whether or not the categories of emotional problems observed in people with intact brains are appropriate to those with injured brains. (For example, see the discussion of depression-like symptoms following right hemisphere stroke in the "Interactions" section below.) Nevertheless, we cannot assume that the emotional problems of those with brain injury will be the same as the problems of those with intact brains. In fact, the clinical case literature suggests that there are good reasons to suppose otherwise.

PSYCHOMETRIC APPROACH

The psychometric approach measures human behavior (usually verbal) through standardized, and often highly structured, questions and stimuli. An element of this approach is dedicated to finding alternative, more objective, ways of classifying psychiatric disorders. In addition, the psychometric approach attempts to measure and describe personality, emotional or behavioral characteristics irrespective of the presence or absence of mental disorders. While the psychiatric and psychometric approaches to personality assessment have relevance for neuropsychology, many of the personality changes resulting from brain injury are now recognized to be distinctive; they cannot be accurately described solely in terms of the psychopathology or personalities of persons with intact brains. Therefore, tests developed for neurologically intact populations may have doubtful or limited relevance and validity for brain-injured populations.

NEUROPSYCHOLOGICAL APPROACH

Psychiatry's categorical, diagnostic, psychopathological orientation to personality assessment contrasts with psychometry's approach measuring noncategorical, normal variations in personality. Similarly, early neuropsychology "categorically" validated a test by demonstrating its capacity to distinguish a mixed group of brain-injured subjects from normals (Reitan, 1955). With the growing influence of cognitive psychology there has been a greater emphasis on tests which illuminate the changes in the thought processes of selected populations of brain-injured subjects. The former diagnostic approach is often applied in assessments which seek to differentiate the presence or absence of brain injury, while the latter qualitative and quantitative feature-oriented approach has found favor in assessments which seek to direct rehabilitation and treatment, usually in individuals with known brain injury. These complementary assessment purposes can also be applied to tests of personality and emotions. That is, a personality test can be considered to be a neuropsychological test to the degree that it either discriminates individuals with brain injury from those without or accurately describes features of personality, emotions, and behavior resulting from brain injury. Only quite recently have assessment tools begun to emerge which can be thought of as true neuropsychological measures of personality and emotions. None of these has yet been fully researched nor received widespread acceptance.

ECOLOGICAL APPROACH

The ecological validity of an assessment tool is its relationship to meaningful daily behavior (a combination of face and criterion validity). Some recent research evaluating changes in personality and emotions following brain injury can be viewed as embodying a more ecological approach than the psychiatric and psychometric models which preceded it. Surveys and catalogs which emphasize psychosocial adjustment specific to home or work environments have emerged from post-acute rehabilitation facilities and out-patient programs with community and vocational experience. This orientation based on social and practical skills is in contrast to the earlier models which emerged from hospitals, out-patient mental health clinics and universities. Of course, the ecological validity of these tools and approaches needs to be established empirically and new test development, or modification of existing assessment tools, is time-consuming and costly. The more ecological neuropsychology approach has also found its way into the practice of many neuropsychologists, particularly in the interview phase of assessment.

Issues of the ecological validity of neuropsychological tests of personality and emotions almost immediately raise corollary questions. Which ecology or environment? Whose validity? What aspects of personality and emotions?

Which ecology or environment?

The concept of ecological validity suggests that the clinician benefits from a working knowledge of the social, cultural, familial, economic, physical, and intellectual contexts from which their clients come and to which they will (hopefully) return. Some behaviors and personality traits are considered acceptable or usual in some cultures and contexts, but deviant in other cultures or contexts. Some knowledge of context can be gleaned from technical expertise and the history taken, but some must come from the life experience of the clinician. To give just one illustration, knowledge which is generally available about psychological aspects of culture often far exceeds what can be obtained from tests or professional literature. As the Salvadoran psychologist, Martín-Baró (1991, p. 320), observed: ". . . one learns considerably more about the psychology of the peoples of Latin America by reading a novel by García Márquez or Vargas Llosa, than by reading our technical works on character and personality."

Not only does "ecological validity" imply a knowledge of environment, but the acquisition of a brain injury often means a significant change in environment. At the extreme it may lead to institutionalization. At intermediate levels it may lead to a change of jobs, schools, homes, family constellations, and relationships. At milder levels it may only introduce an additional social context to a life—a context of therapies, support groups, lawyers, bureaucracies, etc. It may be hard to know if certain behavior changes reflect brain injury or a change of contexts. For instance, "ecological" observations of behavior are often carried out in the context of some sort of rehabilitation program, which generally was not a part of the person's "ecological context" prior to the brain injury. Evaluations in the home are uncommon, although their advantages are coming to be recognized (Starch & Falltrick, 1990).

The question of "Whose environment?" is ultimately a question of the intended and actual use of the assessment tool. For example, a behavioral rating scale designed for use with a chronic, severely impaired population might be legitimately validated in an institutional setting. This would not assure its ecological validity, in other circumstances, however, for example, if the scale was used to rate a hospitalized individual in a state of acute traumatic amnesia, that rating might not be very useful in predicting that person's future behavior upon returning home. Similarly, a tool developed and validated in a Zulu community in South Africa may not generalize to East Asian immigrants in Scotland.

Whose validity?

The common lack of awareness of personality change in persons who have experienced brain injury suggests that they themselves should not necessarily be the ultimate reference point for validity, although it would be a strange type of validity, indeed, that left them out entirely. But in going beyond the individual with the injury, how are informants to be chosen? Most often in clinical practice and in research the informant is whichever family member is willing, able, and available to come to the clinic at an appointed weekday daytime hour. Although such informants of convenience are important and their use is a significant advance over the individual interview, they still generally represent only one component of the individual's social context. It seems fairly likely that there could be significant differences between personality and behavior problems manifested at work and those that might be manifested at home, for example.

Again, the question of "Whose validity?" is ultimately a question of the intended use of the instrument. Predicting whether or not someone will be a safe, reliable, and productive employee may be quite different from predicting divorce, and will most likely address distinct interests of different populations.

Which aspects of personality and emotions?

Medical-legal liability, disability-pension, and current health insurance systems in the U.S. often require categorical diagnoses and ascertainments of employability. Often de-emphasized are personality changes resulting from brain injury which may be positive (Ranseen, 1990), personality and behavior problems which fall short of formal psychiatric diagnoses, which may be manifested primarily outside the workplace, or which may not be clearly attributable to injury. Yet, at times, any of these may have greater ecological significance than diagnosable disorders attributable to injury. The context of demonstrated validity and appropriate use for an instrument, then, may well reflect the social forces which brought about its existence.

Even sweeping these institutional and societal pressures aside, the question of ecological validity has two distinct strains: The clinician wants to know what changes may be present which could give evidence of a brain injury and its nature and which may represent problems requiring intervention. The researcher wants to know what changes are present which may give evidence regarding the nature of brain functioning. Both operate implicitly or explicitly from a conceptualization of the nature of personality following brain injury, as follows.

FACTORS OF PERSONALITY AND EMOTIONS FOLLOWING BRAIN INJURY

Catalogs or lists of personality changes resulting from brain injury (e.g., Pepping & Roueche, 1991; Sohlberg & Mateer, 1989; Williams & Long, 1987; Ylvisaker & Gobble, 1987) can give the impression that these changes are haphazard and chaotic. While a unified and accepted theory of personality changes following brain injury is not yet available (Borod, 1992) (indeed, there is not yet an accepted theory of personality in persons with intact brains), nevertheless, some of the changes can be related to each other in a conceptualization that has more coherence and clinical utility than simple lists.

The following provisional conceptualization does not qualify as a theory. It is simply an attempt to reduce a bewildering number of clinical phenomena into a manageable set of concepts.

PSYCHOLOGICAL FACTORS

Psychological factors which influence the personality, emotions, and behavior or the person with a brain injury are those factors which can be understood from the perspective of the psychology of individuals without brain injury.

Pre-brain-injury Personality

Since anyone can have injury to their brain, the neuropsychologist must be familiar with the full range of human personalities. A common effect of brain injury is that the affected individuals may become conservative in their coping strategies, resorting to the primitive tried-and-true defenses. For this reason a family may report, for example, that the person has always been that way, even when his or her behavior is very unusual. The brain-injured person who adopts this type of regressive coping style is, indeed, just like he or she always was, only more so, becoming a caricature of him- or herself.

The neuropsychologist is interested not only in psychopathology that may have preceded the brain injury. Normal variations in personality may also be relevant to post-injury personality, behavior, and rehabilitation. Other sources of variation in adjustment to a brain injury may include premorbid coping style; family dynamics; religious faith; beliefs regarding brain injury, healing, disability, and causes of illness; and sources of self-esteem.

Some types of brain injury are more likely to occur in some types of personalities than others. The following forms of brain injury have behavioral risk factors associated with them:

1. Traumatic Head Injury—angry, risk-taking, substance-abusing, young adult males
2. Stroke—Type A personality, smokers, people prone to incomplete medical adherence
3. AIDS—homosexual and bisexual males, multipartner heterosexuals, IV drug abusers, risk-takers.

The following lifestyle and behavioral patterns are among those predisposing to brain injury:

1. Substance abusers—at risk for toxicity, trauma, stroke, anoxia, dietary deficiencies
2. Suicide attempters—at risk for trauma, toxicity, anoxia.

Psychological Reactions to Injury or Illness

Most brain injuries are emotionally significant events which can initiate reactive experiences. Typical psychological reactions to such experiences are well known and can be described for a variety of similar human experiences which do not produce brain injury. These reactions in persons with brain injuries, however, are colored or modified by changes in the ability to process emotions and information. Emotional or psychological reactions are also often seen in the relatives or significant others of persons with brain injury as they react to what has happened to the brain-injured person.

Grief Reactions

Acquired brain injury is often experienced as a major loss. The kinds of grief reactions which often occur following the death of a loved one or other major losses also often occur following brain injury. The sequence, intensity, and duration of these reactions varies with the circumstances and the individual's pre-dispositions. Psychological adjustment will be modified by changes in the brain-injured individual's capacity to perceive and experience the losses and their consequences. Types of grief reactions include:

Shock. Although awake and alert, the person in emotional shock may have a limited ability to respond to the environment in any more than routine ways. They may show psychic numbing or extreme emotional reactions. This is usually a relatively short-lived experience, ranging from a few seconds to a few hours.

Denial. This primitive defense mechanism in the brain-injured person often occurs with and is reinforced by a neurogenic lack of awareness of deficits (see "Anosognosia" below).

Anger. This common reaction to loss is also often misdirected. It can be a sign of a healthy ego which is struggling to regain what was unfairly taken or to seek redress.

Depression. This is often the longest-lasting aspect of a grief reaction. It can easily be confused with impaired initiation, diminished emotional reactivity, impaired emotional expressiveness, or reflex crying (see these topics below).

Post-traumatic stress disorder

Individuals who have life-threatening or otherwise emotionally shocking experiences often develop features of a post-traumatic stress disorder (American Psychiatric Association, 1994). These include:

1. Re-experiencing the trauma through nightmares, flashbacks, intrusive thoughts, and/or emotional reactions to reminders of the event.
2. Increased arousal such as hypervigilance, increased startle responses, sleep disturbance, concentration difficulty, or irritability.
3. Avoiding reminders of the traumatic event, amnesia for the event, psychic numbing, lack of interest in life, restricted range of affect, and feelings of detachment and futurelessness.

Frustration

Persons with brain injury may be frustrated as they fail in previously successful endeavors. Such reactions may be modified by impaired ability to anticipate difficulties, impaired ability to perceive alternative solutions, and changes in emotional reactivity (see "Catastrophic reactions" below).

Perplexity

Persons with brain injury are often perplexed by changes in their own abilities, behavior, and emotions that they cannot predict and do not understand (Lezak, 1978). This reaction also depends upon their ability to perceive the changes, their emotional reactivity, their access to information about their brain injury, and their ability to absorb that information and apply it to their experiences.

Paranoia

Loss of control over many aspects of one's life can often result from significant brain injury. Confusion, amnesia, denial, lack of awareness of deficits, difficulty appreciating another person's perspective, and/or misperceiving communication may lead to a paranoid interpretation of these losses and other events (Prigatano, O'Brien, & Klonoff, 1988).

Personal Reformation from Traumatic Experience

Some persons with brain injury experience a personal reformation or religious or spiritual awakening from the realization that they almost died.

Embarrassment

A common reaction to symptoms of brain injury, especially for the person who is well aware of symptoms, is embarrassment. Fear of problems with bladder or bowel incontinence, reflex crying, irritability, memory loss, word-finding difficulties, and/or automatic cursing, for example, can lead some people to isolate themselves socially.

NEUROLOGICAL AND NEUROPSYCHOLOGICAL FACTORS

Many of the changes in personality, emotions, and behavior following brain injury are the direct result of neurological damage. That is, they are the result of injury to the structures responsible for the behavior which is altered, rather than a psychological reaction to loss, trauma, or changes in other aspects of functioning. These alterations may vary in time according to the stage of the disease or recovery process. It is these transformations in personality, emotions, and behavior which are particularly distinctive with brain injury and are often unlike phenomena observed in persons with intact brains.

Emotional Changes

Emotional reactivity. Brain injury can produce modulations in the magnitude of experienced emotional responses. These changes can affect all forms of emotional response equally, or some more or less than others. They are distinct from modifications of emotional communication described below.

Decreased emotional reactivity. The person with a brain injury may have a reduced emotional reactivity, giving the impression of indifference. This is particularly true with lateral dorsal frontal lobe injury. Most often all forms of emotional response are diminished (e.g., joy, sorrow, lust, fear, anger). Such "flatness" may look like depression, but most often the individual feels little emotion, including depression. This reaction may also resemble the psychic numbing sometimes resulting from a post-traumatic stress disorder (Blumer & Benson, 1975; Prigatano, 1992; Stuss & Benson, 1986; Stuss, Gow, & Hetherington, 1992).

Increased emotional reactivity. Some individuals with brain injury may tend to be emotionally over-reactive. This can take many forms including the following:

1. Agitation—people in the acute stages of injury, or emergence from coma, or in the later stages of progressive dementias sometimes become agitated. They may be restless, or abusive, or even assaultive in their poorly directed struggle to escape the threats they perceive from their disorientation (Corrigan & Mysiw, 1988).
2. Irritability/Impulsive anger—This is one of the most commonly reported and problematic personality changes resulting from brain injury. Persons with brain injury often experience and express anger more readily than previously. These reactions are often quite brief and surprising to both the person experiencing them and to those present. The "explosions" may occur following relatively trivial events and may not serve any purpose. Such reactions often are exacerbated by concrete thinking or memory deficits preventing the person from seeing past or current solutions or perspectives (Miller, 1993; Prigatano, 1992).

3. Labile affect—Some persons with brain injury have rapid and intense fluctuations in many types of emotional reactions, sometimes going from intense joy to fear to rage to sorrow within a few minutes (Prigatano, 1992). This is particularly likely to occur when emotional reactions are unmodulated by recent memories or any ability to maintain ongoing plans.

4. Catastrophic reactions—Severe frustration, coupled with overstimulation or a sense of being overwhelmed, and an inability to perceive alternatives can lead to a catastrophic reaction. There is an intense desire to escape, and there may be features of a panic attack (Goldstein, 1952).

5. Personality changes associated with temporal lobe epilepsy—Although controversial, it appears that a small minority of persons with temporal lobe epilepsy, or partial complex seizures, may demonstrate a variety of complex changes in personality (Bear & Fedio, 1977). These include hypermoralism, emotionality, sexual changes, religiosity, hypergraphia, persistence, an exaggerated sense of personal destiny, etc. These may reflect abnormal discharge from the limbic system, yielding an exaggerated emotional valence being attached to benign experiences.

Changes in emotional communication. Brain injury can produce dissociations between internal emotional experiences and outward manifestations of those experiences. These dissociations can often be discovered through interview or observation of verbal or emotional behaviors.

Decreased emotional communication abilities. These impairments can be expressive or receptive:

1. Flat affect (impaired emotional expressiveness)—Brain injury, particularly right frontal lobe damage (Borod, 1992; Cancelliere & Kertesz, 1990; Ross, 1981, 1993) or Parkinson's Disease (Blonder, Gur, & Gur, 1989), may lead to difficulty with emotional expression through tone of voice, facial expressions, and gestures, even though internal feelings may be every bit as intense as previously experienced. As with decreased emotional reactivity, this lack of emotional communication ability can be mistaken for depression.

2. Impaired emotional comprehension—Persons with damage to the posterior portions of the right hemisphere are often found to have difficulty understanding or interpreting the emotions in others'

tone of voice, facial expressions, etc. (Borod, 1992; Ross, 1981, 1993).

Increased involuntary emotional communication. The most common involuntary emotional expressions are the following:

1. Reflex crying and laughing—Persons with various kinds of brain injuries, but particularly with focal damage to the pyramidal portion of the motor system sometimes develop reflex crying or laughing (pseudobulbar affect, emotional incontinence) (Lieberman & Benson, 1977; Ross & Stewart, 1987). This crying and laughing is a response which is usually appropriate in type but out of character and out of proportion to the situation and the person's actual emotions. Again, the crying can be mistaken for depression.

2. Automatic cursing of aphasia and Tourette's Syndrome—Severe aphasics sometimes have a preserved ability to curse, thought by some to be due to right hemisphere mechanisms. This cursing is often involuntary, and can be mistaken for changes in personality. Involuntary cursing is also sometimes seen as part of the tics of Tourette's Syndrome (Devinsky, Bear, Moya, & Benowitz, 1993).

Executive Function Impairments

Impairments in executive functions or the processes of behavioral self-regulation can be conceptualized both as cognitive impairments and as changes in personality. They are most commonly associated with damage to the frontal lobes. Executive functions include the ability to select an undertaking, make a plan, initiate the undertaking, recognize and correct for errors or unexpected events (plan repair), recognize completion, and evaluate outcome (Lezak, 1983). Disturbances in these abilities can occur in various forms and combinations.

Conceptually, experientially, and neuroanatomically, the executive functions stand at the interface of cognition and personality. For example, one executive function impairment is concreteness (see below). Cognitively, this condition includes a loss of ability to shift one's point of view or consider another perspective. In the realm of personality, this is often experienced as a lack of empathy (Grattan & Eslinger, 1989). The neuroanatomical manifestations of this interface are seen in the frontal lobe projections. The frontal lobes have rich reciprocal connections with the posterior cortex, associated with many major cognitive functions, as well as with the limbic system, strongly associated with emotions.

Lack of awareness of deficits (anosognosia). Persons with brain injury often have difficulty recognizing acquired neurological impairments or limitations in their abilities. They may not recognize the presence of a limitation such as a hemiplegia, or they may recognize it but be unable to take it into account when planning even such common activities as standing up. They may have difficulty recognizing when they make mistakes and correcting those mistakes, resulting in impairments in plan repair. Their lack of awareness may be reinforced by a psychological reaction of denial, but the two are also independent processes which can be dissociated (Prigatano & Schacter, 1991).

Disturbances of activation. Disturbances of initiation. Initiation may be inadequate or excessive as follows:

1. Insufficient initiation—Certain types of brain injury, particularly Parkinson's Disease and damage to the basal ganglia or to the dorsolateral frontal lobes, can produce difficulties in initiating movement, activities, and ideas (Prigatano, 1992; Stuss, Gow & Hetherington, 1992). People so affected often show little spontaneity and may be content to follow along with activities suggested or initiated by others. This impairment may also be mistaken for depression.

2. Excessive initiation (Disinhibition/Impulsivity)—Disinhibition is a common problem following brain injury, with impulsive, embarrassing, offensive or even dangerous behavior resulting. Such individuals will often be distractible and stimulus-bound, reacting to the immediate environment without regard for future consequences or social perceptions. They may be offensive to others in some circumstances, or may be more vulnerable to exploitation. Rarely, some overly inhibited individuals become more appropriately assertive. Disinhibition is seen particularly with damage to the orbital frontal cortex (Stuss & Benson, 1986; Stuss, Gow, & Hetherington, 1992).

Disturbances of termination. The ability to end activities appropriately can also take place insufficiently or excessively as follows:

1. Inadequate termination (Perseveration)—Inappropriate repetition of an action, word, or idea may take place over intervals from a fraction of a second up to several hours. The phenomena of perseveration range from stuttering to obsessive-compulsive symp-

toms, and may represent several distinct entities (Hotz & Helm-Estabrooks, 1995; Sandson & Albert, 1984).

2. Excessive termination (Impersistence)—Some individuals have difficulty appropriately maintaining an activity once started (Lopez, Becker, & Boller, 1991). This phenomenon may be due, at least in part, to attention impairments or fatigue.

Impaired planning and judgment. Some persons with brain injury have difficulty planning a complex task or sequence of activities (Stuss & Benson, 1986; Stuss, Gow, & Hetherington, 1992). They may have difficulty thinking of the different possible ways of doing something, what problems may arise, or in what order something needs to be done. They may be poor at evaluating risks and benefits or considering alternatives. Such difficulties often include limitations in social judgment. These impairments can be difficult to detect with structured cognitive tests. Even when verbal judgments are measured to be normal, for example, on the Comprehension subtest of one of the Wechsler Intelligence scales, the person's actual behavior may not reflect the use of good judgment.

Concreteness. Persons with brain injury are often less able to think abstractly (Goldstein, 1952). They may have difficulty understanding the significance of metaphors and stories, or generalizing an experience from one setting to another.

Lack of empathy. Because they have difficulty changing perspectives or points of view, some people with brain injury have difficulty in empathizing with other people, or understanding other people's feelings (Grattan & Eslinger, 1989). They may be seen as self-centered, stubborn, or selfish. This lack of empathy can be particularly devastating to a spouse or other close person, being perceived as a loss of love, yet it may be less apparent to others with whom they may be able to maintain superficial, polite relationships.

Confabulation. The combination of impairments in new learning abilities and disinhibition can produce a tendency to make up memories (Prigatano & Schacter, 1991; Shapiro, Alexander, Gardner, & Mercer, 1981; Stuss, Gow & Hetherington, 1992). Persons with this difficulty often talk about recent events that did not happen, sometimes insisting on their version of events. They can be perceived as lying and unreliable. They may be particularly susceptible to misinterpreting events to suit their own emotional needs.

Impaired communication pragmatics. Persons with executive function deficits or right hemisphere damage are likely to have difficulty in the efficacy or social appropriateness of their communication (McDonald, 1992; McDonald & VanSommers, 1993). There may be disturbances in body language, eye contact, tone of voice, or their assumptions about what the listener knows. They may talk too much or too little, interrupt or fail to respond, not listen, or have difficulty staying on topic.

Cognitively Mediated Changes of Personality

Various cognitive impairments may create false impressions of indifference, deception, or lack of cooperation. For example, the person who, due to attention impairments, does not answer questions, strays from the topic of conversation, or cannot stick with a task is often seen as not caring or as uncooperative (Weber, 1990). The person who cannot remember what they are told or what has happened may be seen as uncooperative, passive-aggressive, or unloving. Sometimes they are thought to be lying.

Aphasics are impaired in one of the major channels by which we manifest personality. It can be more difficult or sometimes impossible for them to communicate how they feel, what they want, what they think, etc. Many people fatigue more easily following brain injury (Lezak, 1978; Weber, 1990). When fatigued, their brain injury symptoms emerge more readily. They may be seen as inconsistent or unreliable. Others may come to regard their symptoms as not real because they are inconsistently present.

Interactions

With so many different factors influencing personality following brain injury the possibilities for combinations and interactions of features are enormous. It cannot be presumed that the various components of personality in an individual with a brain injury can be observed and measured independently, and that their effects will be simply additive. What follows is just a few typical interactions among the three major categories.

A fairly common syndrome among persons with a right middle cerebral artery occlusion involves a left hemiplegia, left neglect, impaired emotional communication including monotone speech and decreased facial expression, reflex crying, a lack of initiation, disinhibition, a lack of awareness of deficits, and distractibility (Gordon et al., 1991). There may be difficulty sleeping due to difficulty turning in bed, decreased sexual activity due to motoric difficulties, and a decreased interest in some foods because facial weakness makes them more difficult to eat. Social disinhibition can lead these individuals to make inappropriate jokes about death. Outside observers may interpret these changes as signs of depression (e.g., disturbances of sleep, appetite, and libido; decreased concentration, interest, and energy; flat affect; increased crying; and suicidal ideation). The outside observer may also reason, "I would be depressed if I had all of those problems." While some such persons are depressed, many are not, as a careful interview can reveal. As the anosognosia resolves itself, the reactive depression that outside observers initially projected may well emerge. Embarrassment over reflex crying and other behavioral changes may lead to social withdrawal.

Someone with a mild to moderate head injury may manifest irritability, impaired planning and judgment, mild impairments in memory and attention, and fatigability. Familiar activities such as work or handling money may result in frustration and perplexity. Memory impairments may make the immediate past less accessible, while planning impairments make the future less accessible. Immediate frustration, magnified by fatigue and irritability, can lead to embarrassing and severe (catastrophic) emotional reactions. For example, one previously very competent woman who had such a head injury described planning a trip downtown with four errands in four shops in sequence. However, the first shop was closed. Not knowing what to do (although the other errands did not depend upon the first one), she sat down on the sidewalk and cried, and then went straight home. Evaluating such interactions accurately presents a daunting challenge both to the experienced clinician and to the developer of tests.

This description of possible reactions and changes in the individual with a brain injury represents only the major and most common features which have been observed influencing personality. More subtle features or rare phenomena and rare interactions are not described. Doubtless this classification will not survive intact the tests of empirical verification and clinical usefulness. However, as a provisional organization of these features it can help in guiding the search for attempts at systematic evaluation.

CONVENTIONAL PERSONALITY TESTS

Most adult neuropsychological assessments are carried out within a few years of an actual or suspected brain injury. Some of the major purposes of such assessments are to determine the effects of the injury on cognition, emotions, personality, and behavior. Most conventional personality tests, such as the MMPI, the California Personality Inventory, the Rorschach, the Thematic

Apperception Test, etc., were not designed to be sensitive to the specific types of personality and emotional change that result from brain injury and which are outlined above. Furthermore, they generally do not distinguish premorbid from postmorbid characteristics. The ability of these tests to distinguish brain-injured from non-injured individuals generally is not impressive (Lezak, 1983).

One of the most common and significant personality changes resulting from brain injury is a lack of awareness of deficits. Since many of these tests rely primarily upon self-report, their validity in the face of a lack of awareness of deficits is questionable. While some such tests are sensitive to psychological denial, their ability to distinguish anosognosia generally has not been demonstrated. For these reasons, these tests cannot be considered to be true neuropsychological tests.

In spite of their shortcomings, some of these tests, particularly the MMPI-II, still play a role in many neuropsychological assessments, in part due to the absence of well-researched neuropsychological tests of personality. These tests can have a legitimate use in neuropsychology, particularly for the client with a mild or questionable injury or the client whose injury was many years previous. Special cautions must be taken in their interpretation, however (Alfano, Finlayson, Stearns, & Neilson, 1990).

More useful are the conventional measures of emotional state, such as the Beck, Hamilton, and Zung Depression Scales, the Beck Anxiety Scale, the Overt Aggression Scale (Yudofsky, Silver, Jackson, Endicott, & Williams, 1986), and others. These measure current emotional state, which can then be compared to the inferred pre-injury emotional status. Nevertheless, interpretation must again proceed with caution due to the effects of lack of awareness of deficits (Hunger, Enkemann, & Kleim, 1983), the tendency of some neuropsychological symptoms to mimic psychopathological symptoms, and the possibility that the concepts upon which these scales are based are not uniformly valid for persons with brain injuries.

TECHNIQUES OF NEUROPSYCHOLOGICAL PERSONALITY ASSESSMENT

Clearly, no one test or assessment technique is adequate for assessing the etiology or nature of emotions and personality following brain injury. Information needed as part of a complete assessment may include (Lezak, 1983; Walsh, 1978):

1. Medical history;
2. Mental health history;
3. Social history;
4. Educational and vocational history;

5. School, military, substance abuse and legal histories when relevant;
6. Interview with the injured person;
7. Interview with a family member or other informant who knew the injured person well both before and after injury;
8. Reports from members of the rehabilitation team, when relevant;
9. Behavioral observations;
10. Cognitive neuropsychological test results;
11. Evaluation of the injured person's environment, including home visit and assessment of family dynamics (Starch & Falltrick, 1990); and
12. Tests of emotions and personality.

Interpreting all this information is difficult. Fortunately, the clinician is not entirely dependent upon research results and the manufacturers of tests. Even in the absence of appropriate commercial products, a clinician can often approximate an ecologically valid evaluation of personality changes resulting from brain injury. Including open-ended questions in the interviews of the affected person and informants increases the chances that unusual or unsuspected changes will be detected. Home visits or community excursions can contribute immensely to the ecological validity of an assessment in selected instances, especially when the home or work setting is unfamiliar to the clinician or informants are not available to come to the clinic (Starch & Falltrick, 1990).

Next, the features that are desirable for neuropsychological tests of personality and emotions (See Table 1) are discussed. This is followed by a review of the tests currently in use or development and a discussion of what still needs to be done.

TABLE 1
DESIRABLE FEATURES OF NEUROPSYCHOLOGICAL PERSONALITY ASSESSMENT TOOLS

- Are reliable
- Are valid in describing and predicting behavior in the person's customary and/or probable contexts
- Have prognostic and treatment value
- Distinguish pre- from post-injury personality
- Distinguish psychological reactions to injury from neurological changes
- Can be applied in spite of cognitive, perceptual or motor impairments
- Measure anosognosia and denial through use of informant
- Are repeatable

DESIRABLE FEATURES OF NEUROPSYCHOLOGICAL PERSONALITY ASSESSMENT TOOLS

Of course, it is critical that neuropsychological tools for the assessment of personality meet conventional standards of reliability and validity (American Psychological Association, 1985). A closely related criterion is that they should have prognostic and treatment value.

Such tests should be designed to probe and distinguish pre-injury personality features, emotional reactions to injury, and neuropsychological features of personality. It is important to distinguish these features for several reasons. First, in the case of a diagnostic assessment it is critical to know if a symptom represents a change in someone's personality. Such evidence increases the likelihood that an event, possibly including neurologic insult, produced that change. It is then important to know if that change is likely to be due to brain injury or if it is an expected psychological reaction to the event(s). This distinction is important not only in determining if there is brain injury but also the nature and localization of damage. Even when there is a known neurological diagnosis it can be important for forensic, prognostic, and therapeutic reasons to know if the symptoms present are due to pre-injury personality or are a result of the injury. Such evaluations are complex and require retrospective analysis. Uncertainties may be particularly prominent in conditions with gradual onset.

It is also desirable that neuropsychological personality assessment tools be available for persons with various cognitive, perceptual, motor, attentional, or language impairments.

Because anosognosia and denial are of central importance in so many of the personality changes resulting from brain injury, these features generally should be accounted for and measured by most neuropsychological tests of personality and emotions. Often, it is necessary to contrast input from the injured person with that from an informant who knows the person well.

These measures should be repeatable.

It is unlikely that a single test will be appropriate for all age ranges, levels of severity, and different disease states. For example, the Temporal Lobe Epilepsy Personality Inventory (Bear & Fedio, 1977) and the Structured Clinical Interview for Complex Partial Seizure-Like Symptoms (Roberts et al., 1990) have been developed to tap disease-specific problems. Alternative instruments may be needed for cases when there is a known disease for which the examiner is seeking prognostic and treatment information versus evaluation of a mental health problem when an organic diagnosis is being considered. Flexibility in choosing neuropsychological tests may be as important for assessing personality as for assessment of cognition.

While there would be some advantage to being able to distinguish individuals with brain lesions from those with intact brains on the basis of personality tests, such discriminating power is not emphasized here as a necessary feature of neuropsychological tests of personality and behavior. There are two reasons for this. First, there is no *a priori* reason to suppose that such a discrimination is consistently possible, and, in fact to date, multiple attempts using existing instruments have failed. Second, many psychiatric disorders, most notably schizophrenia, are increasingly felt to reflect biological and neurological disorders with associated cognitive deficits. The discrimination of "organic" versus "functional" personality features or changes, therefore, is becoming increasingly problematic for some conditions.

STATE OF THE ART

As noted above, there is a relative lack of validated personality assessment methods for the neurologically impaired, though instruments which have great clinical utility are available, for those cognizant of their limitations. This deficit has been recognized and new instruments are being developed. Perhaps the most pragmatic approach at this time is to use some of the developing, more ecologically oriented instruments in tandem with more traditional approaches.

Traditional tests are next reviewed along with more recent instruments, organized according to information gathering approaches. The clinician as well as the researcher should always keep in mind, however, that all such instruments are but one part of a full clinical assessment.

SELF-REPORT

The complexities and difficulties of emotional and personality assessment are perhaps most strongly reflected in the case where brain-injured individuals are asked to analyze their own function. It has long been recognized that there is often little relationship between self-reported function and observed behavior. The meaning of test scores must be demonstrated empirically, through associations with other criteria. The reasons for this are multi-factorial. The enterprise of asking individuals to attend to and report symptoms, feelings, or other internal states can alter their occurrence. This has been repeatedly demonstrated with respect to overt behaviors in cases of self-monitoring during behavioral change attempts. It has also been shown to occur in the case of self-reports of physical symptoms (e.g., Pennebaker, 1982). As previously noted, brain injury can alter self-awareness as well as the neurological foundations of emotional perception, feeling, and expression, further complicating clear understanding of self-report data. Levels of cognitive disturbance and/or premorbid skill level may preclude some individuals from reliably completing some self-report instruments, or more informally describing their emotional experience. The complexities of personality assessment through self-report are well illustrated in attempts to understand post-concussive symptomatology following mild head injury. Several studies have clearly shown that self-reported symptoms can relate in some cases to such non-injury variables as age, sex, education, compensation or insurance status, nature of employment, or existence of pre-injury stressors (e.g., Dencker, 1958; Kelly, 1975; McKinlay, Brooks, & Bond, 1983; Minderhoud, Boelens, Huizenga, & Sann, 1980; Rimel, Giordani, Barth, Boll, & Jane, 1981; Rutherford, 1989; Rutherford, Merrett, & McDonald, 1979).

It is important to note that the biases inherent in self-report data can be evaluated and can serve as important clinical information in their own right, as well as providing a framework for understanding other clinical data. The MMPI recognizes this with its validity scales. Altered self-awareness following brain injury has been investigated by comparing, for example, general ratings of function by brain-injured individuals with similar ratings by interested observers (e.g., Bear & Fedio, 1977; Fordyce & Roueche, 1986; Heaton & Pendelton, 1981). The attained relationships have helped in the interpretation of independent measures of emotional and psychological function.

THE MMPI

Several traditional multidimensional personality inventories are available. Some, like the SCL-90 (Derogatis, Lipman, & Covi, 1973), have been employed with neurologically impaired populations (e.g., Hinkeldey & Corrigan, 1990; Jellinek, Torkelson, & Harvey, 1982). The MMPI (Dahlstrom & Welsh, 1960) continues to be the most commonly employed measure for use among brain-injured individuals. Early attempts at using the MMPI as a diagnostic tool for brain injury have fortunately been largely abandoned (see Lezak, 1983). The absence of any consistent relationship between any measures of emotional function following brain injury (including MMPI results) and independent measures of severity of head injury (Bond, 1975; Levin & Grossman, 1978; Fordyce, Roueche, & Prigatano, 1983) coupled with the previously noted complexities in understanding personality function after brain injury, highlight the reasonableness of not employing tests of emotional functioning as brain injury screening tools. Some authors have recently argued that the neurological content of many MMPI items may artificially inflate profile configuration, yielding invalid interpretations of emotional distress levels. Some investigators have deleted these items from scales and showed a not-unexpected drop in profile elevations (e.g., Alfano et al., 1990; Gass & Russell, 1991). Obviously, care must be taken in interpreting a modified MMPI, or any test scores, within the framework of existing validity data. Modification of original scales seems unnecessary, however, and is perhaps founded in the misconception that self-report responses to MMPI items (or any other verbal test item) are accurate reflections of the test-taker's internal state. The MMPI was constructed with an understanding that the relationship between self-report and internal state are not directly knowable.

While there exists a wealth of information on MMPI scores among brain-injured individuals (e.g., Farr & Martin, 1988) additional validity data is clearly needed. Some regular relationships are tending to emerge, however. For example, levels of emotional distress on the MMPI have been shown to relate lawfully to independent measures of personal awareness (Fordyce & Roueche, 1986; Heaton & Pendelton, 1981), the time since head injury (Fordyce et al., 1983; Gass & Russell, 1991), and independent measures of emotional functioning (e.g., Fordyce et al., 1983). In the hands of an experienced clinician, the MMPI remains a valuable source of data in understanding the full range of factors responsible for a particular individual's general psycho-social function. More reliable interpretation of profile elevations and a further increase in the predictive criterion validity of the MMPI will await further validity studies. It is of interest to note, however, that MMPI profile elevations have predicted gross vocational outcomes at least as accurately as comprehensive neuropsychological test battery scores (e.g. Heaton, et al., 1978; Newman, et al., 1978; Prigatano et al., 1984).

THE SICKNESS IMPACT PROFILE (SIP)

Other structured self-report measures of psycho-social function are available or are being developed, designed specifically for use with medical populations. The SIP exemplifies such an instrument. Created outside of traditional personality theory, it includes dimensions of nonemotional functioning. It is organized into scales which attempt to measure general behavioral dispositions. It assesses the impact of illness on twelve aspects of function including social interaction, communication, alertness behavior, and emotional behavior. These latter scales are combined into a general measure of psycho-social function. Reports of the development and validation of the SIP are readily available (Bergner, Bobbitt, Carter, & Gilson, 1981).

Early results indicate the SIP has some utility with respect to understanding the emotional consequences of head trauma. For example, among a group of head-injured persons with varying levels of injury severity, variability on SIP scales was also large, with more general impairment indicated on psycho-social scales compared to physical scales (Klonoff, Snow, & Costa, 1986). SIP elevations on several of these same scales distinguished a heterogeneous group of people with head injuries (McLean, Dikmen, Temkin, & Wyler, 1983) and people with mild head injuries (Dikmen, McLean, & Temkin, 1986) from peer-matched controls at one month post-injury. SIP elevations tended to normalize at one year for the mildly injured people. Interestingly, Fraser, Dikmen, McLean, Miller, and Temkin (1988) did not demonstrate a relationship between SIP elevations and employment status at one year post-injury for people with head injuries. While the SIP is perhaps not as detailed in its focus on emotional behavior as the MMPI, its validation heritage is excellent and it has been applied to several neurologically impaired populations, such as those with multiple sclerosis (e.g., Rao et al., 1991) and chronic obstructive pulmonary disease (COPD) (McSweeney, Grant, Heaton, Prigatano, & Adams, 1985).

SYMPTOM CHECKLISTS

Less-formalized methods of written self-report of symptoms following brain injury are also available. Symptom checklists are probably the most frequently used method appearing in the head injury literature for assessing psycho-social function. These checklists are almost always developed by the authors of a particular study and, while reflecting common knowledge about the studied clinical entity, are quite often idiosyncratic. They typically ask the informant to note the categorical presence or absence of a wide spectrum of impairments, including those of an emotional and interpersonal nature. Such checklists are frequently used to analyze post-concussive syndrome following mild head injury. Subjects often receive these checklists through the mail (e.g., Cook, 1972; Minderhoud et al., 1980; Edna, 1987), or they may complete them as part of an on-site general clinical evaluation (e.g., Dikmen et al., 1986; McLean et al., 1983). Self-report checklists have also been used with people with more severe head injuries (e.g., Bond, 1975; Lishman, 1968). van Zomeren and van den Burg (1985) also administered a symptom checklist to more severely head-injured people, but actually read the items directly to the individual.

Similarly, a number of investigators have adopted an elegant, if crude, approach to assessing the emotional state of people with severe aphasia. These visual mood scales typically use pictorial representations of moods, such as schematic faces. People with aphasia are asked by whatever means possible to indicate their mood by pointing to a place on a line between two moods. Such measures are often understood by people with aphasia who lack other means of reporting their moods (e.g., Stern & Bachman, 1991).

Asking people to analyze and report on their own problems, is of course, a reasonable method of evaluation. Given the complexities in self-report noted above, however, and coupled with the fact that frequently reported symptoms are common in the general population (e.g., Dikmen et al., 1986; Pennebaker, 1982), the information derived from these instruments would be more meaningful and clinically useful if standardized questionnaires could be employed across studies and if the results of reliability or validity evaluations would accompany such reports.

RATING SCALES OF SPECIFIC EMOTIONS

Rating scales of more isolated emotional functions reflect another form of written self-report that has been utilized in neurologically impaired populations. Typically, scales validated and utilized in psychiatric populations have been employed in studying the emotional consequences of brain injury. More recently, given an increasing understanding of the unique impact of brain injury on emotional behavior, these instruments are being modified, or new instruments developed for use with brain-injured populations. The Beck Depression Inventory (Beck, Ward, Mendelson, Mock, & Erbaugh, 1961), the Zung Depression Scales (Zung, 1965), and the State/Trait Anxiety Inventory (Spielberger, Gorsuch, & Lushene, 1969) are three examples. Note that the same criticisms applied to other self-report measures of emotional function among brain-injured individuals (for example, the MMPI) hold for these more specific self-report inventories.

A number of examples of the use of these instruments with neurologically impaired populations are available. For example, both the Beck and Zung inventories have been used with people recovering from cerebral vascular accident (Robinson & Price, 1982), and multiple sclerosis (Rao et al., 1991; Whitlock & Siskind, 1980). The Zung has also been used in studies of depression among demented individuals (e.g., Knesevich, Martin, Berg, & Danziger, 1983). Often, but not always, brain-injured individuals may under-report impairments in emotional and psycho-social function (e.g., Fordyce & Roueche,

1986 for head injury and Teri & Wagner, 1992 for dementia). It is also well known that depression can often, even in neurologically impaired populations, lead to overestimations of the degree of impairment (Fordyce & Roueche, 1986).

STRUCTURED CLINICAL INTERVIEWS

Another commonly employed method for assessing post-brain injury emotional functions is through a structured clinical interview completed by a professional. These methods provide an opportunity for asking people questions about their perceived functioning. They also provide for direct observation of behavior, mood, and aspects of social functioning. Unfortunately, seldom are the specific aspects of the interview described in detail in published studies and reliability and validity data are available in varying degrees. While this particular methodology may ensure more detailed information, and perhaps circumvent problems associated with level of confusion and the inability to complete written self-report inventories, they are not necessarily more objective.

In the case of mild head injury or post-concussive syndrome, information about the same variables seen on symptom checklists has also been elicited using structured clinical interviews (e.g. Levin, Mattis, et al., 1987; Wrightson & Gronwall, 1981). For more severely involved head injury victims, such interviews usually assess a broader range of social emotional variables (e.g., Fahy, Irving, & Millac, 1967; McKinlay et al., 1983; Oddy, Coughlan, Tyerman, & Jenkins, 1985; Weddell, Oddy, & Jenkins, 1980).

OBSERVER RATING SCALES

Behavior rating scales have been utilized to quantify information obtained in structured interviews. For example, Bond (1975) augmented patient interviews with interview data from a relative or close friend. Both sets of data were used to rate patients on neurophysical, mental, and social rating scales. The reliability or validity of these scales were not provided. Fahy et al. (1967) applied formal psychiatric diagnostic criteria to structured interviews of people with head injuries and their relatives. Again, reliability and validity were not provided. Weddell and colleagues (1980) and Oddy et al. (1985) also utilized rating scales, with some investigation of reliability, to understand the emotional functioning of both head-injured individuals and relatives. Also, McKinlay, Brooks, Bond, Martinage, and Marshall (1981) applied a formal rating scale to a structured interview of the relatives of head-injured victims. They provide some reliability data, too.

More formal psychiatric rating scales have been employed in assessing post-brain injury emotional characteristics. These may be relatively broad in scope, assessing several aspects of emotional function, or relatively focused. They have the advantage of being widely employed, with fairly extensive general reliability and validity information available. Levin and Grossman (1978), for example, utilized The Brief Psychiatric Rating Scale (Overall & Gorham, 1962) in rating post-traumatic psycho-social disturbance following head trauma. Ratings on this instrument, developed in psychiatric populations, were based on clinical observations of patient behavior during interview, testing, and unobtrusive behavioral observations during hospitalization. Excellent reliability and validity data are presented. Levin, High, and colleagues (1987) modified the Brief Psychiatric Rating Scale and added new scales reflecting functional issues specific to problems of traumatic brain injury, including diminished insight and disinhibition. They again present excellent reliability data and early studies of validity.

Rating scales of more specific emotional behavior applied during structured interview settings are also available, and some are now being modified for use in neurological populations. For instance, the Hamilton Rating Scale (Hamilton, 1960) is probably the most commonly employed instrument assessing depression among psychiatric populations. It has also now been employed in the assessment of affective disturbance among brain-injured individuals, though reliability and validity data are limited (e.g., Sunderland et al., 1988).

Because assessing depressive symptomatology in brain-injured individuals can be particularly problematic, new scales are being formulated which are specifically designed for the neurologically impaired. Most of this work has been applied to the analysis of depression in dementia and stroke. The Cornell Scale for Depression and Dementia (Alexopoulos, Abrams, Young, & Shamoian, 1988) and the Dementia Mood Assessment Scale (Sunderland et al., 1988), for example, provide systems for either clinician ratings of depression based on interview of the person with dementia and professional caregivers, or direct observation of affect and behavior of the person with dementia during interview.

The Memory Assessment Clinics—Psychiatric (MAC-P) (Crook, Feher, & Larrabee, 1993) is a clinician-rated instrument for dementia and related disorders. It consists of 25 items based largely on in-clinic behavior. Its eight empirically derived factors include three quasi-affective dimensions: general psychiatric, depression, and somatic complaints. Initial reliability and validity are satisfactory.

The Structured Assessment of Depression in Brain-Damaged Individuals (SADBD) (Gordon et al., 1991) is a structured interview which has been modified both in content and in presentation to account for neurological dysfunction. It incorporates an assessment of the person's awareness of his or her own symptoms of neurological dysfunction, a modified Hamilton Rating Scale for Depression, and a modified Beck Depression Inventory. Self-report and/or clinician ratings are used—depending upon accuracy of self-report, cognitive impairment, and insight—to arrive at DSM-III-R diagnoses. Preliminary reliability and validity data from stroke populations are acceptable, and the SADBD holds promise for generalization to other neurological populations.

The Rancho Los Amigos Scale (Hagen, 1982) is widely employed in rating the level of recovery from traumatic head injury based upon behavior, cognition and, to some extent, emotional state. Reliability and validity data for its eight stages of recovery are not available.

OTHER REPORT

Asking caregivers or cohabiting relatives to assess the characteristics of brain-injured individuals is a useful way to obtain information about psycho-social function. In addition to less formalized checklists as described above, formal psychometric instruments are available by which relatives can describe the emotional function of neurologically impaired patients.

The most commonly employed instrument is the Behavioral Symptoms and Social Behavior scale (R1) of the Katz Adjustment Scale (Katz & Lyerly, 1963). The person with a brain injury is assessed by a relative on 13 scales of general psychological function, not unlike those generated by the MMPI, and comparisons are made to general and psychiatric standardization norms (Hogarty & Katz, 1971). The Katz Adjustment Scale has been employed in several studies of outcome from head injuries (e.g., Fordyce et al., 1983; Goran & Fabiano, 1993; Hinkeldey & Corrigan, 1990; Klonoff et al., 1986; Prigatano et al., 1984) as well as other patient populations such as multiple sclerosis (Rao et al., 1991) or COPD (McSweeney et al., 1985). Data are accumulating to support validity in neurological groups along with findings that augment other sources of psychosocial data. The Katz has also been modified and re-factored for use with a brain-injured population (Jackson, Hopewell, Glass, & Warburg, 1992).

As with other techniques, new instruments of relative-reported psycho-social function are now being designed specifically for use with neurologically impaired populations. Examples are available for specific diagnoses such as dementia (Molloy, McLlroy, Guyatt, & Lever, 1991), frontal lobe impairment (Martzke, Swan, & Varney, 1991), and general neurologically impaired groups (Nelson et al., 1989, see below).

OTHER METHODS

Experimental methods and instruments may also some day assist in the clinical evaluation of the emotional consequences of brain injury. For example, a number of investigators are examining the capacity of brain-injured individuals to generate emotional responses to standardized stimuli or to accurately discriminate various emotional stimuli (Ross, 1981, 1993; Borod et al., 1990). For example, the Victoria Emotion Recognition Test (Mountain & Spreen, 1993) asks subjects to judge the type and intensity of emotion displayed in photographs of faces and taped voice clips. The instruments employed, while highly idiosyncratic, are shown to be reliable, and initial studies suggest the potential for considerable validity and utility in understanding the emotional behavior and communication of brain-injured individuals.

Behavioral observation methods also have tremendous potential with respect to the evaluation of the psycho-social consequences of brain injury. These are time-consuming to develop, administer, and score (a test is always easier), yet in some ways yield the most valid data on specific behaviors of interest. To date, specific functions such as general work skills (e.g., Lewis, Hinman, & Rossler, 1988; Newton & Johnson, 1985), specific work task performance (Butler, Anderson, Furst, Namerow, & Satz, 1989), or pragmatic communication skills (see Kennedy & DeRuyter, 1991 for review) have been assessed using behavioral observation methods. Behavior observation strategies developed to assess the aggressive behavior of children (e.g., Patterson & Cobb, 1973) could likely be fruitfully applied to some adult neurologically impaired patients.

PRE-INJURY PERSONALITY

One of the most difficult evaluation enterprises is to determine what aspects of post-brain injury behavior are reflective of long-standing characteristics. The psychological autopsy literature is concerned with retrospective personality assessment, but it is mostly concerned with determining the reasons for completed suicide, and is of limited relevance to neuropsychology. Methods are now available to estimate pre-lesion intellectual function after brain injury (see several chapters in Rourke, Costa, Cicchetti, Adams, & Plasterk, 1991). Attempts have also been made to distinguish pre- and post-injury emotional and personality functioning. The DSM-IV attempts to distinguish, through categorical criterion-based descriptions, between long-standing emotional disorders (Axis II) and more immediate emotional problems (Axis I), including those related to brain injury. It makes no attempts, however, to qualify personality characteristics which fail to reach the level of a formal disorder.

Early attempts at understanding the long-term emotional consequences of head trauma on the basis of pre-lesion personality characteristics met with only limited success (e.g., Kozol, 1946). More recently, some investigators have had relatives complete behavioral checklists regarding how the person with a brain injury "is now" as well as how they viewed the person "before injury" (e.g., Brooks & McKinlay, 1983; Hartlage & Williams, 1991). Another strategy is to have relatives rate current behavioral/emotional characteristics only if they reflect a change from pre-injury function (e.g., Weddell et al., 1980; McKinlay et al., 1981). All of these studies suggest notable changes in emotional function subsequent to injury, but independent validations are not available.

HYBRID METHODOLOGIES

As noted above, the heterogeneity of the population of persons with neuropsychological deficits suggests that no one test or method will prove appropriate for evaluating all forms of change in personality and behavior. The emergence of hybrid methodologies in instruments specifically designed for a neuropsychological population seems both inevitable and desirable. A notable early experimental example of such is the Temporal Lobe Epilepsy Personality Inventory (Bear & Fedio, 1977), which makes explicit use of comparisons between self-report and family member report. The Behavior Change Inventory (BCI) (Hartlage, 1991) is an adjective checklist which is completed both as a self-report and as a report by an informant, and refers to personality both before and after the brain injury, allowing for (cautious) interpretation of changes in personality and of self-awareness. Its ease of administration and completion makes it useful for evaluating subjects with significant cognitive limitations. While research data on the BCI are limited and there are intrinsic limits to the sophistication possible with an adjective checklist, nevertheless this instrument holds promise to meet some specific needs in the clinical neuropsychological evaluation.

Finally, there are two new instruments that appear to meet all of the desirable features of neuropsychological personality assessment tools listed in Table 1, although validity studies are still being extended. The Neuropsychology Behavior and Affect Profile (Nelson, Satz, & D'Elia, 1994; Nelson et al., 1989) appears to be particularly useful with an older population, and for evaluation of individuals with stroke, dementia, related conditions, and suspicions thereof. This instrument incorporates both before and after ratings and self- and peer-ratings. The lengthy development process has resulted in a scale of tolerable length with acceptable reliability and validity data. Its limitation is that it has only five scales (Indifference, Inappropriateness, Pragnosia (impaired communication pragmatics, depression, mania), which are apparently based on *a priori* choices rather than empirical criteria.

The Head Injury Family Interview (HI-FI) (Kay, Cavallo, Ezrachi, & Vavagiakis, 1995) is really much more than its name implies. It also covers much more than personality, behavior, and affect of the person with the brain dysfunction, but is included here for its value in evaluating those areas. The HI-FI is a state-of-the-art, five-part structured interview, supplemented with a problem checklist. The interviews and checklist are for both the person with the injury and an informant; they allow for easy comparisons of perspectives. There are specific sections in the informant interviews for parents, spouses, siblings, and children. The questions proceed from general and open-ended, to specific. The interviews cover pre-injury background, history of the disability, community integration, and functional competencies. There is considerable detail concerning behavioral and affective changes, interpersonal skills, and actual functioning, as well as impact of the injury on the family. While designed for use with traumatic brain injury, it can be easily and appropriately adapted to many other forms of brain insult.

A drawback for some is that the HI-FI requires 1½ to 2 hours of clinician time to administer. However, when it is not being used for research, a clinician can, with experience, use the HI-FI somewhat selectively, skipping parts of less relevance to the particular circumstances or where the information may have been obtained from other sources, but using the interview as a model and a check on thoroughness. Some parts can also be filled out as a questionnaire instead of an interview, if necessary, but the interview format is preferred. Reliability is acceptable, and preliminary validity data are promising. Results of these studies have been factor analyzed, but the HI-FI has not been used to derive scales. The HI-FI was developed using public funds and is in the public domain. The authors encourage adaptations.

CONCLUSION

At long last the drunk described in the introduction has gotten a flashlight and begun to wander towards where the keys were dropped. Specifically, neuropsychological tests of personality and emotions are beginning to arrive on the scene, although few are commercially available as of yet. While initial results look promising, most of the tests and scales currently in development need to be better researched and validated. These measures will probably continue to be provisional for some years as neuropsychology continues to work out theories and descriptions of personality and emotional changes following brain injury. Yet clinicians cannot afford to wait for theory. As a similar situation, there is as yet no one generally accepted theory of personality in the temporarily able-brained, yet the field of clinical personality assessment has been thriving for many years.

The advance of neuropsychology towards more ecologically valid tests of personality and behavior has barely begun. The progress so far (relative to conventional personality testing) has been primarily in shifting focus onto those personality features which appear to be distinctive to brain injury, in focusing on changes in personality and not just current state, in incorporating relatives' reports, in considering the effects of brain injury on employability, in adapting measures to factor out some of the medical concomitants of injury, and in adapting measures for the cognitive limitations of parts of the neuropsychological population.

Critical research issues remaining include:

1. Developing systematic ways to evaluate lack of awareness and related influences in assessments of emotional functioning;
2. Finding and validating ways of retrospectively evaluating pre-injury personality;
3. More clearly determining what types of changes in personality and behavior may directly result from brain injury (including changes which may not yet have been described);
4. Finding ways to evaluate those changes;
5. Determining ways of discriminating direct effects of brain injury on personality and behavior from emotional reactions to injury or illness (which might well be seen in similar illnesses and losses without brain injury);
6. Determining the effects of those changes on functioning in a variety of settings such as family, work, school, and community;
7. Determining the validity of the measures of those functions in each of those social contexts;
8. Determining the generalizability of those measures to a variety of ages, cultures, languages, and types of neurological disease;
9. Finding ways of systematizing the integration of information from cognitive evaluation, pre-injury personality evaluation, and post-injury personality evaluation;

10. Developing and validating versions of instruments that can be administered in spite of various sensory, motor, linguistic, and cognitive impairments;

11. Researching how to predict further changes in personality features after the time of assessment.

Hopefully, the ecological perspective in neuropsychological assessment of personality, emotions, and behavior will not only improve clinical practice, but also advance theoretical understanding of brain-behavior relationships. Clinical neuropsychology research has contributed richly to cognitive theory. Eventually, it may be able to contribute as fully to personality theory. Ultimately, the ecological perspective may help us to arrive at a better understanding of the evolution of personality, emotions, and behavior.

REFERENCES

Acker, M. (1986). Relationships between test scores and everyday life functioning. In B. Uzzell & Y. Gross (Eds.), *Clinical neuropsychology of intervention* (pp. 85-118). Boston: Martinus Nijhoff Publishing.

Alexopoulos, G., Abrams, R., Young, R., & Shamoian, C. (1988). Cornell scale for depression in dementia. *Biological Psychiatry, 23*, 271-284.

Alfano, D., Finlayson, A., Stearns, G., & Neilson, P. (1990). The MMPI and neurologic dysfunction: Profile configuration and analysis. *The Clinical Neuropsychologist, 4*, 69-79.

American Psychiatric Association. (1987). *Diagnostic and statistical manual,* 3rd. ed.—rev. Washington, DC: Author.

American Psychiatric Association. (1994). *Diagnostic and statistical manual,* 4th ed. Washington DC: Author.

American Psychological Association, American Educational Research Association, and National Council of Measurement Used in Education (Joint Committee) (1954). Technical recommendations for psychological tests. *Psychological Bulletin, 51*, 201-238.

American Psychological Association. (1985). *Standards for educational and psychological testing.* Washington, DC: Author.

Bear, D. M., & Fedio, P., (1977). Quantitative analysis of interictal behavior in temporal lobe epilepsy. *Archives of Neurology, 34*, 454-467.

Beck, A., Ward, C., Mendelson, M., Mock, J., & Erbaugh, J. (1961). An inventory for measuring depression. *Archives of General Psychiatry, 4*, 561-571.

Bergner, M., Bobbitt, R., Carter, W., & Gilson, B. (1981). The sickness impact profile: A development and revision of a health status measure. *Medical Care. 19,* 787-805.

Blonder, L. X., Gur, R. E., & Gur, R. C. (1989). The effects of right and left hemiparkinsonism on prosody. *Brain and Language, 36*, 193-207.

Blumer, D., & Benson, D. F., (1975). Personality changes with frontal and temporal lobe lesions. In D. F. Benson & D. Blumer (Eds.), *Psychiatric aspects of neurologic disease: Vol. 1* (pp. 151-170). New York: Grune & Stratton.

Bond, M. (1975). Assessment of psychological outcome after severe head injury. *CIBA Foundation Symposium, 34,* 141-153.

Borod, J. C. (1992). Interhemispheric and intrahemispheric control of emotion: A focus on unilateral brain damage. *Journal of Consulting and Clinical Psychology, 60,* 339-348.

Borod, J., Welkowitz, J., Alpert, M., Brozgold, A., Martin, C., Peselow, E., & Diller, L. (1990). Parameters of emotional processing in neuropsychiatric disorders: Conceptual issues and a battery of tests. *Journal of Communication Disorders, 23,* 247-271.

Brooks, M., & McKinlay, W. (1983). Personality and behavior change after severe blunt head injury—a relative's view. *Journal of Neurology, Neurosurgery and Psychiatry, 46,* 336-344.

Butler, R., Anderson, L., Furst, C., Namerow, N., & Satz, P. (1989). Behavioral assessment in neuropsychological rehabilitation: A method for measuring vocational-related skills. *The Clinical Neuropsychologist. 3,* 235-243.

Cancelliere, A. E. B., & Kertesz, A. (1990). Lesion localization in acquired deficits of emotional expression and comprehension. *Brain and Cognition, 13,* 133-147.

Cook, J. (1972). The post-concussional syndrome and factors influencing after minor head injury admitted to the hospital. *Scandinavian Journal of Rehabilitation Medicine, 4,* 27-30.

Corey, M. R. (1987). A comprehensive model for psychosocial assessment of individuals with closed head injury. *Cognitive Rehabilitation, 5*(6), 28-33.

Corrigan, J. D., & Mysiw, J. (1988). Agitation following traumatic head injury: Equivocal evidence for a discrete stage of cognitive recovery. *Archives of Physical Medicine and Rehabilitation, 69,* 487-492.

Cronback, L. J., & Meehl, P. E. (1955). Construct validity in psychological tests. *Psychological Bulletin, 52,* 281-302.

Crook, T. H., Feher, E. P., & Larrabee, G. J. (1993). Initial validation of the MAC-P: A new clinician-rated scale for cognitive and affective changes in dementia. *Clinical Neuropsychologist, 7,* 420-429.

Dahlstrom, W. & Welsh, G. (1960). *An MMPI handbook* (Vol I: Clinical interpretation—rev. ed.). Minneapolis: University of Minnesota Press.

Dencker, S. (1958). A follow-up study of 128 closed head injuries in twins using co-twins as controls. *Acta Psychiatrica et Neurologica Scandinavica, 33* (Supplement 123).

Derogatis, L., Lipman, R., & Covi, L. (1973). SCL-90: Outpatient psychiatric rating scale— Preliminary report. *Psychopharmacology Bulletin. 9,* 13-28.

Devinsky, O., Bear, D., Moya, K., & Benowitz, L. (1993). Perception of emotion in patients with Tourette's syndrome. *Neuropsychiatry, Neuropsychology, & Behavioral Neurology, 6,* 166-169.

Dikmen, S., McLean, A., & Temkin, N. (1986). Neuropsychological and psychosocial consequences of minor head injury. *Journal of Neurology, Neurosurgery, and Psychiatry, 49,* 1227-1232.

Edna, T. (1987). Disability 3-5 years after minor head injury. *Journal of Oslo City Hospital, 37,* 41-48.

Fahy, T., Irving, M., & Millac, P. (1967). Severe head injuries: A six year follow-up. *Lancet, ii,* 475-479.

Farr, S., & Martin, P. (1988). The MMPI and neuropsychologic dysfunction. In R. Greene (Ed.), *The MMPI: Use with specific populations* (pp. 214-245). Philadelphia: Grune & Stratton.

Fordyce, D. J., & Roueche, J. R. (1986). Changes in perspectives of disability among patients, staff, and relatives during rehabilitation of brain injury. *Rehabilitation Psychology, 31,* 217-229.

Fordyce, D. J., Roueche, J. R., & Prigatano, G. P. (1983). Enhanced emotional reactions in chronic head trauma patients. *Journal of Neurology, Neurosurgery, and Psychiatry, 46,* 620-624.

Fraser, R., Dikmen, S., McLean, A., Miller, B., & Temkin, N. (1988). Employability of head injury survivors: First year post-injury. *Rehabilitation Counseling Bulletin, 31,* 276-288.

Gass, C., & Russell, E. (1991). MMPI profiles of closed head trauma patients: Impact of neurologic complaints. *Journal of Clinical Psychology, 47,* 253-260.

Goldstein, K. (1952). The effects of brain damage on the personality. *Psychiatry, 15,* 245-260.

Goran, D .A., & Fabiano, R. J. (1993). The scaling of the Katz Adjustment Scale in a traumatic brain injury rehabilitation sample. *Brain Injury, 7,* 219-229.

Gordon, W. A., Hibbard, M. R., Egelko, S., Riley, E., Simon, D., Diller, L., Ross, E. D., & Lieberman, A. (1991). Issues in the diagnosis of post-stroke depression. *Rehabilitation Psychology, 36*(2), 71-87.

Grant, I., & Alves, W. (1987). Psychiatric and psychosocial disturbances in head injury. In H. S. Levin, J. Grafman, & H. M. Eisenberg (Eds.), *Neurobehavioral recovery from head injury* (pp. 232-261). New York: Oxford.

Grattan, L., & Eslinger, P .J. (1989). The relationship between cognitive flexibility and empathy after brain injury. *Journal of Clinical and Experimental Neuropsychology, 11,* 47.

Hagen, C. (1982). Language-cognitive disorganization following closed head injury: A conceptualization. In L. E. Trexler (Ed.), *Cognitive rehabilitation: Conceptualization and intervention.* New York: Plenum.

Hamilton, M. (1960). A rating scale for depression. *Journal of Neurology, Neurosurgery and Psychiatry, 23,* 56-62.

Hartlage, L. (1991). Assessment of behavioral sequelae of traumatic and chemical CNS insult. *Archives of Clinical Neuropsychology, 6,* 279-286.

Hartlage, L., & Williams, B. (1991). Assessment of behavioral sequelae of traumatic and chemical CNS insult. *Archives of Clinical Neuropsychology, 6,* 271-286.

Heaton, R., Chelune, G., & Lehman, R. (1978). Using neuropsychological and personality tests to assess the likelihood of patient employment. *Journal of Nervous and Mental Disease, 166,* 408-416.

Heaton, R., & Pendelton, M. (1981). Use of neuropsychological tests to predict adult patients' everyday functioning. *Journal of Consulting and Clinical Psychology, 49,* 807-821.

Hinkeldey, N., & Corrigan, J. (1990). The structure of head-injured patients' neurobehavioral complaints: A preliminary study. *Brain Injury, 4,* 111-114.

Hogarty, G., & Katz, M. (1971). Norms of adjustment and social behavior. *Archives of General Psychiatry, 25,* 470-480.

Hotz, G., & Helm-Estabrooks, N. (1995). Preservation. Part I: A review. *Brain Injury, 9,* 151-159.

Hunger, J., Enkemann, J., & Kleim, J. (1983). Das Freiburger Persönlichkeitsinventar (FPI) in der Persönlichkeitsdiagnostic hirngeschädigter Patienten (The Freiburger Personality Inventory (FPI) in personality assessment of brain-damaged patients). *Nervenartz, 54,* 316-319.

Jackson, H. F., Hopewell, C. A., Glass, C. A., & Warburg, R. (1992). The Katz Adjustment Scale: Modification for use with victims of traumatic brain and spinal injury. *Brain Injury, 6,* 109-127.

Jellinek, H., Torkelson, R., & Harvey, R. (1982). Functional abilities and distress levels in brain-injured patients at long-term follow-up. *Archives of Physical Medicine and Rehabilitation, 63,* 160-162.

Katz, M., & Lyerly, S. (1963). Methods of measuring adjustment and behavior in the community: I. rationale, description, discriminative validity, and scale development. *Psychological Reports, 13*, 503-535.

Kay, T., Cavallo, M. M., Ezrachi, O., & Vavagiakis, P. (1995). The head injury family interview: A clinical and research tool. *Journal of Head Trauma Rehabilitation, 10*(2), 12-31.

Kelly, R. (1975). The post-traumatic syndrome: An iatrogenic disease. *Forensic Science, 6*, 17-24.

Kennedy, M., & DeRuyter, F. (1991). Cognitive and language bases for communication disorders. In D. Beukleman & K. Yorkston (Eds.), *Communication disorders following brain injury* (pp. 123-190). Austin, TX: Pro Ed.

Klonoff, P., Snow, W., & Costa, L. (1986). Quality of life in patients 2 to 4 years after closed head injury. *Neurosurgery, 19*, 735-743.

Knesevich, J., Martin, R., Berg, L., & Danziger, W. (1983). Preliminary report on affective symptoms in the early stages of senile dementia of the Alzheimer type. *American Journal of Psychiatry, 140*, 233-234.

Kozol, H. (1946). Pretraumatic personality and psychiatric sequelae of head injury: II. *Archives of Neurology and Psychiatry, 57*, 245-275.

Levin, H., & Grossman, R. (1978). Behavioral sequelae of closed head injury. *Archives of Neurology, 35*, 720-727.

Levin, H., High, W., Goethe, K., Sisson, R., Overall, J., Rhoades, H., Eisenberg, H., Kalisky, Z., & Gary, H. (1987). The neurobehavioral rating scale: Assessment of the behavioral sequelae of head injury by the clinician. *Journal of Neurology, Neurosurgery and Psychiatry, 50*, 183-193.

Levin, H., Mattis, S., Ruff, R., Eisenberg, H., Marshall, L., Tabaddor, K., High, W., & Frankowski, R. (1987). Neurobehavioral outcome following minor head injury: A three-center study. *Journal of Neurosurgery, 66*, 234-243.

Lewis, F., Hinman, S., & Roessler, R. (1988). Assessing TBI clients' work adjustment skills: The work performance assessment (WPA). *Rehabilitation Psychology, 4*, 213-220.

Lezak, M. D. (1978). Subtle sequelae of brain damage: Perplexity, distractibility, and fatigue. *American Journal of Physical Medicine, 67*, 9-15.

Lezak, M. D. (1983). *Neuropsychological assessment, 2nd ed.* New York: Oxford University Press.

Lieberman, A., & Benson, D. F. (1977). Control of emotional expression in pseudobulbar palsy: A personal experience. *Archives of Neurology, 34*, 717-719.

Lishman, W. (1968). Brain damage in relation to psychiatric disability after head injury. *British Journal of Psychiatry, 114*, 373-410.

Lopez, O. L., Becker, J. T., & Boller, F. (1991). Motor impersistence in Alzheimers' disease. *Cortex, 27*, 93-99.

Martín-Baró, I. (1991). Towards a liberation psychology. In J. Hassett & H. Lacey (Eds.), *Towards a society that serves its people: The intellectual contribution of El Salvador's murdered Jesuits* (pp. 319-332). Washington, DC: Georgetown University Press.

Martzke, J., Swan, C., & Varney, N. (1991). Post-traumatic anosmia and orbital frontal damage: Neuropsychological and neuropsychiatric correlates. *Neuropsychology, 5*, 213-225.

McDonald, S. (1992). Communication disorders following closed head injury: New approaches to assessment and rehabilitation. *Brain Injury, 6*, 283-292.

McDonald, S., & VanSommers, P. (1993). Pragmatic language skills after closed head injury: Ability to negotiate requests. *Cognitive Neuropsychology, 10*, 297-315.

McKinlay, W., Brooks, D., & Bond, B. (1983). Post-concussional symptoms, financial compensation and outcome of severe blunt head injury. *Journal of Neurology, Neurosurgery and Psychiatry, 46,* 1084-1091.

McKinlay, W., Brooks, D., Bond, M., Martinage, D., & Marshall, N. (1981). The short-term outcome of severe blunt head-injury as reported by relatives of the injured person. *Journal of Neurology, Neurosurgery and Psychiatry, 44,* 527-533.

McLean, A., Dikmen, S., Temkin, N., Wyler, A., & Gale, J. (1984). Psychosocial functioning at one month after head injury. *Neurosurgery, 14,* 393-399.

McLean, A., Temkin, N., Dikmen, S., & Wyler, A. (1983). The behavioral sequelae of head injury. *Journal of Clinical Neuropsychology, 5,* 361-376.

McSweeney, A., Grant, I., Heaton, R., Prigatano, G., & Adams, K. (1985). Relationship of neuropsychological status to everyday functioning in healthy and chronically ill persons. *Journal of Clinical and Experimental Neuropsychology, 7,* 281-291.

Miller, L. (1993*). Psychotherapy of the brain-injured patient: Reclaiming the shattered self.* Norton: New York.

Minderhoud, J., Boelens, M., Huizenga, J., & Sann, R. (1980). Treatment of minor head injuries. *Clinical Neurology and Neurosurgery, 82,* 127-140.

Molloy, D., McLlroy, Guyatt, G., & Lever, J. (1991). Validity and reliability of the dysfunctional behavior rating instrument. *Acta Psychiatrica Scandinavica, 84,* 103-106.

Mountain, M., & Spreen, O. (1993). *Implications of impaired ability in brain damaged patients to recognize emotion.* Paper presented to the International Neuropsychological Society, Funchal, Madiera, Portugal.

Nelson, L., Satz, P., & D'Elia, L. (1994). *Neuropsychology behavior and affect profile.* Palo Alto, CA: Mind Garden.

Nelson, L., Satz, P., Mitrushina, D., Van Gorp, W., Cicchetti, D., Lewis, R., & Van Lancker, D. (1989). Development and validation of the neuropsychology behavior and affect profile. *Psychological Assessment, 1,* 266-272.

Newman, O., Heaton, R., & Lehman, R. (1978). Neuropsychological and MMPI correlates of patients' future employment characteristics. *Perceptual and Motor Skills, 46,* 635-642.

Newton, A., & Johnson, D. (1985). Social adjustment and interaction after severe head injury. *British Journal of Clinical Psychology, 24,* 225-234.

Oddy, M., Coughlan, T., Tyerman, A., & Jenkins, D. (1985). Social adjustment after closed head injury: A further follow-up 7 years after injury. *Journal of Neurology, Neurosurgery, and Psychiatry, 48,* 564-568.

Overall, J., & Gorham, D. (1962). The brief psychiatric rating scale. *Psychological Reports, 10,* 799-812.

Patterson, G., & Cobb, J. (1973). Stimulus control for classes of noxious behaviors. In J. Knutson (Ed.), *The control of aggression* (pp. 145-200). Chicago: Aldine Publishing.

Pennebaker, J. (1982). *The psychology of physical symptoms.* New York: Springer-Verlag.

Pepping, M., & Roueche, D. (1991). Psychosocial consequences of significant brain injury. In D. E. Tupper & K. D. Cicerone (Eds.*), The neuropsychology of everyday life: Issues in development and rehabilitation.* Boston: Kluwer.

Ponsford, J. L. (1990) Psychological sequelae of closed head injury: Time to redress the imbalance. *Brain Injury, 4,* 111-114.

Prigatano, G. P., (1992). Personality disturbances associated with traumatic brain injury. *Journal of Consulting and Clinical Psychology, 60,* 360-368.

Prigatano, G. P., Fordyce, D. J., Zeiner, H. K., Roueche, J. R., Pepping, M., & Wood, B. C. (1984). Neuropsychological rehabilitation after closed head injury in young adults. *Journal of Neurology, Neurosurgery, and Psychiatry, 47,* 505-513.

Prigatano, G. P., O'Brien, K. P., & Kolonoff, P. S. (1988). The clinical management of paranoid delusions in postacute traumatic brain-injured patients. *Journal of Head Trauma Rehabilitation, 3,* 23-32.

Prigatano, G. P., & Schacter, D. L. (Eds.). (1991*). Awareness of deficit after brain injury: Clinical and theoretical issues.* New York: Oxford University Press.

Ranseen, J. (1990). Positive personality change following traumatic head injury: Four case studies. *Cognitive Rehabilitation, 8*(2), 8-12.

Rao, S., Leo, G., Ellington, L., Nauertz, T., Bernardin, & Unverzagt, F. (1991). Cognitive dysfunction in multiple sclerosis: 2. Impact on social functioning. *Neurology. 41,* 692-696.

Reitan, R. (1955). Investigation of the validity of Halstead's measure of biological intelligence. *Archives of Neurology and Psychiatry, 73,* 28-35.

Rimel, R., Giordani, B., Barth, J., Boll, T., & Jane, J. (1981). Disability caused by minor head injury. *Neurosurgery, 9,* 221-228.

Roberts, R. J., Varney, N. R., Hulbert, J. R., Paulsen, J. S., Richardson, E. D., Springer, J. A., Shepherd, J. S., Swan, C. M., Legrand, J. A., Harvey, J. H., & Struchen, M. A. (1990). The neuropathology of everyday life: The frequency of partial seizure symptoms among normals. *Neuropsychology, 4,* 65-85.

Robinson, R., & Price, T. (1982). Poststroke depressive disorders: A follow-up study of 103 patients. *Stroke, 13,* 635-640.

Ross, E. D. (1981). The aprosodias: Functional-anatomic organization of the affective components of language in the right hemisphere. *Archives of Neurology, 38,* 561-569.

Ross, E. D. (1993). Nonverbal aspects of language. *Behavioral Neurology, 11,*9-23.

Ross, E. D., & Stewart, R. S. (1987). Pathological display of affect in patients with depression and right frontal brain damage: An alternative mechanism. *Journal of Nervous and Mental Disease, 175,* 165-172.

Rourke, B., Costa, L., Cicchetti, D., Adams, K., & Plasterk, K. (Eds). (1991). *Methodological and biostatistical foundations of clinical neuropsychology.* Amsterdam: Swets & Zeitlinger.

Rutherford, W. (1989). Postconcussion symptoms: Relationship to acute neurological indices, individual differences, and circumstances of injury. In H. Levin, H. Eisenberg, & A. Benton (Eds.), *Mild head injury* (pp. 217-228). New York: Oxford University Press.

Rutherford, W., Merrett, J., & McDonald, J. (1979). Symptoms at one year following concussion from minor head injuries. *Injury, 10,* 225-230.

Sandson, J. & Albert, M. L. (1984). The varieties of perseveration. *Neuropsychologia, 22,* 715-732.

Shapiro, B. E., Alexander, M. P., Gardner, H. & Mercer, B. (1981). Mechanisms of confabulation. *Neurology, 31,* 1070-1076.

Sohlberg, M. M. & Mateer, C. A. (1989*). Introduction to cognitive rehabilitation: Theory and practice.* New York: Guilford.

Spielberger, C., Gorsuch, R., & Lushene, R. (1970*). The state-trait anxiety inventory (STAI): Test Manual for Form A.* Palo Alto: Consulting Psychology Press.

Starch, S., & Falltrick, E. (1990). The importance of a home evaluation for brain injured clients: A team approach. *Cognitive Rehabilitation, 8*(6), 28-32.

Stern, R. A., & Bachman, D. L., (1991). Depressive symptoms following stroke. *American Journal of Psychiatry, 148,* 351-356.

Stuss, D. T., & Benson, D. F. (1986). *The frontal lobes.* New York: Raven Press.

Stuss, D. T., Gow, C. A., & Hetherington, C. R. (1992). "No longer Gage": Frontal lobe dysfunction and emotional changes. *Journal of Consulting and Clinical Psychology, 60,* 349-

359.

Sunderland, T., Alterman, I., Yount, D., Hill, J., Tariot, P., Newhouse, P., Mueller, E., Mellow, A., & Cohen, R. (1988). A new scale for the assessment of depressed mood in demented patients. *American Journal of Psychiatry, 145*, 955-959.

Teri, L., & Wagner, A. (1992). Alzheimer's disease and depression. *Journal of Consulting and Clinical Psychology, 60*, 379-391.

van Zomeren, A., & van den Berg, W. (1985). Residual complaints of patients 2 years after severe head injury. *Journal of Neurology, Neurosurgery, and Psychiatry, 48*, 21-28.

Walsh, K. W. (1978). *Neuropsychology: A clinical approach.* London: Churchill Livingstone.

Weber, A. M. (1990). A practical clinical approach to understanding and treating attentional problems. *Journal of Head Trauma Rehabilitation, 5*, 73-85.

Weddell, R., Oddy, M., & Jenkins, D. (1980). Social adjustment after rehabilitation: A two-year follow-up of patients with severe head injury. *Psychological Medicine, 10*, 257-263.

Whitlock, F., & Siskind, M. (1980). Depression as a major symptom of multiple sclerosis. *Journal of Neurology, Neurosurgery, & Psychiatry, 43*, 861-865.

Wiggins, J. (1973). *Personality and prediction: Principles of personality assessment.* Reading, MA: Addison-Wesley.

Williams, J. M., & Long, C. J. (Eds.). (1987). *The rehabilitation of cognitive disabilities.* New York: Plenum Press.

Wrightson, P., & Gronwall, D. (1981). Time off work and symptoms after minor head injury. *Injury, 12*, 445-454.

Ylvisaker, M., & Gobble, E. M. R. (Eds.) (1987). *Community reentry for head injured adults.* Boston: Little, Brown & Co.

Yudofsky, S. C., Silver, J. M., Jackson, M., Endicott, J., & Williams, D. (1986). The Overt Aggression Scale: An operationalized rating scale for verbal and physical aggression. *American Journal of Psychiatry, 143*, 35-39.

Zung, W. (1965). A self-rating depression scale. *Archives of General Psychiatry. 12*, 63-70.

17

NEUROPSYCHOLOGY OF DRUG ABUSE:
Ecological Validity

Arthur MacNeill Horton, Jr., Ed.D., A.B.P.P.(CL), A.B.P.N.

INTRODUCTION

The use of psychoactive substances to modify mood, behavior, and perceptions maybe as old as humankind itself. Since the earliest recorded time, people have used natural substances, such as peyote from the cactus and leaves from the opium plant to change their emotions. Over the years, technology enabled raw materials to be processed to produce alcohol, heroin, and cocaine. In more modern times, chemical advances have included LSD, PCP, and a variety of designer drugs.

While societies at various times have prohibited the use of addictive substances, successful prohibition has been rare. For example, in the early 1600s tobacco use was opposed by the government of King James I to no avail. In the 1700s and 1800s, when the use of opium was vigorously opposed in China by the Emperor, the British Empire fought two opium wars to allow the drug to be sold in China. Surprisingly, in the 1700s, chocolate was made illegal in England for a short time. In the U.S, alcohol was prohibited in 1920, but this mandate was later reversed by a Constitutional amendment in 1933.

Recently, substance abuse has been estimated to involve some 10% to 15% of the U. S. population (Tarter & Edwards, 1987). The majority of substance abusers are alcoholics, but drug abusers number in the millions. Simple numbers, however, fail to capture the damage to society that substance abuse causes. Substance abuse in the form of drug abuse has been estimated as costing the U. S. some $60 billion a year (Harwood, Napolitano, Kristiansen, & Collins, 1984). Substance abuse affects society through increased medical illness as well as domestic violence, traffic accidents, crime, and in negative psychological, social, and emotional effects on abusers and their spouses, children, and significant others (Hubbard et al., 1989). At the same time, it should be recognized that the use of certain substances to modify mood is regarded under selected cultural circumstances as normal and appropriate.

Social norms clearly influence decisions as to whether the use of a particular substance is pathological. As is well known, Native American tribes in the southwestern U.S. have long-used peyote in their religious rites. Most adults have used caffeine in the form of coffee, tea, or cola drinks. The limited use of marijuana for certain medical diseases is allowed by legal authorities for selected individuals in the U.S. When prescribed by a physician, narcotics are used for the alleviation of pain in medically ill individuals.

OVERVIEW

A considerable body of literature suggests that there are neuropsychological effects from certain abused drugs (Spencer & Boren, 1990). While this literature is still in its early stages of development, given the extent of drug abuse in the U.S. there are particularly serious implications for the assessment and treatment of drug abusers. As observed by Tarter and Edwards (1987), very little attention has been given to the functional adaptive capacity of individuals with substance abuse problems. They suggested that neuropsychological assessment by measuring an individual's organic integrity can provide a basis for estimating an individual's potential for change as well as their rehabilitation prognosis.

The purpose of this chapter is to make suggestions with respect to the ecological validity of the neuropsychological assessment of drug abusers. This effort requires a brief and selective review of the available literature with respect to the neuropsychological impairment of drug abusers. It should be clearly noted that this review is confined to drug abusers. The topic of alcohol abusers and neuropsychological deficits has been reviewed by Benedict and Horton (1992). In addition, as agreement that drug abuse causes residual neuropsychological impairments has only recently been reached for even a few drugs, studies to assess the ecological validity of these findings in populations of drug abusers for the most part remain to be done. If there were little or no agreement that residual neuropsychological effects of abused drugs were a reality, there would be little motivation to study the ecological validity of these effects. This chapter serves to set the stage for the planning of future studies in this important area of clinical and scientific interest.

ADDICTION

According to the DSM-IV (APA, 1994), the essential features of substance abuse are:

> ...a maladaptive pattern of substance use manifested by recurrent and significant adverse consequences related to repeated use of substances. These may be repeated failure to fulfill major role obligations, repeated use in situations in which it is physically hazardous, multiple legal problems, and recurrent social and interpersonal problems....The individual may repeatedly demonstrate intoxication or other substance-related symptoms when expected to fulfill major role obligations at work, school, or home. (p. 182)

The symptoms of psychoactive substance abuse not only include physiological symptoms of tolerance and withdrawal, but also cognitive and behavioral symptoms which are typically manifested in the individual's workplace, home, schoolwork, and interpersonal interactions with others in a variety of settings.

NEUROPSYCHOLOGICAL ASSESSMENT

Neuropsychological tests have been traditionally regarded as valued measures of brain-behavior relationships (Horton & Wedding, 1984). For a specific neuropsychological test to be accepted as valid it must be empirically proven to be a measure of brain function. For many neurological conditions (e.g., toxic disorders, head injury) performance-based behavioral measures (e.g., neuropsychological testing) are the preferred method of assessing subtle cognitive, memory, and perceptual-motor changes (Horton & Wedding, 1984). Others (Tarter & Edwards, 1987) suggest that neuropsychological assessment might be viewed as comprised of three separate spheres of functioning: cognitive/psychomotor, psychopathological, and social-interpersonal relationships. In this chapter a more narrow approach is taken.

The aspect of neuropsychological evaluation addressed here is the cognitive/psychomotor. The assessment of psychopathology and social-interpersonal relationships will not be specifically addressed due to limitations of space, although this is in no way an attempt to minimize their importance. Also as mentioned by Tarter and Edwards (1987), whether or not the neuropsychologist relies on a screening or full neuropsychological battery depends on a number of circumstances. For example, some of the factors include resources in terms of personnel and technical expertise, the amount of time available for testing, the financial cost of the procedure, the specific referral questions, as well as the patient's receptivity to the completion of an extensive set of procedures. Moreover, the relative importance of each factor may vary depending upon unique setting effects.

SCREENING ASSESSMENTS

Screening assessments can be quite valuable in identifying the presence or absence of neuropsychological deficits in patient populations where the incidence of such impairment is relatively low. A screening assessment approach also works best in situations where there are many patients to be examined. For example, in an outpatient, drug-free, drug abuse treatment program one would not expect gross organic impairment in the majority of the patients. Therefore, a screening procedure that is economical yet effective in identifying patients who are neuropsychologically impaired would be appropriate.

The advantage of using a screening procedure is that those patients who would fail to benefit from a very cognitively oriented treatment approach would be quickly identified and their special needs can be addressed. A number of general screening tests have been developed. One particular measure is a short form of the test made up from the Brain Age Quotient (BAQ) (Reitan, 1973). The BAQ is an actuarial combination of six neuropsychological test scores. These include the Category test, the Tactual Performance test, and the Trail Making test from the Halstead-Reitan Neuropsychological test battery and the Block Design and Digit Symbol subtest of the Wechsler Adult Intelligence Scale (WAIS). Reitan initially proposed using the BAQ as a means of studying age-related cognitive deterioration. An important advantage of the BAQ score is that it is essentially independent of chronological age (Schau & O'Leary, 1977). Interestingly, short forms of the BAQ based on a three subtest set (Trail Making Test Part B, Block Design, and Digit Symbol subtests) or simply the score from Trails B can serve as a possible substitute for the long form of BAQ (Horton & Anilane, 1986). It should be noted, however, that the three subtests short form or the Trails B form must be prorated to approximate the full BAQ and that specific norms available from Reitan (1973) must be used.

COMPREHENSIVE ASSESSMENT

A comprehensive, neuropsychological assessment requires greater expertise and time on part of the examiner, more complex and expensive equipment and a considerable degree of professional expertise to interpret the test data. In terms of applying the neuropsychological test results to address such issues as vocational fitness and employability, social functioning and interpersonal effectiveness, the use of comprehensive neuropsychological assessment can be helpful in many cases.

With respect to comprehensive neuropsychological test batteries, research utilizing the Halstead-Reitan test battery (Parson & Farr, 1981) found that drug users were not grossly impaired on the Halstead-Reitan, with respect to the level of performance criterion (see Reitan & Wolfson, 1985 for discussion of performance level issues). Nonetheless, some specific patterns of impairment were reported. For example, relative to other patients, drug users generally showed particular difficulties in terms of fine motor speed and non-verbal pattern recognition as well as difficulties on tasks involving visual abstraction and set shifting abilities. Although the Luria-Nebraska Neuropsychological Test Battery (LNNB) is also a comprehensive test battery, very few studies have examined the cognitive impairments of substance abusers.

PSYCHOACTIVE SUBSTANCES

The following sections include a brief and very selective review of the neuropsychological test data currently available regarding the residual effects of various psychoactive substances. There are a number of very serious difficulties involved with measuring residual drug abuse effects in human beings, as noted in a review by Reed and Grant (1990).

For example, the issue of multiple substance abuse is particularly difficult to control since many drug addicts are referred to as "garbage can" abusers, meaning most have used a wide variety of psychoactive substances. While some abusers may have a preference for one substance versus others, in actuality their daily consumption of addictive substances is more often a product of drug availability than any major preference on their part.

Accurately determining the quantity of drug taken is another confounding issue. For example, most psychological studies have asked the person, after the fact, how much of a drug or what drugs they had abused. If the short-term memory of these individuals is impaired, their recall of what drugs they used can be confounded with their cognitive deficits.

The method of drug abuse administration raises additional concerns. For example, whether one takes a drug through injection, or orally, or through the nose may have different effects with respect to the action of the drug and may produce different residual neuropsychological impairments. In addition, there are numerous premorbid and concurrent medical risk factors which are of significance in terms of understanding the effects of drugs on a person's mental abilities. For example, Tarter and Edwards (1987) described a number of pre-existing issues which bear on an individual's reactions to various drugs. Such issues include a pre-existing history of learning disabilities, attention deficit disorder, and hyperactivity. In addition, poor nutrition and health combined with impaired organs are likely to significantly affect the substance abuser's cognitive functioning.

MARIJUANA/CANNABIS

While the vast majority of research studies (Mendelson & Meyer, 1972; Grant, Rochford, Flemming, & Stunkard, 1973; Carlin & Trupin, 1977) have not reported significant chronic neuropsychological deficits in marijuana users, some recent studies have reported that short-term memory functions may be impaired after consistent marijuana use (Page, Fletcher, & True, 1988; Schwartz, Gruenewald, Klitzner, & Fedio, 1989). Since the earlier studies relied on relatively poor measures of short-term memory functioning, the new findings might reflect better measures of short-term memory.

HALLUCINOGENS/LSD

In general, the vast majority of research studies have reported some cognitive deficits. For example, McGlothlin, Arnold, and Freedman (1969) and Acord and Baker (1973) both found evidence of deficits in visual abstraction and concept formation. However, these deficits could possibly have been related to one of the many above-mentioned confounding issues.

OPIATES

While early research by Fields and Fullerton (1975) found no clear evidence for neuropsychological deficits with heroin addicts, Rounsaville, Novelly, Kleber, & Jones (1980) found heroin addicts who were also polydrug users to be moderate to severely impaired on a battery of neuropsychological tests. Interestingly, they also found that those heroin addicts who were most impaired tended to have a childhood history of hyperactivity and a poorer academic records. In a follow-up study, however, Rounsaville, Jones, Novelly, and Kleber (1982) found their drug users to perform better than demographically similar controls on specific neuropsychological tests. Thus, it is unclear whether heroin addicts have any neuropsychological impairments.

SEDATIVES

Research clearly suggests that sedative use is associated with certain cognitive deficits. For example, Judd and Grant (1975) reported neuropsychological deficits among sedative abusers. Their conclusions, however, must be taken with caution since many of their patients had also been abusers of stimulants, alcohol, and opiates. Bergman, Borg, and Holm (1980), in a more carefully controlled study, found neuropsychological impairments in subjects who were treated only for illicit sedative abuse.

PHENCYCLIDINE (PCP)

Neuropsychological research studies have not overwhelmingly demonstrated the presence of cognitive impairments in PCP users even though PCP is generally believed to produce organic mental disorder. For example, Carlin, Grant, Adams, and Reed (1979) were unable to detect gross neuropsychological deficit in PCP drug users, but reported subtle deficits in terms of the PCP drug abuser's ability to process rhythmetric patterns. At this time, however, few conclusions can be drawn regarding the potential effects of PCP use on neuropsychological test performance.

COCAINE/STIMULANTS

O'Malley and Gawin (1990) demonstrated mild neuropsychological impairments in chronic cocaine users. Their findings were consistent with the level of deficits reported in research studies for polydrug users. Also, there have been other reports of subtle neuropsychological deficits with respect to cocaine abusers (Strickland et al., 1993) that were confirmed by Single Photon Emission Computerized Tomography (SPECT). Possible mechanisms of action to produce cognitive deficit are that cocaine users are more likely to have strokes and seizures than other patients (Volkow, Mullani, Gould, Adler, & Krajewski, 1988). It is remarkable that there have been relatively few studies of stimulant use in humans as there is considerable animal research suggesting possible neuropsychological deficits (Reed & Grant, 1990).

Investigators in future studies may wish to use tools such as Positron Emission Tomography (PET) (Volkow, Fowler, & Wolf, 1991) in conjunction with neuropsychological testing.

INHALANTS/SOLVENTS

The evidence for neuropsychological impairment on inhalants/solvents is clear. For example, Bigler (1979) observed a generalized pattern of cognitive deficits on the Halstead-Reitan neuropsychological test battery. Korman, Matthews, and Lovitt (1981) also demonstrated neuropsychological impairment by inhalant abusers. Tsushina and Towne (1977) found a sample of glue sniffers were neuropsychologically impaired on the Halstead-Reitan Test Battery. In addition, Berry, Heaton, & Kirley (1977) found a group of chronic abusers were also impaired on sections of the Halstead-Reitan Neuropsychological Test Battery.

POLYDRUG ABUSE

There is also considerable evidence that polydrug abusers have neuropsychological impairments. For example, Judd and Grant (1975) reported that polydrug abusers were impaired on the Halstead-Reitan Neuropsychological Test Battery. Grant, Mohns, Miller, and Reitan (1976) also demonstrated evidence for impairment of neuropsychological functioning. However, the data suggesting polydrug users are suffering neuropsychological impairment in these studies are not free from possible confounds with respect to medical and psychiatric risk factors. For example, it is possible that some of the polydrug users they studied also abused alcohol. Thus, the effects reported may be due to alcohol consumption (Tarter & Edwards, 1987).

ECOLOGICAL VALIDITY

With respect to the above findings, it seems clear that neuropsychological testing when using a level of performance model, may not be able to detect subtle cognitive deficits present in many individuals who abuse drugs due to a variety of confounding factors. The clear exception to this appears to be individuals who engage in inhalant/solvent and/or polydrug abuse. There is the possibility that subtle patterns of deficit could be identified, (Parson & Farr,

1981), but there have been few studies. With respect to the issue of ecological validity, the drug abuser may, like many patients with subtle residual cognitive deficits, perform significantly better in rather artificial test settings than real-world environments since they are well-known to exhibit major difficulties at work, home, or school, particularly when they are required to function in relatively demanding situations.

Also, many substance abusers could have been more able physiologically premorbidly, so there is an ability level/deficit identification problem. This sort of problem is often found when a level of performance model is used in assessment (Reitan & Wolfson, 1985).

Heaton and Pendleton (1981) demonstrated some years ago that neuropsychological testing has a uniquely important role in predicting the likely impact of neuropsychological deficits on everyday functioning. Specific areas of everyday functioning would be vocational functioning, academic achievement, self-care, and independent living. Unfortunately, very little research has been done relating neuropsychological deficits in substance abusers to these areas of functioning and virtually none in terms of relating their functioning to their success in therapy. These are areas that would profit from greatly increased attention. Clearly, there are major clinical questions concerning living arrangements, employability, and the prospects for benefiting from drug abuse treatment as well as the need for specific environmental, vocational, social, and emotional support systems. The definition of ecological validity proposed by Sbordone (Chapter 2) may also be beneficial in the conceptualization and design of such research studies.

SUMMARY

This chapter briefly discussed neuropsychological assessment batteries both from a screening perspective and also in terms of comprehensive neuropsychological functioning with respect to evaluating drug abusers. Attention was devoted to the manifold difficulties of assessing the residual neuropsychological effects of various psycho-active substances. A brief and selective review of neuropsychological test results with drug abusers was presented for a few psychoactive substances. The current research, with respect to the use of neuropsychological tests to predict the behavior/social/vocational functioning of drug abusers, is composed of a small number of studies, all of which are flawed in some way. These studies also suggest future research should examine the functioning of drug abusers in relatively demanding environments to determine their ability to work, attend school, and function in demanding real-world settings. The neuropsychological assessment of drug abusers with respect to its ecological validity, is an area that clearly requires much additional work. Paul Meehl (1955) said many years ago that so little was known about psychotherapy that the only thing to do was to do a great deal of experimentation. The same notion is just as valid today with respect to the ecological validity of neuropsychological testing for drug abusers.

Dr. Horton's contributions to this chapter were performed in his capacity as a private citizen and were neither supported, endorsed or approved by the National Institute on Drug Abuse, The National Institutes on Health, the Public Health Service or the U.S. Department of Health and Human Services, or any other agency or component of the Federal Government.

REFERENCES

Acord, L. D., & Barker, D. D. (1973). Hallucinogenic drugs and cerebral deficit. *Journal of Nervous and Mental Diseases, 156,* 281-283.

American Psychiatric Association. (1994). Diagnostic Statistical Manual of mental Disorders IV.

Benedict, R. H. B., & Horton, A. M., Jr. (1992). Neuropsychology of alcohol induced brain damage: Current perspectives on diagnosis, recovery, and prevention. In D. Templer, L. Hartlage, & W. G. Cannon (Eds.), *Preventable brain damage: Brain vulnerability and brain health* (pp. 146-160). New York: Springer.

Bergman, H., Borg, S., & Holm, L. (1980). Neuropsychological impairments and the exclusive abuse of sedatives or hypnotics. *American Journal of Psychiatry 137,* 215-217.

Berry, G., Heaton, R., & Kirley, M. (1977). Neuropsychological deficits of chronic inhalant abusers. In B. Rumaek & A. Temple (Eds.), *Management of the poisoned patient* (pp. 59-83). Princeton: Sciences Press.

Bigler, E. D. (1979). Neuropsychological evaluation of adolescent patients hospitalized with chronic inhalant abuse. *Clinical Neuropsychology, 1,* 8-12.

Carlin, A., Grant, I., Adams, K., & Reed, R. (1979). Is phencyclidine (PCP) abuse associated with organic mental impairment? *American Journal of Drug and Alcohol Abuse 6,* 273-281.

Carlin, A. S., & Trupin, E. (1977). The effects of long-term chronic cannabis use on neuropsychological functioning. *International Journal of Addiction, 12,* 617-624.

Fields, F. S., & Fullerton, J. (1975). Influences of heroin addiction on neuropsychological functioning. *Journal of Consulting and Clinical Psychology, 43,* 114.

Grant, I., Mohns, L., Miller, M., & Reitan, R (1976). A neuropsychological study of polydrug users. *Archives of General Psychiatry, 33,* 973-978.

Grant, I., Rochford, J., Fleming, T. & Stunkard, A. (1973). A neuropsychological assessment of the effects of moderate marijuana use. *Journal of Nervous and Mental Disease, 156,* 278-280.

Halstead, W. C. (1947). *Brain and intelligence.* Chicago: University of Chicago Press.

Harwood, H. J., Napolitano, D., M., Kristiansen, P. L., & Collins, J. J. (1984) *Economic costs to society of alcohol and drug abuse and mental illness: 1980.* Research Triangle Park, NC: Research Triangle Institute.

Heaton, R. K, & Pendleton, M. C. (1981). Use of neuropsychological tests to predict adult patient's everyday functioning. *Journal of Consulting and Clinical Psychology, 49,* 807-821.

Horton, A. M., Jr., & Anilane, J. (1986). Relationship of Trail Making test-part B and brain age quotients — long and short forms. *Psychotherapy in Private Practices, 21,* 39-43.

Horton, A. M., Jr., & Wedding, D. (1984). *Introduction to clinical and behavioral neuropsychology.* New York: Praeger.

Hubbard, R. L., Marsden, M. E., Rachal, J. V., Harwood, H. J., Cavanaugh, E. R., & Ginzburg, H. M. (1989). *Drug abuse treatment: A national study of effectiveness.* Chapel Hill: University of North Carolina Press.

Judd, L. L., & Grant, I. (1975). Brain dysfunction in chronic sedative users. *Journal of Psychedelic Drugs, 7,* 143-149.

Korman, M., Matthews, R. W., & Lovitt, R. (1981). Neuropsychological effects of abuse on inhalants. *Perceptual & Motor Skills, 53,* 547-553.

McGlothlin, W. H., Arnold, D. D. & Freedman, D. X. (1969). Organicity measures following repeated LSD ingestion. *Archives of General Psychiatry, 21,* 704-709.

Meehl, P. E. (1955). Psychotherapy. *Annual Review of Psychology, 6,* 357-378.

Mendelson, J. H., & Meyer, R. E. (1972). Behavioral and biological concomitants of chronic marijuana smoking by heavy and casual users. In *Marijuana: A signal of misunderstanding,* Vol. 1, Washington, DC: U.S. Government Printing Office.

O'Malley, S. S., & Gawin, F. H. (1990). Abstinence symptomatology and neuropsychological deficits in chronic cocaine abusers. In J. W. Spencer & J. J. Boren, *Residual effects of abused drugs on behavior* (pp. 179-190). National Institute on Drug Abuse Research Monograph 101, OHHS Pub. No. (ADM) 90-1719. Washington, DC: Superintendent of Documents, U.S. Government Printing Office.

Page, J. B., Fletcher, J., & True, W. P. (1988). Psychosociocultural perspectives on chronic cannabis use: The Costa Rican follow-up. *Journal of Psychoactive Drugs, 20,* 57-65.

Parson, O. A., & Farr, S. P. (1981). The neuropsychology of alcohol and drug use. In S. Filskov & T. J. Boll (Eds.), *The handbook of clinical neuropsychology* (pp. 320-365). New York: Wiley.

Reed, R., & Grant, I. (1990). The long term neurobehavioral consequence of substance abuse: conceptual and methodological challenge for future research. In J. W. Spencer & J. J. Boren (Eds.), *Residual effects of abused drugs on behavior.* Research Monograph 101 (pp. 10-56). Rockville, MD: National Institute on Drug Abuse.

Reitan, R. M. (1955). Investigation of the validity of Halstead's measure of biological intelligence. *Archives of Neurology and Psychiatry, 73,* 280-35.

Reitan, R. (1973). *Behavioral manifestations of impaired brain functioning in aging.* Paper presented at the Annual Meeting of the American Psychological Association, Montreal, Canada.

Reitan, R. M., & Wolfson, D. (1985). *The Halstead-Reitan Neuropsychological Battery.* Tucson, AZ: Neuropsychology Press.

Rounsaville, B. J., Novelly, R. A., & Kleber, H. D. (1980). Neuropsychological impairments in opiate addicts: Risk factors. *Annals of the New York Academy of Science, 362,* 79-80.

Rounsaville, B. J., Jones, C. Novelly, R. A., & Kleber, H. D. (1982). Neuropsychological functioning in opiate addicts. *Journal of Nervous and Mental Diseases, 170,* 209-216.

Schau, E. J., & O'Leary, M. R. (1977). Adaptive abilities of hospitalized alcoholics and matched controls: The brain-age quotient. *Journal of Studies on Alcohol, 38,* 403-409.

Schwartz, R. H., Gruenewald, P. J., Klitzner, M., & Fedio, P. (1989). Short-term memory impairment in cannabis-dependent adolescents. *American Journal of Diseases of Children, 143*(100), 1214-1219.

Spencer, J. W., & Boren, (1990). *Residual effects of abused drugs in behavior.* Research Monograph 101. Rockville, MD: National Institute on Drug Abuse.

Strickland, T. L., Mena, I., Villanueva-Meyer, J., Miller, B., Mehringer, C. M., Satz, P., & Myers, H. (1993). Cerebral perfusion and neuropsychological consequences of chronic cocaine use. *Journal of Neuropsychiatry and Clinical Neuroscience, 5,* 419-427.

Tarter, R. E., & Edwards, K. L. (1987). Brief and comprehensive neuropsychological assessment of alcohol and substance abuse. In L. C. Hartlage, J. L. Hornsby, & M. J. Asken (Eds.), *Essentials of neuropsychological assessment* (pp. 138-162). New York: Springer.

Tsushina, W., & Towne, W. (1977). Effects of paint sniffing on neuropsychological test performance. *Journal of Abnormal Psychology, 86,* 402-407.

Volkow, N. D., Fowler, J. S., & Wolf, A. P. (1991). Use of positron mission tomography to study cocaine in the human brain. In R. S. Rapaka, A. Makriyhnnis, & M. J. Kuhar (Eds.), *Emerging technologies and new direction in drug abuse research* (pp. 168-179). National Institute on Drug Abuse Research Monograph 112, DHHS Pub. No. (ADM) 91-1812. Washington, DC: Superintendent of Documents, U.S. Government Printing Office.

Volkow, N. D., Mullani, N., Gould, K. L., Adler, S., & Krajewski, K. (1988). Cerebral blood flow in chronic cocaine users: A study with positron emission tomography. *British Journal of Psychiatry, 152,* 641-648.

18

NEUROPSYCHOLOGY AND REHABILITATION COUNSELING:
Bridging the Gap

Brian T. McMahon, Ph.D., C.R.C.
Linda R. Shaw, Ph.D., C.R.C.

INTRODUCTION

On most traumatic brain injury (TBI) rehabilitation teams, neuropsychologists (whether as full-time staff members or consultants) are generally cast in positions of leadership or (at a minimum) significant influence. This occurs in large part due to their degree of graduate education relative to other team members, the documented importance of specialized knowledge in the area of brain-behavior relationships (Dial, Chan, Gray, Tunick, & Marme, 1991), and the involvement of neuropsychologists at all levels of care which bridge medical and non-medical environments.

Most vocational rehabilitation counselors, whose primary interest is to return the client with TBI to the highest possible level of vocational functioning, are cognizant of the fact that the primary impediments to vocational re-entry are the cognitive and psychosocial barriers experienced by most clients (Fraser, McMahon, & Vogenthaler, 1988). For example, neuropsychological findings such as problems in thinking and reasoning, information processing speed, attention, concentration, and short-term memory are recognized by the vocational specialist as formidable vocational barriers. The implications of a severe memory impairment in relation to new learning ability are particularly devastating in a world of work in which "re-careering" is the order of the day (i.e., "...process of repeatedly acquiring marketable skills and changing careers in response to the turbulent job market of the high-tech society") (Krannich, 1988, p. 14).

Similarly, those typical sequalae which one encounters in a psychosocial assessment (e.g., problems in assuming responsibility, initiation, social isolation) directly impact such work adaptive behaviors such as coworker relations, the primary cause of most job terminations in America. Because these same issues are the primary purview of neuropsychologists, there is an obvious need for strong communication and collaboration between rehabilitation counselors and neuropsychologists in the interest of maximizing return to work. Competent program managers will encourage and provide regular opportunities for such cooperation.

It is all the more regrettable, then, that there continues to be significant misunderstanding and miscommunication between the disciplines of vocational rehabilitation counseling and neuropsychology (Kay & Silver, 1988). From the authors' perspective this is partially rooted in the stark reality that basic neuropsychological training does not provide exposure to vocational issues such as the importance of understanding an individual's work repertoire; occupational information regarding 20,000 distinct American occupations; the requirements of various work environments; or even the basic nature of the vocational rehabilitation process. Conversely, the training of rehabilitation counselors in brain-behavior relationships, which is so vital to the understanding of individuals with TBI, is equally deficient.

In summary, the mastery by members of each discipline of the body of knowledge of the other is not much greater than that of the layperson. This chapter is intended to begin to bridge this knowledge deficit by providing neuropsychologists with a basic primer of vocational rehabilitation and related issues in order to enhance the effectiveness of their leadership role vis-a-vis the clients' vocational re-entry objectives.

WORK REPERTOIRE AND THE VOCATIONAL REHABILITATION PROCESS

The primary benefit of vocational rehabilitation (VR) programming to the interdisciplinary team and the overall operation of the TBI treatment program may be its capacity to provide traction, focus, and meaning to other therapies or services. Ultimately, effective job placement at the highest possible level is more likely when all therapies can be related to work, and vice-versa. Fraser, McMahon, and Vogenthaler (1988) provided specific suggestions regarding ways in which all interdisciplinary team members might approach their respective duties to maximize the level and stability of ultimate job placement. Such a pervasive VR approach seeks to distribute responsibility for VR outcomes among all interdisciplinary team members. This is typically accomplished only by a strong management commitment and consistent staff training. If successful, however, the program is able to achieve an effective VR effort without the expenditure of significant funds for what is regarded, regrettably and often erroneously, as a non-reimbursable service component.

VR is also more effective when all interdisciplinary team members understand that the primary impediments to vocational recovery are the clients' cognitive and psychosocial deficits (McMahon & Fraser, 1988a). Accordingly, those team members whose primary responsibilities are for cognitive and psychosocial remediation generally experience more interaction with VR personnel than other team members, and appropriately so. Fawber and Wachter (1987) argue that traditional VR which typically occurs at the end of the treatment continuum is insufficient for effecting successful placement for persons with TBI. Rather, they argue for a "treatment oriented placement process (with) concomitant treatment of cognitive and psychosocial sequaelae of severe head injury" (p. 28).

It is also generally agreed that VR interventions should be directed at the entire work repertoire including work behaviors (skill proficiency, work rate, work quality, work endurance); work adaptive behaviors; work values; work interests; learning style; and motivation. Perhaps the single largest explanation for the failure of most VR programs with TBI clients is their excessive emphasis on the development of skill proficiency, typically manifest by elaborate training services. On balance, greater benefits will be realized when services are focused on work adaptive behaviors, especially the abilities to relate to coworkers and supervisors.

In each step of the VR process there exist unique considerations which, if implemented, can significantly enhance the effectiveness of VR interventions with persons with TBI (Fraser, McMahon, & Vogenthaler, 1988; McMahon & Fraser, 1988b). In work evaluation, for example, these include:

- the avoidance of group interventions;
- the minimal use of commercially available work samples;
- the expectation of frustration and anger;
- the testing of limits;
- the flexibility of test administration;
- the avoidance of attribution of all errors to neurogenic causes;
- the need to evaluate all areas of the work repertoire, especially work-adaptive behaviors;
- the focus on known correlates of vocational success;
- the pre-eminence of situational assessment, on-the-job evaluation, and occupational trials.

Regarding job placement, a decision-tree has been described which delineates how vocational and neuropsychological evaluation results may be used to prescribe the appropriate job placement approach (Fraser, Clemmons, & McMahon, 1990). More traditional job placement approaches (e.g., selective placement and job-seeking skills training) have many inherent limitations when applied to persons with TBI. Specifically, the inefficiency of the former and the didactic nature of the latter are problematic. The "systems selling" approach (McMahon & Spencer, 1979) is likely to experience a resurgence of interest in the post-ADA era (Americans with Disabilities Act). This approach involves a straightforward exchange of VR consultation and technical assistance to employers in exchange for preferential hiring considerations for a segment of rehabilitation clientele.

In the near future, traditional job placement approaches will most likely be used in tandem with supported employment interventions. Supported employment is defined as paid work, typically in a variety of settings, in which disabled workers are integrated with nondisabled workers, and in which supports are provided to ensure that the disabled worker will succeed. Eligible workers are those who would not otherwise succeed without such supports, defined as any activity designed to improve client competitiveness.

To be maximally effective, certain aspects of supported employment require more emphasis than others. The individual supported jobs model appears most effective, but it is sometimes difficult to extend this approach to clients with more serious behavioral or cognitive involvement. An affirmative industry approach has been found effective, but only when used in a complementary fashion as transitional to the supported jobs model. The failure of supported employment interventions is most often traced to an overreliance on job coaching, a narrow range of supports utilized, and the failure to emphasize natural supports which will receive far greater attention in the decade ahead (Fraser, 1991). It is the authors' opinion that all interdisciplinary team members should participate as job coaches and the utilization of categorical job coaches should be avoided.

Increasingly it appears that vocational interventions are generally most effective when the workplace is utilized as a primary site of all (not just vocational) rehabilitation activity. The employer can be considered as a primary community resource with all assessment, work skills training, and work adjustment training occurring in normalized environments such as employer OJT programs, occupational trials, neighboring vocational-technical schools, projects with industry, apprenticeship programs, and the like. As noted earlier, this is the fundamental approach of employer-based disability management programs (Schwartz, Watson, Galvin, & Lipoff, 1989; Shrey & LaCerte, 1995) which are becoming increasingly popular in the present decade. Rehabilitation facilities as centers of vocational rehabilitation, especially sheltered workshops, should be utilized only as a last resort, as none can compare to the workplace for face validity and the broadest possible range of occupational and training experiences.

One might consider that when a child becomes disabled, there follows automatically every effort to reintegrate that child into the school environment at the earliest possible moment and to expect that school to accommodate that child and become the logical site and vehicle of redevelopment (not just educational redevelopment). So too with the TBI adult, the preinjury worksite should perform a similar role whenever possible.

McMahon and Shaw (1991b) have described how outpatient day programming is naturally consistent with these recommendations because the "face validity" of the evaluation experience is naturally improved and the range of occupational opportunities considered is typically expanded beyond what is available in remote residential settings. Conversely, one potential danger of day programming is the tendency to subcontract vocational evaluation services to extant VR facilities in which reliance on prepackaged, commercially available work samples is a common practice. This approach often leads to the underestimation of vocational potential for individuals with TBI.

PHILOSOPHICAL ORIENTATION

It is the authors' impression that another key issue in the lack of meaningful communication between the two professions lies in the matter of philosophical orientation. Rehabilitation counselors who have graduated from CORE accredited programs have completed mandatory training in rehabilitation philosophy. This is, by design, a value-processing experience in which professionals become guided by such concepts as whole person, interdisciplinary team functioning, normalization, least restrictive environment, criterion of ultimate functioning, outcome orientation, emphasis on residual assets, client involvement in rehabilitation planning, emphasis on compensatory and coping mechanisms, and the like.

These are not matters of rhetoric to CRCs; they establish parameters which influence clinical, management, and case management decisions. These principles are strongly reinforced through several professional associations (e.g., National Rehabilitation Counseling Association, American Rehabilitation Counseling Association, National Council on Rehabilitation Education); credentialling bodies (e.g., Commission on Rehabilitation Counselor Certification, 1990; Council on Rehabilitation Education, 1991); and a unified Code of Ethics for Rehabilitation Counselors (Tarvydas & Pape, 1988). As the professional rehabilitation community interfaces with the community of people with disabilities, the importance of these philosophical tenets is emphasized to an even greater degree. Those CRCs who are themselves disabled or whose professional roots are in the independent living movement, for example, tend to be even more outspoken regarding these values (Bowe, 1978; McMahon, 1991; McMahon & Shaw, 1991a; Shapiro, 1993;).

In order to facilitate a clear understanding of the orientation of the rehabilitation counselor toward neuropsychology, several of these philosophical principles are discussed in greater detail:

1. **Holistic Approach.** Rehabilitation counselors tend to ascribe to the perspective that rehabilitation efforts should be directed toward the whole person within an ecological context. They view the tendency of many rehabilitationists to divide people into convenient parts (e.g., physical, psychological, spiritual) as harmful and instead emphasize a more integrated approach to evaluation and treatment.

2. **Interdisciplinary Team Process.** Coming from a holistic framework, rehabilitation counselors firmly believe in a coordinated, integrated team approach. In TBI rehabilitation, the rehabilitation counselor's emphasis on integration of treatment components often results in a transdisciplinary approach with deliberate blurring of discipline boundaries. While rehabilitation counselors are certainly not the only specialty that ever stresses interdisciplinary or transdisciplinary team functioning, they tend to be one of the disciplines most emphatically committed to it, due in part to their general holistic philosophy. This emphasis is also due, however, to an historical tradition wherein the rehabilitation counselor is cast in the role of a coordinator of services (Whitehouse, 1975). Since the inception of the profession, rehabilitation counselors have been challenged with the task of coordinating and integrating the activities of many professionals with various philosophical orientations and cultures. They have, for many years, been in a key position to view the problems created by turfguarding and the lack of communication among disciplines, and have frequently assumed the role of case manager to resolve communication problems.

3. **Criterion of Ultimate Functioning.** This principle is almost universally ascribed to by rehabilitation counselors. It is defined as the belief that persons with disabilities have a right and rehabilitation professionals have a responsibility to promote opportunities "...to function as productively and independently as possible in socially, vocationally, and domestically integrated community settings" (Pancsofar & Blackwell, 1986, p. 9). Key words contained within this

definition include "productively," emphasizing the rehabilitation counselor's underlying belief in the importance of work to all persons; "independently," stressing the rehabilitation counselor's emphasis on promoting independence rather than engaging in a care-giving model which may foster dependence; and "domestically integrated settings," illustrating the importance of normalized community life.

4. **Normalization**. Normalization was defined by Wolfensburger as "...the use of means which are culturally normative to offer a person life conditions at least as good as the average citizen" (Pancsofar and Blackwell, 1986, p. 6). This principle stresses the importance of striving to afford persons with disabilities the opportunity to live, work, and function in as "normal" an environment and manner as possible.

5. **Functional Approach**. The principle of normalization is a primary philosophical underpinning for the strong conviction generally held by rehabilitation counselors that the primary goal of rehabilitation is to assist the client in regaining the functional ability to become as fully reintegrated as possible into ordinary adult pursuits within the home, the workplace, and the community. The very heavy emphases of most rehabilitation counselors on functional approaches often causes them frustration in traditional clinic settings which they may perceive as "abnormal" environments far removed from the person's normal sphere of activity (e.g., home, work, community).

Similarly, rehabilitation counselors often feel that the emphasis on diagnosis and treatment within the clinical setting lacks validity, occurring as it does outside of more normalized settings. They note problems with motivating clients who may have difficulty understanding the relevance of lengthy clinical diagnostic and treatment procedures to their own goals (i.e., getting back to "normal life"). Additionally, rehabilitation counselors frequently express concerns about the difficulty of generalizing skills learned in clinical environments to settings in which clients ultimately must learn to function successfully. Such concerns about generalization are particularly acute among rehabilitation counselors in TBI rehabilitation (Durgin, Cullity, & Devine, 1991).

Consequently, many rehabilitation counselors have adopted a general feeling that lengthy, clinically based diagnostic and treatment procedures have little utility for them in effecting the kinds of functional outcomes desired (Hart & Hayden, 1986). This orientation has fueled the growth of the disability management movement (Habeck, Shrey, & Growick, 1991), wherein rehabilitation services are provided within the work setting.

6. **Emphasis on Residual Assets**. Rehabilitation counselors tend to strongly emphasize ability vs. disability in their approach to rehabilitation. This may be related to the fact that rehabilitation counselors have historically operated within

related to the fact that rehabilitation counselors have historically operated within the "real-world" environment of the workplace where they often confront attitudinal and architectural barriers to employment. There is a natural tendency for nondisabled persons to perceive persons with disability as disabled in all ways because of certain discrete limitations, a phenomenon termed "spread" (Wright, 1960). Rehabilitation counselors, charged with overcoming such attitudinal barriers in order to achieve successful vocational outcomes, have consistently sought to contain this "spread" by emphasizing the individual's abilities rather than disabilities. Rehabilitation counselors have become further convinced of the importance of not dwelling on disability as technological advances have begun to make it possible for persons previously termed "severely disabled" to live and work independently (Rubin & Roessler, 1995).

Disability has come to be perceived as an impairment that can be minimized by creativity, initiative, and by focusing upon the individual's residual assets and abilities. This "can do" attitude has become endemic to the field of rehabilitation counseling, reinforced by everincreasing successes in assisting persons previously deemed "too disabled" in becoming independent, productive citizens. Consequently, many rehabilitation counselors have little patience with pessimistic diagnoses and dire predictions of rehabilitation potential, particularly when such conclusions have been reached based upon clinical models of assessment rather than in community or workbased functional assessment environments (Bowe, 1978; Shapiro, 1993).

How is neuropsychology regarded through the eyes of such rehabilitationists? On balance, it is perceived as being too preoccupied with the evaluation, diagnosis, and measurement of deficits; as too preoccupied with identifying deficits rather than areas of cognitive and psychological strengths; as too soft or general regarding treatment recommendations (particularly of a vocational nature); as conducted in a clinic or laboratory too far removed from the real-life situation of the client; and as too focused upon the brain component of the brain-behavior relationship. The authors acknowledge that this is a colloquial, noncomplementary generalization or depiction. CRCs tend to hold this perception to some extent about most TBI team members. The point is that this is a perception which is rooted in the CRC's philosophical bias which is not necessarily imparted, as a matter of training, to any other member of the TBI team. CRCs often feel that their sensitivity to these values is perceived by others as quasi-evangelical, naive, or simplistic, particularly in the for-profit climate in which most TBI rehabilitation ensues (Mullins, 1989).

Most importantly, although CRCs do not equate the meaning of life to the meaning of work, they do elevate vocational objectives to a higher level of importance than most other team members. CRCs are very interested in the extent to which work is a central life interest and in the individual meaning of work for each client. Most believe that vocational services are unlike any others provided to the TBI client in that they are "pull factors," that is, they reach in from the community to restore the identity of the client as a worker, engage the client in a life-style which includes gainful activity, and sustain the client in a productive lifestyle long after the other "push therapies" (i.e., those from which the client will hopefully become completely independent) have been terminated.

Work is perceived by CRCs as both an outcome and a means to continued rehabilitation and integration. Work is a primary means by which at least 20 independent human needs are met (Loftquist & Dawis, 1969) and without maximizing vocational gain it is difficult to regard the business of rehabilitation as complete. CRCs are usually strong advocates for early vocational intervention, including in TBI rehabilitation (Fraser, McMahon, & Vogenthaler, 1988), and perhaps no expression so irritates the CRC as ..."He has completed rehabilitation now, let's refer him for vocational services."

HISTORY AND SYSTEMS ORIENTATION

A brief overview of the history of vocational rehabilitation is presented to facilitate an understanding of rehabilitation counseling. Although this history may be organized according to various themes, the most useful one is federal legislation. Vocational rehabilitation is a small but very proud profession which some have described as the oldest human service profession in America. Its legislative roots go back to the Smith-Fess Act (Soldiers Rehabilitation Act) of 1917 which provided for basic vocational rehabilitation assistance to World War I veterans. Through a long series of key pieces of federal laws and amendments, including the Civilian Rehabilitation Act, the Social Security Act, the Randolph-Sheppard Act, the Community Mental Health Act, and the Rehabilitation Act of 1973, a partnership was formed between the federal Rehabilitation Services Administration and the vocational rehabilitation agency in each state/territory. Within this partnership approximately $1.5 billion annually of federal funds is matched by approximately $0.5 billion of state money to provide vocational rehabilitation services to disabled Americans who meet certain criteria. This state-federal program is administered through state vocational rehabilitation agencies (Rubin and Roessler, 1995).

The long-standing relationship between vocational rehabilitation and landmark federal legislation has been viewed both as a blessing and a curse, but no one can argue the impact. For example, among other key provisions the Rehabilitation Act of 1973 required the state-federal program to prioritize services to the severely disabled. While seemingly a noble endeavor, this often left the less-than-severely disabled without access to the state-federal program due to funding limitations. The majority of these clients were industrially injured workers with back injuries. Workers' compensation insurance companies responded by developing their own medical management, vocational rehabilitation, and case management services, giving birth to over 7,000 private sector insurance rehabilitation companies in the 1970s, perhaps the fastest growing area of the human services economy (McMahon & Matkin, 1982).

Rehabilitation counselors and their associations are very active politically. They were instrumental in the lobbying and passage of the Americans with Disabilities Act of 1990, unequivocally the most significant piece of civil rights legislation since 1964. The employment provisions alone (Title I) will forever change the way human resources in American businesses are managed, and all TBI team members should be educated regarding the basic provisions of this law (Hablutzel & McMahon, 1991).

It is worth noting that in an era of strict accountability to both financial providers, legislators, and persons with disabilities, rehabilitation counselors responded with the development of certification and accreditation mechanisms and a unified code of ethics. These now-sophisticated processes have provided an historical basis for similar movements (including counselor licensure) by counselors, mental health counselors, and marriage and family counselors.

It is useful to understand that there are profound differences in the professional activities of CRCs who work in the public (state-federal, nonprofit) and private (for-profit) sector (McMahon, 1979). Few are so important as the fact that in the public sector, caseloads are very high, often in excess of 125 severely disabled clients per counselor. Maximization of vocational goals is generally encouraged, and the state-federal system is relatively training-oriented. In the private sector, immediate return to work with the same employer is usually the first priority. This is a service delivery system oriented toward expeditious job placement. Unfortunately, in some settings, ethical conflicts and court appearances are the prices paid for manageable caseloads and higher salaries (Matkin & May, 1981).

CREDENTIALLING

The issues of the proper identification, training, and credentialling of clinical neuropsychologists have been problematic for those inside as well as outside the profession. Vocational rehabilitation counselors, who frequently refer to and purchase neuropsychological services from psychologists, have learned through experience that their time and monies have been wasted on those who purport to be what they are not. Similarly, it is not unusual to hear expressions of disappointment from neuropsychologists regarding the training and expertise of rehabilitation counselors, especially as they relate to individuals with TBI. To be sure, these impressions are often valid, and as with neuropsychology the root of the problem lies in credentialling.

There are perhaps 75,000 individuals who hold such job titles as rehabilitation counselor, rehabilitation specialist, rehabilitation consultant, vocational specialist, and the like. These are not legally protected terms in most states and can be used by anyone. In terms of competence, the neuropsychologists' interests are best served by seeking dialogue with a master's degreed Certified Rehabilitation Counselor (C.R.C.), preferably a graduate from a rehabilitation counselor training program accredited by the Commission on Rehabilitation Education (C.O.R.E.). The minimum demonstrated proficiencies and curriculum requirements of the Commission on Rehabilitation Counselor Certification (C.R.C.C.) and C.O.R.E. are given in Tables 1 and 2 respectively.

Occupational therapists are well trained at the bachelor's degree level in matters of vocational skill proficiency, but tend to lack awareness of the complete work repertoire, case management processes, and the overall vocational rehabilitation process. The hospital-based work-hardening programs which they typically direct may be giving way to worksite disability management programs in the decade ahead (Habeck et al., 1991).

A brief examination of Table 1 and Table 2 yields yet another interesting finding (i.e., not all rehabilitation counselors are vocational experts). Indeed, vocational issues comprise but a minority of their training, and many CRCs pursue careers in mental health, substance abuse, independent living, advocacy, facility management, and other areas as far removed from vocational issues as neuropsychology, physical therapy, or cognitive remediation. Indeed, the authors have personally hired CRCs in TBI settings as behavior specialists, personal adjustment counselors, case managers, life skills counselors, and even cognitive specialists (McMahon, Shaw, & Mahaffey, 1988). Such specializations are developed through independent research, electives, fieldwork, internship, and post-graduate education and experience (McMahon & Growick, 1988).

Those CRCs who are vocationally oriented may be proficient in one or more aspects of the vocational rehabilitation process (e.g., work evaluation, vocational counseling, vocational training, work adjustment training, job placement, supported employment, injured worker issues).. Few have a mastery of most of these areas. Finally, those vocationally proficient CRCs who have a working knowledge of TBI and its sequalae are a minority indeed. The modi-

---

TABLE 1
CERTIFIED REHABILITATION COUNSELOR EXAMINATION CONTENT CLASSIFICATION CHART
(COMMISSION ON REHABILITATION COUNSELOR CERTIFICATION, 1990)

I. FOUNDATIONS OF REHABILITATION: (includes basic principles of rehabilitation; history of rehabilitation philosophy and legislation; rehabilitation counseling ethics; and disability conditions).

II. CLIENT ASSESSMENT: (includes all major areas of client information; principles, types and techniques of assessment; interpreting assessment results; and resources for assessment).

III. PLANNING AND SERVICE DELIVERY: (includes synthesis of client information; rehabilitation plan development; knowledge of services delivery; identification of community resources; and case management).

IV. COUNSELING AND INTERVIEWING: (includes theories and techniques in vocational and affective counseling; foundations of interviewing; principles of human behavior, and behavior change modalities).

V. JOB DEVELOPMENT AND PLACEMENT: (includes occupational and labor market information; job development; job-seeking skills; placement and follow-up).

---

fication by advisement of the CORE accredited curriculum for rehabilitation counseling students interested in a TBI rehabilitation career has been outlined in detail by McMahon et al. (1988). This article provides useful guidelines for the orientation of many disciplines to TBI.

As illustrated in Figure 1, the identification of a vocationally proficient CRC with a working knowledge of TBI is about as difficult as the identification of a true neuropsychologist certified by the American Board of Professional Psychologists with a working knowledge of vocational issues. The point is that the failure to properly conduct the search has resulted in misperceptions about the professional validity and usefulness of one profession by the other.

BRIDGING THE GAP

Neuropsychologists and rehabilitation counselors ultimately share similar goals. They are united in their commitment to facilitating the TBI client's re-entry into active, productive lives within their homes, workplaces, and communities. Yet problems arise between the two professional groups due to differ-

TABLE 2
**GRADUATE CURRICULUM REQUIREMENTS OF THE COUNCIL
ON REHABILITATION EDUCATION, 1991**

    I. FOUNDATIONS OF REHABILITATION COUNSELING: (includes history and philosophy of rehabilitation and legislation affecting individuals with disabilities; organizational structure of the vocational rehabilitation systems, including public, private for profit, and not-for-profit service settings; laws and ethical standards affecting rehabilitation counseling practice, with examples of their application; societal issues, trends, and developments as they relate to rehabilitation).

   II. COUNSELING SERVICES: (includes behavior, personality, human growth and development; individual, group and family counseling theories and practices; multicultural and gender issues; environmental and attitudinal barriers to individuals with disabilities; services to a variety of disability populations, including multiple disabilities, in diverse settings).

  III. CASE MANAGEMENT: (includes case management process, including case finding, service coordination, referral to and utilization of other disciplines, and client advocacy; planning for the provision of independent living services and vocational rehabilitation services; identification and use of community resources and services in rehabilitation planning; computer applications and technology for caseload management, functional assessment, job matching, etc.)

  IV. VOCATIONAL AND CAREER DEVELOPMENT: (includes vocational aspects of disabilities, including theories and approaches to career development and exploration; occupational information, labor market trends, and the importance of meaningful employment).

   V. ASSESSMENT: (includes medical aspects of disabilities, functional capacities of individuals with disabilities, and appropriate intervention resources (e.g. assistive technology); psycho-social aspects of disabilities, including the impact of disability on the individual and family, and personal, social and cultural adjustment to life; evaluation approaches, techniques, interpretation, available resources, and vocational evaluation).

  VI. JOB DEVELOPMENT AND PLACEMENT: (includes job analysis, work-site modification and restructuring, including the application of appropriate technology; job development, job placement, employer contacts, supported employment, follow-up and/or follow-along services).

 VII. RESEARCH: (includes rehabilitation research literature; statistics, methods, and types of research analyses; design of research projects and consultation on survey procedures and needs assessment approaches).

VIII. CLINICAL EXPERIENCE: (includes 100 clock hours of practicum and 600 clock hours of internship experience under the supervision of a CRC)

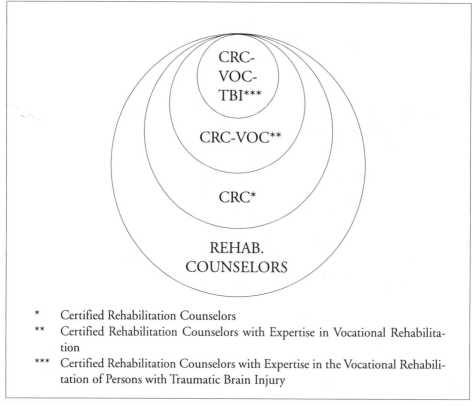

Certified Rehabilitation Counselors

*   Certified Rehabilitation Counselors
**   Certified Rehabilitation Counselors with Expertise in Vocational Rehabilitation
***   Certified Rehabilitation Counselors with Expertise in the Vocational Rehabilitation of Persons with Traumatic Brain Injury

Figure 1. Professional subdivisions within the rehabiltiation counseling profession.

ences in philosophy, lack of knowledge, and lack of communication. Such problems inhibit the development of the close, collaborative relationships needed to maximize the probability of achieving their common goals.

This chapter has attempted to identify some of the issues surrounding the problem and to provide neuropsychologists with information relative to the vocational rehabilitation history and process, and the philosophy and credentialling of rehabilitation counselors. Additional suggestions for facilitating cooperation between the two professions include: 1) formal cross-discipline training; 2) ensuring opportunities for formal (e.g., participation in staffings) and informal (e.g., general discussion, consultation) information sharing (Tankle, 1988; Morse & Morse, 1988); and 3) facilitating awareness among rehabilitation counselors of the need for precise referral questions when requesting neuropsychological evaluation.

Neuropsychologists may at times find themselves anticipating the informational needs of rehabilitation counselors who (because of their unfamiliarity with the neuropsychological evaluation process, its potential, and its limitations) may not even be aware of what questions to ask. The issue of referral questions is discussed in greater detail below.

REFERRAL QUESTIONS FOR THE NEUROPSYCHOLOGIST

It is our frequent experience that when many rehabilitation counselors complain about the lack of usefulness of a given neuropsychological report, they have themselves overlooked a critical step in the information-gathering process that is, they have failed to ask any (or at least appropriate) referral questions. Fraser, Clemmons, and McMahon (1990) recommended clearly that neuropsychologists can be more helpful when provided with a job description of the potential job in question (rooted in a recent and professionally conducted job analysis). This job description should identify only essential job functions per the Americans with Disabilities Act (Hablutzel and McMahon, 1991).

Additionally, the neuropsychologist should be asked relevant referral questions such as:

1. Please comment upon the full complement of work behaviors including proficiency, rate, quality, and endurance.
2. Please comment upon work adaptive behaviors (e.g., concentration and attention to task, capacity to get along with coworkers, response to authority, punctuality, attendance, grooming, hygiene)
3. Please comment upon learning style, with specific impressions regarding the type of training (e.g., formal academic or on-the-job) which may be possible.
4. Please comment upon self-awareness of cognitive strengths and deficits, and response to feedback or correction.
5. Please identify as many areas of strength as possible, and provide suggestions for the compensation of deficits where indicated.
6. Please indicate what level of supervision is required to perform the targeted job with proficiency.
7. Please provide any impressions regarding the client's expressed vocational interests, or motivation for the testing sequence.

The lack of familiarity with pertinent TBI issues by many rehabilitation counselors is reflected in the absence of referral questions. The seven items above might be regarded as "standing" referral questions which, if answered in whole or part, will render the entire evaluation report markedly more useful.

Indeed, the entire TBI rehabilitation movement would be better served if neuropsychologists insisted on specific referral questions with each request for evaluation services.

CONCLUSION

The neuropsychological evaluation can and should assist the rehabilitation counselor in successfully reintegrating the TBI client into the work environment. Conversely, the efforts of the neuropsychologist are a useless academic exercise unless they are perceived as being useful by the rehabilitation team, and more specifically to the rehabilitation counselor. It is incumbent on both professions to take positive steps to ensure that their areas of expertise are available and readily accessible to one another.

REFERENCES

Bowe, F. G. (1978). Handicapping America. New York: Harper and Row Publishers. Commission on Rehabilitation Counselor Certification. *Guide to rehabilitation counselor certification (Rev.)*. Rolling Meadows, IL: Author.

Council on Rehabilitation Education, Inc. (1991). *Accreditation manual for rehabilitation counselor education programs*. Rehabilitation Services Administration grant no. 44-P-81259/5-01. Washington, DC: Author.

Dial, J., Chan, F., Gray, S., Tunick, R., & Marme, M. (1991). Neuropsychological evaluation: A functional and behavioral approach. In B. T. McMahon, & L. S. Shaw, (Eds) *Work worth doing: Advances in brain injury rehabilitation*. Delray Beach, FL: St. Lucie Press, Inc.

Durgin, C. J., Cullity, L., & Devine, P. (1991). Programming for skill maintenance and generalization following brain injury rehabilitation. In B. T. McMahon & L. R. Shaw (Eds.) *Work worth doing: Advances in brain injury rehabilitation*. Delray Beach, FL: St. Lucie Press, Inc.

Fawber, H. L., & Wachter, J. F. (1987). Job placement as a treatment component of the vocational rehabilitation process. *Journal of Head Trauma Rehabilitation, 2*, 27-33. Fraser, R. T. (1991). New avenues to job placement: The advantages of natural supports. In B. T. McMahon & L. R. Shaw (Eds.) *Work worth doing: Advances in brain injury rehabilitation*. Delray Beach, FL: St. Lucie Press, Inc.

Fraser, R. T., Clemmons, D. C., & McMahon, B. T. (1990). Vocational rehabilitation. In J. S. Kreutzer (Ed.), *Community integration following traumatic brain injury*. Baltimore: Paul H. Brookes.

Fraser, R. T., & McMahon, B. T. (1989). *Rehabilitation psychology: Special issue on traumatic brain injury*. Washington, DC: American Psychological Association.

Fraser, R. T., McMahon, B. T., & Vogenthaler, D. R. (1988). Vocational rehabilitation counseling with head injured persons. In S. Rubin (Ed.), *Contemporary challenges to the rehabilitation counseling profession*. Baltimore: Paul H. Brookes.

Habeck, R. V., Shrey, D. E., & Growick, B. S. (1991) *Rehabilitation counseling bulletin: Special issue on disability management and industrial rehabilitation*. Alexandria, Virginia: American Association for Counseling and Development.

Hablutzel, N., & McMahon, B. T. (1991) *The Americans with Disabilities Act: Reasonable Accommodations.* Delray Beach, FL: St. Lucie Press.

Hart, T., & Hayden, M. (1986). Issues in the evaluation of rehabilitation effects. In M. Miner & K. Wagner (Eds.) *Neuro-trauma: Treatment, rehabilitation and related issues* (pp. 197-212). Boston: Butterworth Press.

Kay, T., & Silver, S. M. (1988). The contribution of the neuropsychological evaluation to the vocational rehabilitation of the head injured adult. *Journal of Head Trauma Rehabilitation, 3*(1), 65-76.

Krannich, R. L. (1988). *Careering and re-careering for the 1990's.* Manassas, Virginia: Impact Publications.

Loftquist, L. H., & Dawis, R. V. (1969). *Adjustment to work: A physiological view of man's problems in a work-oriented society.* New York: Appleton-Century-Crofts.

Matkin, R. E., & May, V. R. (1981). Potential conflicts of interest in private rehabilitation: Identification and resolution. *Journal of Applied Rehabilitation Counseling, 12*(1), 15-18.

McMahon, B. T. (1979). Private sector rehabilitation: Benefits, dangers, and implications for education. *Journal of Rehabilitation, 45*(3), 56-58.

McMahon, B. T. (1991). Ethics in business practices. In B. T. McMahon & L. R. Shaw (Eds.), *Work worth doing: Advances in brain injury rehabilitation.* Delray Beach, FL: St. Lucie Press, Inc.

McMahon, B. T., & Fraser, R. T. (1988). Basic issues and trends in head injury rehabilitation. In S. Rubin & N. Rubin (Eds.) *Contemporary challenges to the rehabilitation counseling profession.* Baltimore: Paul H. Brookes.

McMahon, B. T., & Fraser, R. T. (1988) Vocational rehabilitation. In P. Deutsch (Ed.), *Innovations in head injury rehabilitation.* New York: Ahab Press.

McMahon, B. T., & Growick, B. S. (1988). Rehabilitation counseling bulletin: Special issue on traumatic brain injury. Alexandria, VA: American Association for Counseling and Development.

McMahon, B. T., & Matkin, R. E. (1982). *Rehabilitation counseling bulletin: Special issue on private rehabilitation.* Alexandria, VA: American Association for Counseling and Development.

McMahon, B. T., Shaw, L. R., & Mahaffey, D. P. (1988). Career opportunities and professional preparation in head injury rehabilitation. *Rehabilitation Counseling Bulletin, 31*(4), 344-354.

McMahon, B. T., & Shaw, L. R. (Eds.) (1991). *Work worth doing: Advances in brain injury rehabilitation.* Delray Beach, FL: St. Lucie Press, Inc.

McMahon, B. T., & Shaw, L. S. (1991). The Outpatient setting: The preferred context for post-acute rehabilitation. In B. T. McMahon and L.R. Shaw (Eds.), *Work worth doing: Advances in brain injury rehabilitation.* Delray Beach, FL: St. Lucie Press, Inc.

McMahon, B. T., & Spencer, S. A. (1979). A systems selling approach to job development. *Journal of Rehabilitation, 45*(2, 68-70.

Morse, P. A., & Morse, A. R. (1988). Functional living skills: Promoting the interaction between neuropsychology and occupational therapy. *Journal of Head Trauma Rehabilitation, 3*(1), 33-44.

Mullins, L. L. (1989). Hate revisited: power, envy, and greed in the rehabilitation setting. *Archives of Physical Medicine and Rehabilitation, 70,* 740-744.

Pancsofar, E., & Blackwell, R. (1986). *A user's guide to community re-entry for the severely handicapped.* Albany, NY: State University of New York Press.

Rubin, S. E., & Roessler, R. T. (1995). *Foundations of the vocational rehabilitation process* (4th ed.). Austin, Texas: Pro-Ed.

Schwartz, G. E., Watson, S. D., Galvin, D. E., & Lipoff, E. (1989). *The disability management sourcebook*. Washington, DC: Washington Business Group on Health.

Shapiro, J. P. (1993). *No Pity: People with disabilities forging a new civil rights movement.* New York: Times Books.

Shrey, D., & LaCerte, M. (1995) *Principles and practices of disability management.* Delray Beach, FL: St. Lucie Press, Inc.

Tankle, R. S. (1988). Application of neuropsychological test results to interdisciplinary cognitive rehabilitation with head-injured adults. *Journal of Head Trauma Rehabilitation, 3*(1), 24-32.

Tarvydas, V., & Pape, D. (1988). A unified code of ethics for rehabilitation counselors. *Rehabilitation Counseling Bulletin, 31*, 249-254.

Whitehouse, F. A. (1975). Rehabilitation clinician. *Journal of Rehabilitation, 41*, 24-26.

Wright, B. A. (1960). *Physical disability: A psychological approach.* New York: Harper and Row.

19

THE PREDICTION OF VOCATIONAL FUNCTIONING FROM NEUROPSYCHOLOGICAL DATA

Thomas J. Guilmette, Ph.D., A.B.P.P.
Marianna Pinchot Kastner, M.A.

INTRODUCTION

A recent survey of neuropsychology practitioners (Guilmette, Faust, Hart, & Arkes, 1990) revealed that the prediction of work behavior was the second most frequent reason (out of eight listed) for performing a neuropsychological evaluation. This finding contrasts with the primary focus of neuropsychological assessments and the field in general decades ago. Until recently, efforts were directed at developing tests that could separate brain-damaged from normal individuals and at localizing the lesioned brain area. An article entitled, "The question of organicity: Is it still functional?" (Leonberger, 1989) is an example of an emerging trend. The added focus for neuropsychologists on predicting work behavior comes as both a burden and a challenge given that our procedures and techniques have not prepared us well to answer the clinical questions that often confront us in this area. This is not to suggest that the field of neuropsychology is wholly unprepared to address the issue of predicting vocational capabilities, but rather, that adequate empirical studies and guidelines to assist neuropsychologists in this difficult task are only beginning to emerge.

In order to present the many facets of this problem, this chapter is divided into sections which address the history of the prediction of work behavior in psychology in general, the impediments to clinical judgment in the prediction of occupational success, consideration for forensic cases, relevant literature in the prediction of vocational capabilities from neuropsychological data, and finally conclusions and recommendations.

A BRIEF HISTORY ON THE PREDICTION OF WORK BEHAVIOR IN PSYCHOLOGY

Attempting to predict occupational success from psychological tests is a task as old as applied psychology itself. In World War I, for example, Robert Yerkes developed two group tests of intelligence (Army Alpha and Beta) to help place recruits in the most appropriate job within the military. The advent of World War II again renewed interest in job selection within the military environment. For example, psychologists were called upon to determine who would make good officers and pilots. Psychologists were also employed by the Office of Strategic Services to select recruits who could act as secret agents, parachuting behind enemy lines to engage in sabotage and organizing guerrilla forces (Schultz, 1979).

Further efforts to predict occupational success through psychological tests, and eventually neuropsychological measures, were facilitated by the growth of rehabilitation in the 1940s and the post-World War II era. In 1943, Public Law 78-113 was passed by Congress to broaden the limited vocational program inaugurated in 1920 to provide a program of rehabilitation for physically disabled civilians following World War I (the Smith-Fess Act of 1920). Initially, the appropriations were temporary but were to be used to provide vocational guidance, training, and occupational adjustment to disabled citizens (McGowan & Porter, 1967). The 1943 law, however, for the first time extended services to the mentally handicapped and the mentally ill. By also guaranteeing payment of these services, PL 78-113 created an important role for psychologists in the assessment and training of individuals with other than physical handicaps to enter the world of work.

In 1954, rehabilitation professionals received additional support from the federal government with the enactment of Public Law 83-565. This law effected major changes in vocational rehabilitation programs and allowed states to broaden their rehabilitation services by appropriating federal funds to support research and training of more rehabilitation professionals. These legislative acts, in addition to the influx of returning World War II soldiers, increased the importance of the relationship between psychology and the work world. Slightly more than a decade later in 1965, Public Law 333 again broadened the legal and financial base to allow these federal-state programs to reach increasing numbers of disabled people. The need for a psychological evaluation was clearly outlined by the Vocational Rehabilitation Act Amendments of 1965 (Section 401.22 [e]) which stated, "In all cases of mental retardation a psychological evaluation will be obtained which will include a valid test of intelligence and an assessment of social functioning and educational achievement...in all cases of behavioral disorders a psychiatric or psychological evaluation will be obtained, as appropriate." Thus, by the mid-1960s psychologists in the field of rehabilitation counseling and counseling psychology were deeply engaged in issues of appraising vocational fitness and predicting success in the work environment for individuals with disabilities.

At that time most neuropsychological research was not aimed at vocational issues but was directed toward validating assessment methods to determine the presence or absence of organic brain damage. These differential diagnostic and lesion location questions were of little use to vocational psychologists who were more concerned with how a patient's impairments affected their ability to survive in the workplace. How is it, then, that more than 30 years later neuropsychologists have become much more interested in these vocational questions? Might we have something to learn from assessment methods utilized three to four decades ago?

One relevant factor in the integration of vocational and neuropsychological disciplines is that the nature of the population with disabilities has changed in such a way that assessing neuropsychological functioning has become more important. A review of a National Health Survey conducted between 1961 and 1963 (McGowan & Porter, 1967) revealed that brain injuries, strokes, and seizure disorders were absent from a list of the most common disabling conditions. Of the 16 chronic conditions reported as limiting work capacity, neoplasms were 11th and "nervous or mental disorders" were fifth. The category for stroke was labeled "paralysis of extremity or trunk," emphasizing the effects of a stroke as primarily a motor or sensory impairment. Heart disease, arthritis/rheumatism, visual impairments, hearing impairments, asthma/hayfever, and orthopedic conditions were a sample of the chronic conditions limiting work activity. One could infer from that list that greater emphasis was placed on physical rather than cognitive impairments.

The change in the rehabilitation population over the last 20 to 30 years is partly due to the increased survival rate of people with severe traumatic brain injuries. Advances in medical technology, including more expedient rescue services and neurodiagnostic imaging techniques, have resulted in significantly reduced mortality due to traumatic brain injuries and other neurologic disorders. It has become apparent that these survivors often exhibit cognitive and psychosocial deficits which cause significant problems for vocational reintegration (Brooks, McKinlay, Symington, Beattie, & Campsie, 1987). Ben-Yishay, Silver, Piasetsky, and Rattok (1987), for example, reviewed the relationship between employability and head injuries and concluded that "the residual cognitive, emotional, and behavioral sequelae of head injury greatly exceed the physical as a cause of difficulties in a person's long-term vocational rehabilitation" (p. 37). The rapid proliferation of rehabilitation centers over the last 10 to 15 years is a testament to the need for rehabilitation services for brain-injured survivors and this need has not been lost on neuropsychologists whose numbers have increased significantly in those centers over the recent past (Guilmette et al., 1990; Hartlage & Telzrow, 1980). In addition, although ruling out an organic etiology for symptoms remains an important area for neuropsychological assessments, there is less of a need for these kinds of evaluations given advances in neurodiagnostic imaging procedures. Neuropsychologists now have the opportunity to apply their skills and knowledge to other clinically meaningful endeavors.

While neuropsychologists were concentrating on developing tests to assess brain damage, vocational and counseling psychologists were developing tests designed specifically to access skills germane to the workplace (for an excellent historical review, see Super & Crites, 1962). There are now a number of measures with occupational- or vocationally-based norms. These include measures of motor functioning such as the Purdue Pegboard, the Minnesota Rate of Manipulations Test, and the Crawford Small Parts Dexterity Test. Specific tests have been developed to assess clerical aptitude such as the Minnesota Clerical Test and the Clerical Aptitude Test. Mechanical and spatial abilities, with specific occupational norms, can be measured with such instruments as the Bennett Mechanical Comprehension Test and the Spatial Relations and Reasoning subtest of the Differential Aptitude Test (DAT), which is a multiple aptitude test battery.

Since neuropsychologists are becoming more involved in the prediction of vocational functioning, the need to establish ecological validity of neuropsychological measures is becoming clear (Heaton & Pendleton, 1981; Heinrichs, 1990). Unfortunately, relating neuropsychological test measures to vocational functioning is a difficult endeavor as is illuminated later in this chapter. We are bound, however, by the limits of our test measures which have been developed to answer other diagnostic questions (Heinrichs, 1990). Because our measures were not developed specifically to predict vocational outcome, neuropsychologists must be current in their understanding of both the strengths and limitations of their field as they relate to predicting work behaviors.

RELEVANT ISSUES IN CLINICAL JUDGMENT AND FORENSIC NEUROPSYCHOLOGY

Neuropsychologists who attempt to make statements about work behavior from neuropsychological test instruments may be hindered not only by unavailable norms for specific occupational groups, although this is not necessarily insurmountable, but also by limitations in their own clinical judgment and reasoning. Meehl (1954) outlined 40 years ago the relationship between clinical and actuarial prediction, with the latter nearly always outperforming the former. This has generally been supported in subsequent research (Dawes, Faust, & Meehl, 1989) although it is of little help to neuropsychologists because there are no known actuarial formulas derived from neuropsychological test data to accurately predict work functioning. By default, therefore, neuropsychologists must rely on their clinical judgment in integrating test data to make predictions about work functioning. This is a task that should be approached with caution (Wedding & Faust, 1989). Clinical judgment research has generally revealed that integration of complex data is a daunting task and can be difficult to accomplish proficiently. Unfortunately, neuropsychologists frequently adhere to the dictum, "more is better" in spite of most research which suggests that "less is more." Wedding (1983), for example, found that neuropsychologists' diagnostic accuracy was better when provided with limited rather than complete neuropsychological test profiles. Similar research in other areas of psychology has supported this finding (Faust, 1989; Golden, 1964; Oskamp, 1965; Sawyer, 1966). Thus, it appears that the more clinicians try to incorporate large amounts of data into their decision-making strategies, the more they may be prone to making errors. However, this issue has not been empirically tested when attempting to predict work or vocational functioning. Typically, research has centered around making specific decisions about diagnoses.

Within the medico-legal arena, neuropsychologists are playing an increasing role in personal injury litigation, particularly in cases of mild to moderate head trauma (Barth, Gideon, Sciara, Hulsey, & Anchor, 1986; Golden & Strider, 1986). In this role, neuropsychologists are not only offering their diagnostic impressions about the causality of the patient's deficits but questions about vocational impairments are frequently asked as they pertain to the issue of damages. Vocational impairment may contribute significantly to the monetary compensation awarded to a plaintiff both in terms of potential lost wages and for the psychological devastation of being unemployable and unproductive. In a forensic evaluation, where the client has a financial stake in the outcome, special consideration needs to be given to the issue of malingering or exaggeration of symptomatology. When referred for a forensic neuropsychological evaluation, a plaintiff who performs so poorly that the neuropsychologist believes that he or she will be unable to work, is often entitled to greater damages than the plaintiff whose vocational impairment is less profound.

The relevant neuropsychological literature in this area casts some doubt that neuropsychologists are able to detect malingering solely from standard neuropsychological measures with adults (Heaton, Smith, Lehman, & Vogt, 1978), with adolescents (Faust, Hart, Guilmette, & Arkes, 1988), with children (Faust, Hart, & Guilmette, 1988), or from clinical interviews (Rogers, 1984). Although the base rates of malingering in disability and forensic evaluations are unknown, studies have suggested rates up to 64% in personal injury cases (Heaton, Chelune, & Lehman, 1978), 26% in compensable minor head injuries (Binder & Willis, 1991); 47% in workers' compensation (Youngjohn, 1991) and 18% in Social Security Disability claimants (Guilmette, Whelihan, Sparadeo, & Buongiorno, 1994). However, special precautions can be undertaken and should be incorporated in each vocational assessment when legal or forensic issues are relevant.

The MMPI, which is also discussed later in this chapter, has utility in the assessment of exaggerated response sets (Rogers, 1984). The F minus K Index, the Gough Dissimulation Scale (Gough, 1957), and the Obvious and Subtle subscales (Wiener, 1948) have all been used with varying success to rule out symptom exaggeration (Anthony, 1971; Gallucci, 1984; Walters, White, & Greene, 1988). Another technique designed specifically to assess feigned memory impairment is a procedure known as Symptom Validity Testing (Binder & Pankratz, 1987; Pankratz, 1979, 1983). Symptom Validity Testing (SVT) incorporates forced-choice questions in which the patient must respond to one of two alternatives. Those procedures typically appear more difficult than they are and are often performed very easily even by patients with severe cognitive dysfunction. Some researchers have used digit recognition procedures (Binder & Willis, 1991; Guilmette, Hart, & Giuliano, 1993; Guilmette, Hart, Giuliano, & Leininger, 1994), word lists (Iverson, Franzen, & McCracken, 1991), and words and faces (Millis, 1992). At this juncture it would appear that these two techniques (MMPI, SVT) can be far more helpful in determining the presence of symptom exaggeration, poor effort, or malingering than standardized neuropsychological measures. For this reason, any forensic vocational appraisal should include a formal assessment of client motivation.

REVIEW OF RELEVANT LITERATURE

The available literature suggests that neuropsychological test data can contribute to the prediction of vocational functioning, in some cases. However, the scientific literature is difficult to interpret because the existing studies have examined a wide spectrum of patient populations and a wide variety of neuropsychological measures, sometimes with conflicting results. Some investigators have looked at large heterogeneous samples, including all of the patients referred for neuropsychological testing at a given hospital (Heinrichs, 1989), while others have looked at much smaller, more homogeneous samples such as a group of young adults with closed head injury (Prigatano et al., 1984). Neuropsychological measures used have ranged from standard batteries (e.g., the Halstead-Reitan, Luria-Nebraska) to a wide variety of individually designed batteries.

In addition to the variability in populations and measures studied, there is also considerable variation in the vocational outcome measures used. In many studies subjects were classified as either employed or not employed, but criteria used to make the distinction varied; some investigators required full-time work, others included part-time or intermittent full-time work as employment. Some investigators have looked at vocational functioning three months after injury (Barth, Macciocchi, Giordani, Rimel, Jane, & Boll, 1983), two years after injury (Bayless, Varney, & Roberts, 1989), seven years after injury (Brooks et at., 1987), or 15 years after injury (Schwab, Grafman, Salazar, & Kraft, 1993). Most studies have looked at employment in the workplace but at least one has used work quality ratings by supervisors in simulated work settings as an outcome measure (Butler, Anderson, Furst, Namerow, & Satz, 1989).

This variety of populations and measures used has made it difficult to generalize results from one study to another. In addition, within group variability in such subject characteristics as age, type and extent of impairment, previous job history, type of current employment, and financial incentive to work make the task of predicting vocational functioning more difficult since all of these factors are known to affect employability (Humphrey & Oddy, 1980; Weddell, Oddy, & Jenkins, 1980). Measures like the Halstead-Reitan Impairment Index which has considerable predictive power in one group (Newman, Heaton, & Lehman, 1978), may fail to predict when applied to another population (Prigatano et al., 1984).

These conflicting results do not necessarily mean that the measures in question lack validity as predictors for any individual patient, but suggest that patients with different characteristics may need to be tested with different batteries tailored to investigate the specific cognitive abilities needed for their type of work. Test batteries may need to be normed separately for workers in different types of occupations. Ryan, Morrow, Bromet, and Parkinson (1987) have normed a battery (The Pittsfield Occupational Exposures Test Battery) designed to be sensitive to brain injury resulting from exposure to toxic substances. They tested 182 blue-collar workers employed in a heavy industry plant. The battery is made up of subtests from the WAIS-R, Visual Reproduction from the Wechsler Memory Scale-Revised (WMS-R), the Boston Embedded Figures Test, Trails A and B from the Halstead-Reitan, Grooved Pegboard, as well as measures of verbal associate learning, memory for recurring words, symbol digit learning, and incidental memory designed by the investigators. As batteries like this are normed on other occupational groups neuropsychologists should have firmer grounds for prediction.

Few studies have looked at how specific neuropsychological tests predict functioning in specific types of jobs. In one study of 19- to 65-year-old males referred for neuropsychological assessment, which did take into account the different kinds of abilities required by different kinds of jobs, Newman et al., (1978) found that the abilities required by the type of job held by employed patients were related to their specific subtest scores. These investigators looked at subtest scores on the WAIS, the Halstead-Reitan, and the MMPI. They looked at differences between employed and chronically unemployed patients, and also at the requirements of different types of jobs held by the employed patients. While the best predictors of chronic unemployment were measures known to be sensitive to brain damage in general (e.g., Average Impairment Rating, the Halstead Impairment Index, Tactual Performance Test, Trail Making Test and Category Test), the scores on specific subtests varied among employed patients according to the kind of job requirements they had. Those working in clerical, administrative, and professional jobs had high correlations between the verbal, numerical, and clerical skills required by their jobs and their WAIS IQ scores, while those whose jobs required perceptual motor skills scored high on spatial relations skills and low on the MMPI depression scale. For the latter group of patients there was no significant correlation between perceptual motor requirements of the jobs they were holding and their scores on the major tests of brain damage. The authors hypothesized that given a threshold level of general job-holding ability, specific and different test measures are needed to predict performance on different kinds of jobs.

In traumatic brain injury, injury characteristics and severity have been shown to be related to vocational outcome. For example, Paniak and colleagues (Paniak, Shore, Rourke, Finlayson, & Moustacalis, 1992) found that 33 days of post-traumatic amnesia (PTA) was the optimal cutoff point in predicting vocational outcome. In their study, no patient with PTA greater than 33 days who was gainfully employed premorbidly was able to regain his or her premorbid socioeconomic status level. Schwab et al. (1993) found that total lesion volume in brain injury, which reflects the degree of diffuse brain damage, was a valuable predictor of work status. Other injury parameters, such as length of unconsciousness and admitting Glasgow Coma Scales, which reflect to at least some degree severity of trauma, are also likely related to vocational outcome, although the relationship is far from perfect (Dresser et al., 1973; Fordyce, 1991). All these factors reflect the degree of brain insult which, all things being equal, is positively related to vocational impairment. Thus, analysis of injury severity will also aid the neuropsychologist in predicting vocational aptitude.

With regard to neuropsychological test data specifically, four main approaches have been taken in attempting to use neuropsychological test results to predict vocational functioning:

1. Using scores from standardized tests or batteries or summary scores.
2. Regression and discriminant function analyses of neuropsychological data.
3. Integration of neuropsychological with psychosocial data.
4. Assessment of executive and behavioral functions.

STANDARDIZED BATTERIES

Scores on measures of intelligence have been related to a variety of achievement measures in many populations. There is considerable literature on the relationship of IQ scores to academic success and to occupational attainment in normal subjects. In an extensive review of IQ studies, Matarazzo (1972) found a correlation of about .50 between measures of academic success and measures of intelligence. He also found strong correlations between IQ and level of income and type of occupation. In a classic study, Yoakum and Yerkes (1920), for instance, studied Army Alpha scores and military performance in over 100,000 World War I soldiers. They found that intelligence was probably the single most important factor in predicting military efficiency. With impaired subjects, Webster (1979) studied vocational workshop performance in 160 psychiatric outpatients, some of whom were neurologically impaired. He found a correlation of .51 between benchwork skills and the WAIS Performance IQ. In a group of 125 mentally retarded subjects, Malgady, Barcher, Davis, and Towner (1980) found a correlation of .36 between level of functioning in a vocational workshop and overall IQ.

Summary measures of the Halstead-Reitan Battery have been used in several studies as a predictor of whether or not an individual with cognitive impairments is employed. In some cases these have proved to be powerful predictors. In a study of 19- to 65-year-old males referred for neuropsychological assessment, Newman et al. (1978) found that the Russell Average Impairment Rating (based on an extended Halstead-Reitan Battery) correlated .47 with chronic unemployment. Using a cutoff score of 1.61, they were able to correctly classify 78% of subjects as employed or unemployed. Similarly, in a sample of 71 patients aged 15 to 56 with mild head injury, who were tested three months after injury, problems returning to work correlated .41 with the Halstead Impairment Index (Barth et al., 1983). McSweeney, Heaton, Prigatano, and Adams (1985) administered an expanded Halstead-Reitan Battery including the Russell modification of the WMS, the Grooved Pegboard Test and the WAIS to 303 patients with chronic obstructive pulmonary disease and to 99 healthy controls. They correlated the Russell Average Impairment Index with measures of life quality including work, and found that it had a low but significant correlation with ability to work both in impaired patients and in normals.

In a study of the Luria-Nebraska Battery, Heinrichs (1989) found that the mean T-score, a summary measure of the entire battery, correlated -.49 with the patient's employment status at the time of testing. This study was conducted on a sample of general and psychiatric hospital patients referred for neuropsychological assessment whose mean age was 58.8. With some exceptions (Prigatano et. al., 1984), it appears that results from these two standard batteries are about equal.

The McCarron Dial System (MDS) (Blackwell, Dial, Chan, & McCollum, 1985; McCarron & Dial, 1972), a battery which includes neuropsychological, sensory, motor, and psychosocial measures has been used successfully to predict independent living levels (the higher of which include employment) in mentally retarded subjects. These workers found that the strongest predictor in this population was a gross motor measure, but the second strongest was a neuropsychological measure most of whose predictive power was derived from the Peabody Picture Vocabulary Test. Recently, Dial, Chan, and Norton (1990) used the MDS to discriminate brain-damaged from normal subjects, correctly classifying 93% of subjects. Further work with the instrument may demonstrate the usefulness in predicting vocational outcomes in these subjects as well.

Although it is clear from these studies that there is usually a correlation between scores on standard neuropsychological batteries and vocational status, an important question remains—do the neuropsychological data contribute unique information—do they improve prediction over the use of demographic and neurological status data alone? To answer this question several studies have used a regression or discriminate function approach to assess the contribution of neuropsychological variables and to determine which ones have the most predictive power.

REGRESSION AND DISCRIMINANT FUNCTION APPROACHES

Heinrichs (1989) looked at how the Luria-Nebraska added predictive power to demographic variables. He calculated a regression equation using the patient's age, years of education, and neurological diagnosis as demographic variables and the summary measure of the Luria-Nebraska described above. He found that a four variable equation explained 29% of the variance in employment status and the Luria-Nebraska summary contributed 8%. He did not enter individual subtest scores. This would have made it possible to eliminate variables which had low correlations with the outcome measure, and might have resulted in a higher percent of unique explained variance. Nevertheless, he did demonstrate that neuropsychological data added information useful in predicting vocational status.

In a study of 108 adult outpatients with epilepsy, Dikman and Morgan (1980) administered an extensive neuropsychological battery consisting of the WAIS, the Halstead-Reitan, the Stroop, and Logical Memory and Visual Reproduction from the Wechsler Memory Scale. They clustered the subtests into six groups on the basis of face validity: a verbal skills group, a visual-spatial problem-solving group, a flexibility of thinking group, a memory and alertness group, a concept formation group, and a motor function group. When they attempted to predict vocational outcome (employed versus not employed) with a discriminant function analysis using summary measures of each group, they found that only the flexibility of thinking category had discriminatory power. However, when they divided their subjects into two occupational status groups, they found that verbal skills and concept formation groups contributed to the prediction of higher occupational status. This study supports the concept that batteries may need to be tailored to predict specific occupational categories.

Prigatano et al. (1984) found that neuropsychological data alone were not sufficient to predict post-rehabilitation vocational status (employed versus unemployed) in 18 young adults with severe closed head trauma. However, the employed patients did show greater improvement in some neuropsychological scores following rehabilitation than did the nonworking patients. Particularly significant were changes in the WAIS Digit Symbol subtest, the Wechsler Memory Quotient, Visual Reproduction from the WMS, and the number of difficult paired associates learned in the Associate Learning subest from the WMS. However, these investigators found that relatives' ratings of social and emotional functioning on the KATZ Adjustment Scale were a more powerful discriminator than the neuropsychological variables.

In a large ($\underline{n}$ = 520), 15-year follow-up of Vietnam veterans who sustained penetrating head injuries in combat, a logistic regression model of neurologic, neuropsychologic, and social functioning found that seven systematically defined impairments proved most correlated with work status (Schwab et al., 1993). These included post-traumatic epilepsy, paresis, visual field loss, verbal memory loss, visual memory loss, psychological problems, and violent behavior. These disabilities had a cumulative and nearly equipotent effect upon work failure. The authors suggest that a summation of these seven disabilities can yield a "disability score" which can have a practical effect on predicting the likelihood of returning to work .

Several investigators have combined psychosocial data and neuropsychological data in order to increase accuracy in predicting employment status. This has proved to be a fruitful approach as the addition of psychosocial variables has in most cases improved the accuracy of prediction over what can be obtained with neuropsychological data alone.

INTEGRATION OF PSYCHOSOCIAL AND NEUROPSYCHOLOGICAL VARIABLES

Personality and psychosocial dysfunction, particularly irritability and social isolation, are common sequelae in brain damage. This has been demonstrated consistently in traumatic brain injury (Brooks, Campsie, Symington, Beattie, & McKinlay, 1986; Prigatano, 1992; Stuss, Gow, & Hetherington, 1992). Quite obviously, these psychosocial factors can have a significant effect on a patient's ability to function within the workplace, get along well with co-workers, accept criticism, etc. Thus, the need to assess these symptoms in a vocational assessment is intuitively appealing and for which there is also empirical justification.

In a study of a large diverse sample of patients referred for neuropsychological assessment, Heaton, Chelune and Lehman (1978) found that including data from the MMPI added to the power of a discriminant function in predicting employment status. They examined the WAIS Verbal and Performance IQs, the Average Impairment Index of the Halstead-Reitan, the Reading Comprehension and Spelling subtests from the Peabody Individual Achievement Test and Story Memory from the Wechsler Memory Scale as well as the MMPI clinical and validity scales. They found that using an equation that included MMPI variables correctly classified 81% of unemployed and 86% of full-time employed patients. When they used a function based on neuropsychological variables alone, they could correctly classify only 75% of the sample.

In an extensive study of epileptics Schwartz, Dennerll, and Lin (1968), also found that psychosocial as well as neuropsychological scores were important predictor variables. They administered the California Personality Inventory and the Edwards Personal Preference Schedule in addition to the WAIS and the Halstead-Reitan. The former two provided psychosocial measures. Using a discriminant function analysis they found that a combination of neuropsychological and psychosocial variables best predicted current employment status in their sample, allowing them to correctly classify 77% of the employed group and 80% of the unemployed group. Using a stepwise regression analysis they found that the best predictors were WAIS Comprehension, CPI Social Presence, WAIS Digit Symbol, WAIS Similarities, CPI Self Acceptance, CPI Capacity for Status, and Halstead Tapping (dominant hand). All three batteries were needed to get the best prediction.

In Newman, Heaton and Lehman's (1978) study described above, the investigators found psychosocial variables more helpful in predicting job performance than in predicting unemployment. The Average Impairment Index of the Halstead-Reitan was responsible for most of the effect in predicting chronic unemployment. However, when they looked at the prediction of average wages in the subjects who were able to work, they found that among the important predictor variables was the Lie Scale from the MMPI as well as WAIS, WMS, and Halstead-Reitan variables. Total hours worked was predicted almost entirely by MMPI variables, with a contribution also by spatial relations errors (gleaned from the Halstead-Reitan).

Brooks et al. (1987) looked at how specific neuropsychological and psychosocial variables predicted return to work within the first seven years after severe head injury. They administered a nonstandard battery consisting of Progressive Matrices and the Mill Hill Vocabulary Scale to assess intelligence; Logical Memory from the WMS, learning of three verbal paired associates, and the Buschke Procedure (repeated presentation and selective reminding of 12 words) to assess verbal retention; the Rey Complex Figure to assess visual retention; and the Paced Auditory Serial Addition Task (PASAT) to assess attention. In this challenging task, the subject is presented with a series of numbers and after each number is presented, is asked to add the number just presented to the one presented immediately before. Numbers are presented in four series; first 2.4 seconds apart, then 2.0 seconds apart, third 1.6 seconds apart, and finally 1.2 seconds apart. These investigators used a nonstandard scoring procedure, counting the longest string correct as the subject's score. In a regression analysis only Logical Memory and the PASAT contributed explanatory power. Together they explained 29% of the variance in employment status.

Psychosocial variables were derived from interview with relatives of the patient assessing deficits in four areas, subjective (mainly anxiety and depression), control of emotion (mainly anger), self-care (ability to assume responsibility for the household and for personal hygiene) and behavior (deficits included "difficult, disturbing, embarrassing, or puzzling behavior"). In a regression equation the best predictors were the self-care and emotional control variables which together explained about 30% of the employment outcome. These investigators did not attempt to combine the neuropsychological and psychosocial variables into a single equation, which might have had even greater predictive power.

Although combining neuropsychological and psychosocial variables has been a promising approach in predicting vocational functioning, some investigators have felt that a more direct measure of work-related abilities would have greater predictive power than instruments originally developed to assess personality or detect brain damage. Their research has focused on creating direct behavioral measures on which work-related behavior could be directly observed. In addition, executive or frontal lobe functions likely exert some influence over employability. Specific assessment of these capabilities has yielded some positive results.

ASSESSMENT OF EXECUTIVE AND BEHAVIORAL FUNCTIONS

Lezak (1987), in a five-year follow-up of 42 adults who had sustained severe brain injuries found that the cognitive and emotional impairments exhibited by these patients were more disabling than their physical limitations. She concluded that the most significant residual impairments in this group were those functions "required for pursuing a course of study or getting or keeping a job, filling in unscheduled and unstructured time satisfactorily, and making and maintaining close social relationships—the executive functions" (p. 64). Executive functions, associated with the frontal and prefrontal cortex, have been associated with a wide range of emotional and self-regulatory abilities including self-awareness, drive, motivation, organization/problem-solving, emotional stability, impulse control, and memory impairment (Malloy, Bihrle, Duffy, & Cimino, 1993; Prigatano, 1992; Stuss & Gow, 1992; Stuss, Gow, & Hetherington, 1992). In addition to Lezak's (1987) study, other research revealed that frontal lobe impairment is related to poor vocational outcome. Varney (1988) found that 92% of patients with total anosmia (inability to smell/taste), a sign of orbital frontal damage, suffered chronic employment problems at least two years after they had been medically cleared for work. In another group of mild head-injured anosmic patients with above average intelligence and memory, 80% suffered chronic unemployment (Martzke, Swan, & Varney, 1991).

In spite of the crucial importance and often disabling effects of frontal lobe deficits, objective assessment of these functions may be difficult due to the structure of testing itself (Stuss & Benson, 1984; Varney & Menefee, 1993). That is, patients may be capable of inhibiting inappropriate behavior during testing or giving adequate responses to social judgment questions, particularly if of high average intelligence. However, their "real-world" behavior on frontal lobe dimensions may be quite disparate from their performance on formal testing. Obtaining reports from relatives or friends about daily functioning may be necessary.

With regard to formal testing, Bayless et al. (1989) administered Lezak's Tinker Toy Test (Lezak, 1983) to 50 patients who had suffered closed head injury and had been cleared by their physicians to return to work, and to 50 normal controls. In this test the patient is given a selection of tinker toy parts and asked to build anything she or he likes. The authors feel that this test assesses frontal lobe executive functions such as the spontaneous formulation of goals, planning and the carrying out of plans, deficits which have been implicated as a significant impediment to independent employment (Lezak, 1987). Subjects were scored by an observer and points were awarded for such things as the creation of a free-standing structure, complexity and symmetry, the number of pieces used, the presence of working wheels, appropriate naming of the structure, etc. Controls and all but one of the employed head-injured subjects scored over six, while half of the unemployed patients scored six or below. A high score therefore reflected little about the likelihood of employment, but a score below six virtually guaranteed that the patient did not work. Although there are many measures of frontal lobe functions, few have been empirically tested to determine their relationship to work potential.

Butler et al. (1989) gave 20 brain-injured subjects in an outpatient rehabilitation clinic a different behavioral task—they were required to assemble a wooden wheelbarrow using printed instructions. During the task subjects were intentionally interrupted, asked to work for several minutes on another task, and at some point offered criticism when an error was made. On this Behavioral Assessment of Vocational Skills (BAVS), subjects were rated by trained observers on such skills as following directions, organization, range of attention, ability to tolerate frustration, problem solving, judgment and relations with authorities. Subjects also received a neuropsychological battery consisting of the WAIS-R, Trails A and B from the Halstead-Reitan, Logical Memory and Visual Reproduction from the WMS and the Wisconsin Card Sorting Test. These instruments were related to three measures of job performance during a three-month trial of volunteer work which was part of the rehabilitation program. In a multiple regression analysis, the BAVS was the only significant predictor of vocational performance. Butler is now developing another behavioral measure, the Behavioral Evaluation of Frontal Functions (BEFF), designed to assess frontal lobe behaviors in patients undergoing a mock job interview (R.W. Butler, personal communication, July 1, 1991). Further research is necessary to determine the efficacy of those procedures although this appears to be a promising area of investigation.

Another behavioral approach is the Functional Assessment Inventory (FAI) developed by Crewe and Athelston (1981) to describe patients' potential for vocational rehabilitation. The instrument consists of 30 four-point scales of limitations and a 10-point checklist of assets and strengths. Clients are rated on these scales after interviews by vocational counselors. A factor analysis of the scales yielded eight clusters: cognitive functioning, motor functioning, personality and behavior, vocational qualification, medical condition, vision, economic disincentives, and hearing. Mysiw, Corrigan, Hunt, Cavin, and Fish (1989) compared results on the FAI with counselors recommendations on clients' readiness for vocational rehabilitation. Patients were classified into four groups: (1) ready to return to competitive employment, (2) in vocational training, (3) doing supported work, and (4) needing continued remedial therapy. The investigators found that FAI composite scores were closely correlated to the subjects' group placement .

JOB CRITERIA AND ANALYSIS

The United States Department of Labor identified 12,854 for occupations in the U.S. economy (U.S. Department of Labor, 1986). These occupations require various levels of specific aptitudes, many of which may be assessed in vocational neuropsychological evaluations. Lees-Haley (1990) listed these aptitudes, as required of U.S. occupations, derived by the U.S. Department of Labor. The 11 aptitudes are defined as follows (Lees-Haley, 1990, pp. 1,383-1,384):

> Intelligence: General learning ability. The ability to "catch on" or instructions and underlying principles, the ability to reason and make judgments.

> Verbal Aptitude: The ability to understand the meaning of words and to use them effectively. The ability to comprehend language, to understand relationships between words and to understand meanings of whole sentences and paragraphs.

> Numerical Aptitude: The ability to perform arithmetic operations quickly and accurately.

> Spatial Aptitude: Ability to think visually of geometric forms and to comprehend the two-dimensional representation of

three-dimensional objects. The ability to recognize the relationship resulting from the movement of objects in space.

Form Perception: Ability to perceive pertinent detail in objects or in pictorial or graphic material. Ability to make visual comparisons and discriminations and see slight differences in shapes and shadings of figures and widths and lengths of lines.

Clerical Perception: Ability to perceive pertinent detail in verbal or tabular material. Ability to observe differences in copy, to proofread words and numbers, and to avoid perceptual errors in arithmetic computation. A measure of speed of perception is required in many industrial jobs even when the job does not have verbal or numerical content.

Motor Coordination: Ability to coordinate eye and hand or fingers rapidly and accurately in making precise movements with speed. Ability to make movement response accurately and swiftly.

Finger Dexterity: Ability to move fingers, and manipulate small objects with fingers, rapidly or accurately.

Manual Dexterity: Ability to move hands easily and skillfully. To work with hands in placing and turning motions.

Eye-Hand-Foot Coordination: Ability to move the hand and foot coordinately with each other in accordance with visually stimuli.

Color Discrimination: The ability to match or discriminate between colors in terms of hue, saturation, and brilliance. To identify a particular color or color combination from memory and be able to perceive harmonious or contrasting color combinations.

The U.S. Department of Labor has further identified the number of occupations in the U.S. economy that require various levels of these aptitudes. That is, the U.S. Department of Labor has estimated the number of jobs that require more proficient or less proficient functioning in each of these 11 aptitudes among the 12,854 jobs in the economy (for a more complete description see Lees-Haley, 1990).

Reviewing the 11 aptitudes listed above, it is obvious that many neuropsychological measures would directly or indirectly assess these skills. Aptitudes or abilities such as intelligence, verbal skills, numerical abilities, and motor coordination are assessed routinely as part of many neuropsychological assessments. The U.S. Department of Labor recognizes the importance of these aptitudes as they relate to vocational fitness. Other capabilities, such as eye-hand-foot coordination and color discrimination may be less routinely assessed as part of neuropsychological assessments. However, when performing vocational neuropsychological assessments, the clinician may wish to consider these basic aptitudes when describing the client's vocational fitness.

Absent from this list of job aptitudes are more complex and integrated cognitive functions, such as executive skills, as well as psychosocial and psychological variables. Quite obviously, even a person with high levels in each of the 11 aptitudes may be a very poor employment risk if he or she is disinhibited, irritable, socially isolated, and lacks drive/motivation to follow through on plans. When these deficits exist, the impediment to vocational success will likely be substantial.

Given the large number of jobs (over 12,000), the task of predicting success in the U.S. economy becomes quite burdensome. However, assessing each of the aptitudes listed above and determining the patient's level of functioning within each aptitude will help the neuropsychologist determine the possible number of jobs available to the client or patient.

As indicated previously, predicting job success to a specific job is an easier task. Obtaining job descriptions may assist with the analysis of the work to be performed although it is important to recognize that job descriptions do not always reflect the employee's functioning on a daily basis. An analysis of the daily tasks to be performed described by both the employee and the employer may assist in making more accurate predictions about job success. The nature of the job environment (e.g., quiet, distracting, chaotic) also impacts on job performance, particularly for patients who are inattentive, impulsive, etc. Predictive accuracy can be enhanced if the neuropsychologist knows the psychological demands and stressors of the job, the need to interact with others and under what circumstances, how much help or supervision is available, and the importance that interpersonal skills may have in the position.

When possible, observing the patient under conditions that replicate job demands may ultimately provide the greatest amount of ecological validity. As indicated previously, using tests designed for specific occupations will allow the vocational neuropsychologist to better interpret test scores as they relate to job performance. The neuropsychological assessment will need to take into account the underlying cognitive capabilities required of the patient for the job and then tailor the battery or measures used to best assess those functions. From a rehabilitation perspective, the use of job coaches and on-site evaluation of the job environment by the neuropsychologist and/or another professional, such as an occupational therapist, will also provide highly useful information about what skills the patient must possess to be successful.

CONCLUSIONS AND RECOMMENDATIONS

As may be obvious from reading this chapter, predicting occupational success from neuropsychological data is frequently a complicated task. However, in the authors' opinions, the obstacles to making statements about occupational functioning are not insurmountable and the available literature can provide some broad guidelines to follow. What follows is a summary of the literature and suggestions for practitioners utilizing neuropsychological data to predict work functioning. None of the conclusions listed below are to be taken as fact, but rather, only as principles, which in the authors' opinions, may provide some guidance to clinicians working in this emerging area.

1. In general, the greater the level of cognitive dysfunction (brain impairment) the less likely the individual will be employable.

2. The assessment of work capabilities is generally more valid for specific jobs than when trying to predict someone's employability in general. Whenever possible, the neuropsychologist should attempt to determine if the referral source has questions about a specific occupation rather than any occupation.

3. If required to make judgments about a person's ability to perform in a specific job, determine which skills are most necessary and tailor the test battery accordingly. Use those measures which tap skills most related to those necessary in the job.

4. As a corollary to number three above, if an evaluation is designed for a specific occupation for which specific tests are available, use them. Examples have already been cited in the text. In general, such areas as clerical aptitude, manual and motor proficiency, and spatial abilities can be assessed through measures with norms for specific occupational groups.

5. Intelligence and "pure" neuropsychological measures are generally more applicable to the prediction of higher cognitively demanding occupations.

6. Neuropsychological measures tend to be better at "predicting failure" than success. That is, an impaired performance on neuropsychological tests is usually more predictive of work failure than is a normal performance of work success.

7. Do not test indiscriminately, administering measure after measure. This will only result in decreased judgmental accuracy. Rather, assess those cognitive areas generally found to be more predictive of occupational success. In many cases, mental speed/rate of information processing (e.g., PASAT, Digit Symbol, Trail Making Test), memory (e.g., Logical Memory, Paired Associate Learning), and conceptual ability/reasoning (e.g., Comprehension, Similarities, Category Test) have been found to be important in some studies relating neuropsychological test results to work functioning. In addition, for clerical, managerial, and professional occupations, numerical and verbal abilities are especially important. Visual-motor speed and perceptual functioning are often necessary for assembly or jobs requiring constructional skills. Physical skills are crucial for many jobs. Paresis and impaired vision will significantly limit vocational options.

8. Psychosocial and psychological functioning seem to explain unique variance not accounted for by neuropsychological measures alone. The use of psychological self-report measures, such as the MMPI, can be quite helpful in determining the psychosocial functioning of a patient. In addition, interviews with a patient's family regarding how well the patient interacts with others, manages frustration, evidences signs of depression, anxiety, irritability, substance abuse, etc. can provide valuable insights into how the individual is likely to interact with others on the job site.

9. An important trend in the vocational neuropsychological area is the assessment of behavioral, particularly executive, functions. Observing a patient undertake a nonstructured task or role playing job-like interactions or activities can provide qualitative information about the patient's behavior not always available through other neuropsychological measures. Assessment of executive skills is encouraged, although neuropsychological measures in this area are not always sensitive enough to detect subtle impairments, particularly with brighter, more intact individuals .

10. Demographic factors play an important role in the prediction of work behavior, particularly years of education, age, occupational history, incentive to work, and premorbid personality functioning. Establishing injury severity is also an important component in estimating degree of brain damage. Seizure disorders, particularly if poorly controlled, can be a significant obstacle to obtaining and keeping a job.

11. If conducted as part of a forensic evaluation, the use of Symptom Validity Testing and the MMPI are highly recommended.

12. In the field as a whole, greater consensus is necessary in deciding which instruments will be consistently studied to determine their power to predict occupational success. One reason why the research is so fragmented in this area

is because so few investigators use the same neuropsychological measures. This has made it difficult to compare one study with another and resolve differences in research outcome.

13. An additional area of research that would be of great help to clinicians would be the norming of abbreviated but standardized batteries with different occupational groups. For example, IQ, memory functioning, and other neuropsychological indices of successful individuals in specific occupational groups would be of great importance to clinicians practicing in the field of vocational neuropsychology.

The above recommendations are meant neither to frighten nor console the neuropsychologist involved with predicting vocational success. Rather, they are the authors' interpretations of the current literature and are meant as guidelines which may assist practitioners. It is obviously important for clinicians to remain abreast of developments in this emerging area and for them to stay within their professional boundaries by admitting when the data are inconclusive or when they are unable to make a determination about occupational functioning. Because the relationship between neuropsychological data and vocational abilities is not a perfect one, one must be cautious with how the data are interpreted. Lastly, practitioners are encouraged to maintain their own file or log of individuals for whom they have evaluated work capabilities and then to monitor those individuals for months to perhaps years to learn and refine one's approach based on previous successes and failures. It is only in this way that we can avoid our past mistakes and advance not only the field as a whole but our own expertise in this important area.

REFERENCES

Anthony, N. (1971). Comparison of clients' standard, exaggerated, and matching MMPI profiles. *Journal of Consulting and Clinical Psychology, 36,* 100-103.

Barth, J. T., Gideon, D. A., Sciara, A. D., Hulsey, P. H., & Anchor, K. N. (1986). Forensic aspects of mild head trauma. *Journal of Head Trauma Rehabilitation, 1,* 63-70.

Barth, J. T., Macciocchi, S. N., Giordani, B., Rimel, R., Jane, J. A., & Boll. T. J. (1983). Neuropsychological sequelae of minor head injury. *Neurosurgery, 13,* 529-533.

Bayless, J. D., Varney, N. R., & Roberts, R. J. (1989). Tinker Toy Test performance and vocational outcome in patients with closed head injuries. *Journal of Clinical and Experimental Neuropsychology, 11,* 913-917.

Ben-Yishay, Y., Silver, S. M., Piasetsky, E., & Rattok, J. (1987). Relationship between employability and vocational outcome after intensive holistic cognitive rehabilitation. *Journal of Head Trauma Rehabilitation, 2,* 35-48.

Binder, L. M., & Pankratz, L. (1987). Neuropsychological evidence of a factitious memory complaint. *Journal of Clinical and Experimental Neuropsychology, 9,* 167-171.

Binder, L. M., & Willis, S. C. (1991). Assessment of motivation after financially compensable minor head trauma. *Psychological Assessment: A Journal of Consulting and Clinical Psychology, 3,* 168-174.

Blackwell, S., Dial, J., Chan, F., & McCollum, P. (1985). Discriminating functional levels of independent living: A neuropsychological evaluation of mentally retarded adults. *Rehabilitation Counseling Bulletin, 29*, 42-52.

Brooks, N., Campsie, L., Symington, C., Beattie, A., & McKinlay, W. (1986). The five year outcome of severe blunt head injury: A relative's view. *Journal of Neurology, Neurosurgery, and Psychiatry, 49*, 764-770.

Brooks, N., McKinlay, W., Symington, C., Beattie, A., & Campsie, L. (1987). Return to work within the first seven years after severe head injury. *Brain Injury, 1*, 5-19.

Butler, R. W., Anderson, L., Furst, C. J., Namerow, N. S., & Satz, P. (1989). Behavioral assessment in neuropsychological rehabilitation: A method for measuring vocational-related skills. *The Clinical Neuropsychologist, 3*, 235-243.

Crewe, N. M. & Athelstan, G. T. (1981). Functional assessment in vocational rehabilitation: Systemic approach to diagnosis and goal setting. *Archives of Physical Medicine and Rehabilitation, 62*, 299-305.

Dawes, R. M., Faust, D., & Meehl, P. E. (1989). Clinical versus actuarial judgment. *Science, 243*, 1668-1674.

Dial, J. G., Chan, F., & Norton, C. (1990). Neuropsychological assessment of brain damage: Discriminative validity of the McCarron-Dial System. *Brain Injury, 4*, 239-246.

Dikman, S., & Morgan, S.F. (1980). Neuropsychological factors related to employability and occupational status in persons with epilepsy. *Journal of Nervous and Mental Disease, 168*, 236-240.

Dresser, A. C., Meirowsky, A. M., Weiss, G. H., McNeel, M. L., Simon, G. A., & Caveness, W. F. (1973). Gainful employment following head injury: Prognostic factors. *Archives of Neurology, 29*, 111-116.

Faust, D., Hart, K., & Guilmette, T.J. (1988). Pediatric malingering: The capacity of children to fake believable deficits on neuropsychological testing. *Journal of Consulting and Clinical Psychology, 56*, 578-582.

Faust, D., Hart, K., Guilmette, T. J., & Arkes, H. R. (1988). Neuropsychologists' capacity to detect adolescent malingerers. Professional Psychology: *Research and Practice, 19*, 508-515.

Faust, D., (1989). Data integration in legal evaluations: Can clinicians deliver on their premises? *Behavioral Sciences and The Law, 7*, 469-483.

Fordyce, D. J. (1991). Traumatic brain injury in adults: Recovery and rehabilitation. In H. O. Doerr & A. S. Carlin (Eds.), *Forensic neuropsychology: Legal and scientific bases* (pp. 175-213). New York: The Guildford Press.

Gallucci, N. T. (1984). Prediction of dissimulation on the MMPI in a clinical field setting. *Journal of Consulting and Clinical Psychology, 52*, 917-918.

Golden, M. (1964). Some effects of combining psychological tests on clinical inferences. *Journal of Consulting Psychology, 28*, 440-446.

Golden, C. J., & Strider, M. A. (Eds.) (1986). *Forensic neuropsychology.* New York: Plenum Press.

Gough, J. G. (1957). *California Psychological Inventory Manual.* Palo Alto, CA: Consulting Psychologists Press.

Guilmette, T. J., Faust, D., Hart, K., & Arkes, H. R. (1990). A national survey of psychologists who offer neuropsychological services. *Archives of Clinical Neuropsychology, 5*, 373-392.

Guilmette, T. J., Hart, K. J., & Giuliano, A. J. (1993). Malingering detection: The use of a forced choice method in identifying organic versus simulated memory impairment. *The Clinical Neuropsychologist, 7*, 59-69.

Guilmette, T. J., Hart, K. J., Giuliano, A. J., & Leininger, B. (1994). Detecting simulated memory impairment: A comparison of the Rey Fifteen Item Test and the Hiscock Forced-Choice Procedure. *The Clinical Neuropsychologist, 8,* 283-294..

Guilmette, T. J., Whelihan, W., Sparadeo, F., & Buongiorno, G. (1994). The validity of neuropsychological test results in disability evaluations. *Perceptual and Motor Skills, 78,* 1179-1186.

Hartlage, L. C., & Telzrow, C. F. (1980). The practice of clinical neuropsychology in the U.S. *International Journal of Clinical Neuropsychology, 2,* 200-202.

Heaton, R. K., Chelune, G. J., & Lehman, A. W. (1978). Using neuropsychological and personality tests to assess the likelihood of patient employment. *Journal of Nervous and Mental Disease, 166,* 408-416.

Heaton, R. K., & Pendleton, M. G. (1981). Use of neuropsychological tests to predict adult patients' everyday functioning. *Journal of Consulting and Clinical Psychology, 49,* 807-821.

Heaton, R. K., Smith, H. H., Lehman, R. A., & Vogt, A. T. (1978). Prospects for faking believable deficits on neuropsychological testing. *Journal of Consulting and Clinical Psychology, 46,* 892-900.

Heinrichs, R. W. (1989). Neuropsychological test performance and employment status in patients referred for assessment. *Perceptual and Motor Skills, 69,* 899-902.

Heinrichs, R. W. (1990). Current and emergent applications of neuropsychological assessment: Problems of validity and utility. Professional Psychology: *Research and Practice, 21,* 171-176.

Humphrey, M., & Oddy, M. (1980). Return to work after head injury: A review of post-war studies. *Injury, 12,* 107-114.

Iverson, G. L., Franzen, M. D., & McCracken, L. M. (1991). Evaluation of an objective assessment technique for the detecting of malingered memory deficits. *Law and Human Behavior, 15,* 667-676.

Lees-Haley, P. (1990). Vocational neuropsychological requirements of U.S. occupations. *Perceptual and Motor Skills, 70,* 1383-1386.

Leonberger, F. T. (1989). The question of organicity: Is it still functional? *Professional Psychology: Research and Practice, 20,* 411-414.

Lezak, M. D. (1983). *Neuropsychological Assessment* (2nd ed.). New York: Oxford University Press.

Lezak, M. D. (1987). Relationships between personality disorders, social disturbances, and physical rehabilitation following traumatic brain injury. *Journal of Head Trauma Rehabilitation, 2,* 57-69.

Malgady, R. G., Barcher, P. R., Davis, J., & Towner, G. (1980). Validity of the Vocational Adaptation Rating Scale: Prediction of mentally retarded workers' placement in sheltered workshops. *American Journal of Mental Deficiency, 84,* 633-640.

Malloy, P., Bihrle, A., Duffy, J., & Cimino, C. (1993). The orbitomedial frontal syndrome. *Archives of Clinical Neuropsychology, 8,* 185-201.

Martzke, J., Swan, C., & Varney, N. (1991). Post traumatic anosmia and orbital frontal damage: Neuropsychological and neuropsychiatric correlates. *Neuropsychology, 5,* 213-225.

Matarazzo, J. D. (1972). *Wechsler's measurement and appraisal of adult intelligence* (5th ed.). Baltimore, MD: Williams and Wilkins.

McCarron, L., & Dial, J.G. (1972). Neuropsychological predictors of sheltered workshop performance. *American Journal of Mental Deficiency, 77,* 244-250.

McGowan, J.F., & Porter, T.L. (1967). *An introduction to the vocational rehabilitation process.* Washington, DC: U.S. Department of Health, Education and Welfare.

McSweeney, A. J., Heaton, R. K., Prigatano, G. P., & Adams, K. M. (1985). Relationship of neuropsychological status to everyday functioning in healthy and chronically ill persons. *Journal of Clinical and Experimental Neuropsychology, 7,* 281-291.

Meehl, P. (1954). *Clinical versus statistical prediction: A theoretical analysis and a review of the evidence.* Minneapolis, MN: University of Minnesota Press.

Millis, S. R. (1992). The Recognition Memory Test in the detection of malingered and exaggerated memory deficits. *The Clinical Neuropsychologist, 6,* 406-414.

Mysiw, W. J., Corrigan, J. D., Hunt, M., Cavin, D., & Fish, T. (1989). Vocational evaluation of traumatic brain injury patients using the Functional Assessment Inventory. *Brain Injury, 3,* 27-34.

Newman, O. S., Heaton, R. K., & Lehman, R. A. W. (1978). Neuropsychological and MMPI correlates of patients' future employment characteristics. *Perceptual and Motor Skills, 46,* 635-642.

Oskamp, S. (1965). Overconfidence in case-study judgments. *Journal of Clinical Psychology, 29,* 261-265.

Paniak, C. E., Shore, D. L., Rourke, B. P., Finlayson, M. A. J., & Moustacalis, E. (1992). Long-term vocational functioning after severe closed head injury: A controlled study. *Archives of Clinical Neuropsychology, 7,* 529-540.

Pankratz, L. (1979). Symptom validity testing and symptom retraining: Procedures for the assessment and treatment of functional sensory deficits. *Journal of Consulting and Clinical Psychology 47,* 409-410.

Pankratz, L. (1983). A new technique for the assessment and modification of feigned memory deficit. *Perceptual and Motor Skills, 57,* 367-372.

Prigatano, G. P. (1992). Personality disturbances associated with traumatic brain injury. *Journal of Consulting and Clinical Psychology, 60,* 360-368.

Prigatano, G. P., Fordyce, D. J., Zeiner, H. K., Roueche, J. R., Pepping, M., & Wood, B. C. (1984). Neuropsychological rehabilitation after closed head injury in young adults. *Journal of Neurology, Neurosurgery, and Psychiatry, 47,* 505-513.

Rogers, R. (1984). Towards an empirical model of malingering and deception. *Behavioral Sciences and the Law, 2,* 93-111.

Ryan, C. M., Morrow, L. A., Bromet, E. J., & Parkinson, D. R. (1987). Assessment of neuropsychological dysfunction in the work place: Data from the Pittsburgh Occupational Exposures Test Battery. *Journal of Clinical and Experimental Neuropsychology, 9,* 665-679.

Sawyer, J. (1966). Measurement and prediction, clinical and statistical. *Psychological Bulletin, 66,* 178-200.

Schultz, D. P. (1979). *Psychology in use: An introduction to applied psychology.* New York: MacMillan Publishing Company.

Schwab, K., Grafman, J., Salazar, A. M., & Kraft, J. (1993). Residual impairments and work status 15 years after penetrating head injury: Report from the Vietnam Head Injury Study. *Neurology, 43,* 95-103.

Schwartz, M. L., Dennerll, R. D., & Lin, Y. (1968). Neuropsychological and psychosocial predictors of employability in epilepsy. *Journal of Clinical Psychology, 24,* 174-177.

Stuss, D. T., & Benson, D. F. (1984). Neuropsychological studies of the frontal lobes. *Psychological Bulletin, 95,* 3-28.

Stuss, D. T., & Gow, C. A. (1992). "Frontal dysfunction" after traumatic brain injury. *Neuropsychiatry, Neuropsychology, and Behavioral Neurology, 5,* 272-282.

Stuss, D. T., Gow, C. A., & Hetherington, C. R. (1992). "No longer Gage": Frontal lobe dysfunction and emotional changes. *Journal of Consulting and Clinical Psychology, 60,* 349-359.

Super, D. E., & Crites, J. O. (1962). *Appraising vocational fitness by means of psychological tests* (rev. ed.). New York: Harper & Row.

U.S. Department of Labor (1986). *Dictionary of occupational titles.* (4th ed. suppl.). Washington, DC: Superintendent of Documents.

Varney, N. (1988). The prognostic significance of anosmia in patients with closed head trauma. *Journal of Clinical and Experimental Neuropsychology, 10,* 250-254.

Varney, N. R., & Menefee, L. (1993). Psychosocial and executive deficits following closed head injury: Implications for orbital frontal cortex. *Journal of Head Trauma Rehabilitation, 8,* 32-44.

Walters, G. D., White, T. W., & Greene, R. L. (1988). Use of the MMPI to identify malingering and exaggeration of psychiatric symptomatology in male prison inmates. *Journal of Consulting an Clinical Psychology, 56,* 111-117.

Webster, R. E. (1979). Utility of the WAIS in predicting vocational success of psychiatric patients. *Journal of Clinical Psychology, 35,* 111-116.

Weddell, R., Oddy, M., & Jenkins, D. (1980). Social recovery during the first year following severe head injury. *Journal of Neurology, Neurosurgery, and Psychiatry, 43,* 798-802.

Wedding, D. (1983). Clinical and statistical prediction in neuropsychology. *Clinical Neuropsychology, 5,* 49-55.

Wedding, D., & Faust, D. (1989). Clinical judgment and decision making in neuropsychology. *Archives of Clinical Neuropsychology, 4,* 233-265.

Wiener, D. N. (1948). Subtle and obvious keys for the MMPI. *Journal of Consulting Psychology, 12,* 164-170.

Yoakum, C. S., & Yerkes, R. M. (1920). *Army mental tests.* New York: Holt.

Youngjohn, J. R. (1991). Malingering of neuropsychological impairment: An assessment strategy. *A Journal for the Expert Witness, the Trial Attorney, the Trial Judge, 4,* 29-32.

20

THE ECOLOGICAL VALIDITY OF NEUROPSYCHOLOGICAL ASSESSMENT AFTER SEVERE BRAIN INJURY

Barbara A. Wilson, M.Phil., Ph.D., F.B.Ps.S.

THE NATURE OF NEUROPSYCHOLOGICAL ASSESSMENT

A question which is particularly relevant to those responsible for assessing patients who have sustained severe brain damage is how much information about a subject's ability to perform normal everyday tasks can be gained from neuropsychological assessment. This chapter considers some of the answers that might be given to this question.

First, we need a definition of assessment that is likely to be acceptable to psychologists. One that seems to fit this role would be that offered by Sundberg and Tyler, and quoted by Jones (1970, p. 1): "...the systematic collection, organization and interpretation of information about a person and his (her) situations." Jones suggests that we could add "...and the prediction of his (her) behaviour in new situations."

Lezak (1983) points out that neuropsychological assessment is more particularly concerned with assessing changes in behavior following brain dysfunction. Reasons for conducting neuropsychological assessment have shifted in emphasis over the past 20 or so years, from being primarily concerned with diagnosis of behavior that indicated the presence or absence of brain damage and localization of lesions, to being more concerned with identifying deficits resulting from brain injury that may turn out to be treatable or manageable (Hart & Hayden, 1986). In an imaginative and thought-provoking chapter, Hart and Hayden argue that neuropsychologists must now be able to (a) predict how problems resulting from brain injury will affect the activities of daily living (ADL), educational performance, and vocational success of their brain-injured patients; (b) convey these predictions to the patient, the family, and others in terms they will understand; and (c) plan rehabilitation programs to deal with the neuropsychological deficits as they are expressed in real-life activities.

Although these precepts are welcomed by some neuropsychologists, and may indeed form part of the guiding principles in their own assessment practice. However, it would not be true to say that they form general guidelines for neuropsychological assessment that are accepted by all neuropsychologists, many of whom may follow more traditional guidelines in their assessment practice. The implication here is not that more traditional forms of assessment are irrelevant to the daily lives of patients. Indeed, those who have no difficulty in taking on board ecologically valid assessment procedures such as those implied by Hart and Hayden (1986) would be mistaken if they did not recognize that other forms of neuropsychological assessment have been influential in alleviating some of the problems patients have encountered in their daily lives. The distinction to be made is one of emphasis rather than practice, or, more accurately, one of indirectness as opposed to directness. What distinguishes more traditional forms of neuropsychological assessment from the kind implied by Hart and Hayden is that the former's influence on the daily lives of patients is indirect rather than direct.

Neuropsychologists who would not regard their work in rehabilitation as being ecologically valid in the sense offered by Hart and Hayden (1986) have used information from their neuropsychological tests to estimate a person's general level of intellectual functioning, predict that person's premorbid level, and identify cognitive strengths and weaknesses. They have also used information to determine the precise nature of a particular cognitive deficit: for example, whether reading problems following brain injury are more typical of deep dyslexia, surface dyslexia, or some other acquired dyslexic syndrome. Furthermore, neuropsychological assessments that are not directly ecologically valid can ensure that the cognitively impossible is not expected from a patient by finding out whether that patient can understand, remember, read, or perceive material that is offered, and then using this information to identify strengths that can be employed to bypass weaknesses.

Important as this information is, and accepting that it can influence the planning of treatment programs, it offers little in the way of *direct* guidance to therapists involved in the actual treatment of a patient. While it might highlight a problem faced by a patient, it does not indicate a path or treatment program to follow that might lead to that patient overcoming the problem. Indeed, by its very nature, traditional neuropsychological assessment has no brief for saying, "This is the way you might tackle this problem so that the patient may no longer be troubled by it in his or her daily life." Put another way, traditional forms of neuropsychological assessment cannot, in general, directly inform treatment because the information it supplies is usually concerned with a patient's inability to perform a test or task, and this in itself does not usually amount to a "suitable case for treatment."

A caveat is necessary because there are cases, when a particular test is directly tapping a real-life skill, that enables us to treat a patient's inability to perform a particular neuropsychological test. An example would be the case of L.T. (Wilson, 1987) who was unable to read letters of the alphabet. This problem was identified during neuropsychological assessment, and treatment consisted of reteaching L.T. these letters, which in turn enabled her to read words and sentences until she eventually read for pleasure. However, such examples do not affect the general observation that most neuropsychological tests do not directly inform treatment. The items in these tests are not analogous to the everyday tasks encountered by brain-injured people, yet these are the tasks that therapists working in rehabilitation will concentrate on in their attempts to rehabilitate patients.

If we wish to make our neuropsychological assessments more ecologically valid then we must devise tests that do map directly onto everyday behavior and predict real-life problems. The following descriptions of two such tests, designed by the author and colleagues, will illustrate how this can be achieved.

THE RIVERMEAD BEHAVIOURAL MEMORY TEST

Sunderland, Harris, and Baddeley (1983) questioned the usefulness of traditional memory tests for predicting difficulties in everyday life. They argued that although tests such as the prose recall passages from the Wechsler Memory Scale (Wechsler, 1945) are sensitive in detecting organic impairment, such tests are not sensitive in detecting the nature of everyday problems. Because there was a need to devise a test that would overcome such limitations, Wilson, Cockburn, and Baddeley (1985) designed the Rivermead Behavioural Memory Test (RBMT). This test was designed to predict which people would experience everyday memory problems, and to monitor change in memory functioning over time. The test combines features from both traditional and behavioral assessments. It is a standardized test and is administered and scored like any other standardized test but instead of including clinical or experimental material such as paired-associates or abstract drawings, it includes analogs of everyday tasks. It replaces tasks decontextualized from the real world with tasks similar to those required for functioning in the real world. The 12 components or subtests were selected on the basis of (a) observations of brain-injured patients at Rivermead Rehabilitation Centre in Oxford, and (b) memory difficulties reported in a study of head-injured people (Sunderland et al., 1983).

The subtests include remembering a new name, recalling a new route (immediate and delayed), remembering a newspaper article (immediate and delayed), remembering to ask about the next appointment at a predetermined time during the test, remembering to deliver a message, face and picture recognition tasks, and orientation questions. There are four parallel versions of the test. Inter rater and alternate form reliability are very high (Wilson, Cockburn, Baddeley, & Hiorns, 1989).

The original study, funded by the British Medical Research Council, involved 176 brain-injured subjects and 118 control subjects aged between 14 and 69 years. The test was validated in three ways. The first, a rather crude measure, was simply to see whether brain-injured subjects scored worse than controls. This was indeed the case. The brain-injured subjects scored a mean of 6.43 (from a maximum of 12) on the screening score, with a standard deviation of 3.42, while the controls scored a mean of 10.60 with a standard deviation of 1.41.

The second way the RBMT was validated was to see whether the test correlated with other tests of memory (Recognition Memory for Words and Faces) (Warrington, 1984); digit span, spatial span, and the paired associate learning test from Randt, Brown, and Osborne (1980). All correlations were significant at the p .001 level, ranging from 0.24 for backward digit span to 0.60 for Recognition Memory for Words. From this it was concluded that the RBMT, broadly speaking, was a valid measure of memory performance when this was assessed by existing tests.

Ecological validity was determined by correlating performance on the RBMT with memory failures observed by therapists during patients' daily rehabilitation. For a two-week period, occupational, physical, and speech therapists completed a checklist at the end of each session for each patient they were treating. The 19-item checklist was adapted from one designed by Sunderland et al. (1983). Therapists observed 80 patients in this way for a mean of 35 hours per patient (range 16 - 55 hours). The correlation between therapists' observations and RBMT score was -0.75 (p < 0.001). These results suggest the RBMT is a good and ecologically valid measure of everyday memory performance.

These findings have since been corroborated in other studies. Wilson (1991b) in a long-term (5 - 10-year) follow-up study of 54 patients referred for memory therapy between 1979 - 1985, found that the RBMT discriminated between patients who were independent and those who were dependent ($x2$ = 24.72, p<0.001); whereas the Wechsler Memory Scale Revised (WMS-R) (Wechsler, 1987) did not discriminate. Independence was operationally defined as either being in paid employment or in full-time education or living alone.

Schwartz and Macmillan (1989) found that the RBMT correlated with employment status whereas a memory questionnaire did not. They concluded that the RBMT was a more objective measure of functional ability. Kotler-Cope (1990) found the WMS-R was not as valid a measure of everyday memory and had less ecological validity than the RBMT.

From these studies it would be fair to say that the RBMT is indeed an eco-logically valid measure of prediction of everyday memory problems. The fact that there are four parallel versions makes the test a useful tool to monitor change over time. Norms currently exist for all ages from 5 to 96 years. Children aged between 5 and 10 years are given slightly different versions of the test, more suitable to their ages. When planning memory therapy programs, however, the neuropsychologist needs to use additional measures to identify those problems considered important by memory-impaired people and their families (see Wilson 1989, 1991a for further discussion of this issue).

THE BEHAVIOURAL INATTENTION TEST

Wilson, Cockburn, and Halligan (1987) designed the Behavioural Inatten-tion Test (BIT) to predict everyday problems arising from unilateral visual ne-glect (UVN). UVN is a heterogeneous and often transitory phenomenon in which patients fail to report, respond, or orient to stimuli on one side of space (Heilman, Watson, & Valenstein, 1985). The condition is commonly associ-ated with right hemisphere stroke. Diller and Gordon (1981) suggest that ap-proximately 40% of right hemisphere stroke patients show evidence of UVN. The condition is less frequently encountered after left hemisphere stroke and is less severe in these circumstances. Patients with other conditions, such as cere-bral tumor or severe head injury, may also exhibit UVN. Several studies have shown that UVN is one of the major factors impeding functional recovery and rehabilitation success (Denes, Semenza, Stoppa, & Lis, 1982; Kinsella & Ford, 1985).

There was no single standardized battery for the assessment of UVN prior to the development of the BIT, and investigators had to rely on a variety of unstandardized, often cross-modal test procedures, such as the line crossing test (Albert, 1973), indented reading (Caplan,1987), and position bias on Ravens Coloured Matrices (Costa, Vaughan, Horwitz, & Ritter, 1969). Such single tests of neglect are inappropriate because (a) patients often vary in the way the neglect presents itself, and (b) an individual patient may show great variability in the degree of neglect, depending on such factors as fatigue, position of the tester, and presence or absence of distinctive stimuli in the testing room. A red curtain, for example, on the left side may draw the patients' attention to that side and reduce the neglect, whereas a red curtain on the right side may increase the amount of neglect.

Like the traditional memory tests referred to earlier, these single tests of neglect do not map onto the everyday demands faced by patients with UVN. Patients with severe neglect often collide with objects, ignore food on one side of the plate, and attend to only one side of the body. They may experience difficulty with reading, writing, and drawing, activities not always included in these tests of neglect.

The items in the BIT were selected partly as a result of observing right hemisphere stroke patients experiencing everyday problems such as those mentioned above, partly through examining reports from other studies (e.g., Diller and Gordon, 1981), and partly through discussions with health service staff who worked with neglect patients. The complete BIT battery comprises nine behavioral subtests reflecting aspects of daily life, and six simple pencil-and-paper measures of neglect, which we call "conventional" subtests. In the former are picture scanning, telephone dialing, menu reading, article reading, telling and setting the time, coin sorting, address and sentence copying, map navigation, and card sorting. The conventional subtests include line crossing, letter cancellation, figure and shape copying, line bisection, and representational drawing.

The BIT was standardized on 80 patients with unilateral brain damage secondary to stroke. Of these, 26 had a left CVA and 54 a right CVA. The mean age for the former group was 54.6 years and for the latter it was 57.7 years. The age difference was not significant. The patients were, on average, two months post-stroke. Neglect behavior persisting to this stage is likely to present as a serious rehabilitation problem. Fifty control subjects were also tested to establish normative data for the test items. Further details of the standardization procedure can be seen in Halligan, Cockburn, and Wilson (1991). Using the control data to determine cut-off scores, 48% of the right hemisphere stroke patients showed visual neglect compared with 15.4% of the left hemisphere stroke patients.

Like the RBMT, the BIT was validated in three ways. First, we expected brain-damaged patients to score substantially poorer than controls, and this was in fact the case (p <.001). The second was to compare performance on the conventional subtests with performance on the behavioral subtests, given that the conventional tests were used to define the presence of neglect. The correlation coefficient was 0.79 (p <0.01), suggesting that the behavioral items are good measures of neglect. Finally, because the BIT was designed to predict problems with daily functional tasks, we obtained occupational therapists' ratings of the ADL problems of our patient sample together with scores on the Rivermead Activities of Daily Living Scale (Whiting & Lincoln, 1980). The correlation between occupational therapists' ratings and BIT scores was -0.67 p <0.01, while correlation between the RADL and BIT scores was 0.53 (p<0.01), suggesting that the BIT is an ecologically valid measure of everyday problems arising from neglect.

Another study (Shiel, 1990) investigated the relationship between WEI and ADL. She found that patients with neglect as measured by the BIT were significantly more likely to have problems with ADL tasks (p<0.001). She also found (a) that the behavioral subtests correlated higher with ADL scores than the conventional subtests, (b) that the highest correlations were with indoor mobility, transfer from bed to chair, and using the lavatory, and (c) that the results were not due to hemianopia or motor problems.

There are a few other ecologically valid neuropsychological assessments available. Holland's Test of Functional Communication for Aphasic Adults has been available since 1980. Wang and Ennis (1986) produced the Cognitive Competency Test, which assesses skills required for everyday life, and Saxton's Severe Impairment Battery (Saxton, McGonigle, Swihart, & Boller, 1993) promises to be an ecologically valid tool for assessing everyday skills of dementing patients.

FUNCTIONALLY RELEVANT ASSESSMENT PROCEDURES FOR PATIENTS SURVIVING SEVERE HEAD INJURY

The remainder of this chapter describes an ongoing study that is attempting to develop new and ecologically valid assessment procedures for severely head-injured patients. The history of this study began in 1980 when I was asked to assess a woman who had sustained an anesthetic accident. She was left blind, dysphasic, hemiplegic, and dyspraxic so she could not see or speak, could not move her right arm or leg, and could not make her left arm do what she wanted. As the neuropsychologist on the team, I was asked to provide staff with an understanding of the patient's intellectual functioning. My initial reactions were of concern and bewilderment. I could assess people who could not see, speak, or move, but it was necessary for a patient to be able to do one of these things to complete any of the neuropsychological tests with which I was familiar. Following my training maxim that dictated that no patient is untestable I began to look for solutions.

I turned to another part of my earlier training, when I worked with people who were mentally retarded, and considered an assessment and treatment procedure known as "Portage," named after the town of Portage, Wisconsin where it was developed as a home-based teaching technique for parents of mentally retarded children (Shearer et al., 1972). In the Portage method, children are assessed on five developmental scales: motor, language, self-help, socialization, and cognition. Gaps in functioning are pinpointed and treated. Specific objectives (that will almost certainly be achieved within a week) are set, and a treatment program worked out between the home advisor and the parents. In the assessment stage items on each checklist are completed through observation or through eliciting the behavior. For example, the first item on the cognitive scale is "cloth on face." A cloth is put on the child's face and if he or she removes it by any means, the item is passed.

The Portage scales were administered to the anoxic patient described above. Occupational, speech, and physical therapists helped to complete the forms, thus replacing the role of parents in the typical Portage program. The woman's functioning on each of the scales was below a two-year-old level. This does not mean, of course, that she was like a two year old in every way but that in terms of what she could achieve in her everyday life she was more akin to that age group. Her first failure on the self-help scale was item 15, "Eats with a spoon independently." Performance here was unreliable because of her dyspraxia (she could only use her left hand as her right was paralyzed). It was decided to use this item as the first treatment objective.

The programs for this woman and other patients are described in Wilson (1985). In some ways Portage fulfilled the need for an objective assessment of the woman's intellectual functioning. An objective and ecologically valid description of her current levels of functioning was provided. In other ways Portage was inappropriate because many of the items are unsuitable for adults. Included "waves good-bye in imitation of an adult," and "drinks from a bottle alone."

The next stage in the story was an attempt to modify Portage for use with adults. More adult-oriented items can be found in assessments designed for mentally retarded adults: see, for example, Bereweeke (Felce, Jenkins, de Kock, & Mansella, 1983), the Hampshire Assessment for Living with Others, or HALO (Shackleton-Bailey & Piddock, 1982). The developmental approach to measuring recovery after severe head injury is not new (see, for instance, Eson, Yen, & Bourke, 1978), nor necessarily appropriate, but in the absence of firm evidence on whether recovery follows a developmental pattern we decided to pursue this direction. A pilot study was carried out with a physiotherapist, Annelies

Hartman, at Charing Cross Hospital in London, and this is described in Wilson (1988).

Our view at this stage was that we needed to develop our own items independently of, although influenced by, the Portage model. A grant was obtained from the British Medical Research Council to undertake an observational study of 100 patients sustaining severe head injury (defined as in coma for at least six hours) in order to develop functionally relevant assessment procedures. The research team comprises Barbara Wilson, Lindsay McLellan, Mike Campbell, Sandra Horn, Martin Watson, Agnes Shiel, and Tina Perry.

THE SOUTHAMPTON HEAD INJURY PROJECT

(a) Background and Rationale: The rationale behind the project is to provide useful assessment procedures for monitoring recovery from severe head injury. The long-term aim is to use these assessments to (i) pinpoint areas for treatment, and (ii) provide sensitive outcome measures.

There is a considerable gap in our knowledge about the natural history of recovery from traumatic brain injury. This imposes limitations on our ability to assess recovery, especially in regard to the functional and practical skills needed to cope with everyday life. The Glasgow Coma Scale (Teasdale & Jennett, 1974) is widely used for measuring the level of consciousness in early head-injured patients. Indeed it is an integral part of the neurological observation chart for patients with impaired consciousness on many wards. A recent study at Southampton shows, however, that even this relatively straightforward scale is not always used consistently or accurately (Watson, Horn, & Curl, 1992). Furthermore, it is not always a straightforward matter to ascertain when someone is "in" coma.

Several scales exist for monitoring recovery after coma but these often prove less useful than the (often abused) Glasgow Coma Scale. The most widely used of the later scales is perhaps the Glasgow Outcome Scale (Jennett & Bond, 1975), which comprises a short (five category) form and two expanded (eight and ten category) forms. Other well-known scales are the Disability Rating Scale (Rappaport, Hall, Hopkins, Belleza, & Cope, 1982), the Stover and Zeiger Scale (1976), the Ranchos Los Amigos Scales, otherwise known as the Levels of Cognitive Functioning Scales (Hagen, Malkmus, & Durham, 1979), and the Neurobehavioural Rating Scale (Levin et al., 1987). Apart from the last mentioned, which contains 28 items, the others are comprised of eight items or categories that are too broad to detect subtle changes in recovery. These scales may also cross behavioral dimensions such as motor ability, cognitive function, and social awareness, so it is difficult to identify improvements in a specific area. On occasions a patient's behavior may fit into more than one category (for example, "confused - agitated" and "confused non-agitated") over a time. Again, fine gradations of behavior are lost.

Furthermore, these scales rate behaviors rather than observing or measuring them, and so are subject to personal interpretations by staff. One nurse, for example, scored a patient lower than she should on the Glasgow Coma Scale, explaining that the accurate score did not truly reflect her opinion of the patient's condition.

Most importantly, the existing scales do not specify changes in sufficient detail. On the Glasgow Outcome Scale, for example, item 4 is "can travel by public transport and work in a sheltered environment and can therefore be independent in so far as daily life is concerned." This implies that traveling on public transport and working in a sheltered environment always go together. Clearly these are separate skills. Gross measures may be satisfactory for some purposes such as predicting the percentage of patients who will require long-term care but they are insufficient for the therapist planning an individual treatment program, and too broad to identify subtle changes in the patient's abilities or behavior. Potentially avoidable problems will be missed if staff do not have fairly specific means of categorizing, measuring, or comparing observable changes. When staff are supplied with these means they are less likely to disregard potentially important changes, and more likely to record or document them. For example, fewer falls may occur when staff have been supplied with a detailed method of observing slight changes in mobility. Similarly, behavior problems might be avoided if alternative means of communication are provided between staff and patients who cannot communicate normally.

A major aim of the Southampton team was to develop a reliable and valid method of assessing patients who are too impaired for more conventional neuropsychological assessment. It would also have to be more detailed and sophisticated than the conventional neuropsychological methods that Diller (personal communication) suggests cannot test 27% of patients admitted to his center in New York.

The Southampton team believed it ought to be possible to design assessments that are free from the weaknesses discussed above. We were interested in behavioral assessments because they can record and measure things a person does rather than simply confirming or recording impairments or states of being. For example, a behavioral assessment can show that a patient asks the same question 15 times every 10 minutes rather than confirming that the patient has post-traumatic amnesia. Equipped with the first piece of information, it will be possible to organize a treatment program that might reduce the behavior, thus bringing about a more tolerable everyday atmosphere for both the patient and the people with whom he or she communicates. Here we can see the ecological potential of behavioral methods of assessment. Of course it has also been possible to combine a psychometric and behavioral approach in one assessment procedure as we have seen earlier in the discussion of the RBMT and BIT.

(b) Subjects and Procedure: At the time of writing, 88 head-injured patients have been identified from two district general hospitals. All had a coma of at least six hours. Length of coma ranged between one and 36 days, with a median of six days. Ages ranged from 14 to 67 years, with a mean of 26.72 years and a standard deviation of 16.40 years. There were 73 males and 15 females. Of these, eight did not emerge from coma and five of these died. A further three died after emerging from coma.

The principal aim was to record spontaneous behavior and develop assessment procedures to plot courses of recovery in the following areas: motor ability, cognitive skills, self-care, and social behavior. In addition to observed spontaneous responses some behaviors were elicited by appropriate stimuli: for example, a red ball was used to see whether a subject looked at a brightly colored stimulus, and a narrow-beam flashlight was used to see if a subject could track a moving light. Certain items were taken from existing ADL and motor scales, and a few from the Portage checklists. Patients were observed from the day of admission. Where possible, observations were carried out daily. Intervals between observations were longer at the more distant hospital, and where recovery itself was slow.

(c) Problems en Route: The first problem to overcome was to redefine coma. As mentioned earlier, the GCS was not always completed accurately, consistently, or even correctly. Second, using the widely accepted eight or less on the GCS as "in coma" and nine or more as "out of coma" led to anomalies. The original studies by Teasdale and Jennett (1974) totaled scores from the three sections of the GCS (eye opening, motor response, and verbal response) as a convenient means for accommodating data on the computer. Clinically, such totaling is less useful, for although patients who achieve the same score through a different combination show similar outcomes (Teasdale et al., 1979), the total scores for patients undergoing clinical care can be misleading. This point was acknowledged by Jennett and Teasdale in 1977. In addition, patients can score nine and be "in coma" according to other criteria or, conversely, score eight and be out of coma. For example, a patient may score nine in the following manner: (a) Eyes open spontaneously equals four, (b) verbal incomprehensible sounds equals two, (c) motor flexes abnormally to pain equals three. Spontaneous eye opening, however, has little or no relationship with coma, and an appropriate verbal response may not occur for weeks or months after consciousness has been regained. So the patient might be in or out of coma with a score of nine. Similarly a conscious patient, unable to move or speak, can score eight or less.

We chose to define the end of coma operationally as "consistently able to obey a command," which means that information has been received, understood and acted upon. Others have also suggested this definition (for example, Bricolo, Turazzi, and Ferlotti, 1980; Levin, Grossman, Rose, and Teasdale, 1979). By "ability to obey a command" we have to be certain that we are not measuring some other behavior. We have seen patients described as "opening eyes to command" when they are in reality opening their eyes to speech. Other patients have been described as "squeezing tester's hand on command" when the patient is in fact exhibiting a grasp reflex. An unequivocal response must be observed, such as lifting an arm or turning one's head towards the door. The command, of course, must be within the patient's motor ability. For further discussion see Horn, Watson, Wilson, and McLellan (1992).

It also became apparent early on that we should not assume a patient was incapable of a response before incorporating personal or highly motivating stimuli in our testing procedures. One 36-year-old man, for example, first seen 91 days post-injury, was opening his eyes spontaneously, making incomprehensible sounds, and localizing to painful stimuli. He had a dense right hemiplegia and no speech. It was difficult to know whether he was capable of obeying a command. When asked to lift his arm, for example, he sometimes responded perhaps after 30 seconds or more but his responses were inconsistent. On the 103rd day post-injury he was offered a £10.00 note. The tester said, "A..., would you like this?" The patient looked up?, reached out his hand and took the note. The tester said, "Good A..., but that was only a test. It's my £10.00 note and I'm afraid I need it back." The patient smiled broadly and gave the note back. See Watson and Horn (1991) for a further description.

(d) Some Preliminary Results: Observations produced 162 items of behavior observed at different stages during recovery. In order to examine more closely which behaviors were observed during coma a subgroup of 12 patients was observed daily from admission. This group comprised nine men and three women, aged 17 to 67 years (mean 29.5 years, S.D. 16.38 years). Time in coma ranged from one day to 86 days. Three items of behavior were identified that appeared to have little significance as all patients, even those who died subsequently, displayed them. These items were (i) eyes open briefly, (ii) eyes open for an extended period, and (iii) eyes open and move. This left a list of 17 items that were always observed before the end of coma (using our operational definition). The rank order of occurrence was as follows: eyes open but do not focus, eyes focus momentarily, attention held by dominant stimulus, patient looks at person giving attention, focuses briefly on moving object, shows agitated behavior when wet or soiled, makes eye contact, vocalizes to express need or want, tracks source of sound, frowns/grimaces to show dislike, smiles, cloth on face - becomes quiescent, focuses briefly on person or object, turns head/ eyes to look at person talking, watches person moving in line of vision, expletive speech, makes eye contact for five seconds.

Five further items of behavior that sometimes occurred during coma and sometimes after coma were also identified and placed in rank order of occurrence. These were: moves spontaneously to facilitate dressing, cloth on face causes distress, cloth on face patient removes three consecutive times, tracks sound for five seconds, shows a selective response to preferred people. Operational definitions were determined for each of these behaviors to ensure inter rater reliability.

Following these developments, a visual awareness scale has been developed from observations of 84 patients. The scale comprises 16 items analyzed by a paired-preference technique to determine the best fit for order of recovery. This techniques generates a matrix of order of recovery from all items across all patients.

Similar scales have been developed to assess cognition, communication and speech, social behavior, self-care, continence, and motor recovery. We asked members of the child health team to rank the items on each scale according to the developmental sequence they would expect. Correlations between these "blind" rankings and our results showed good agreement. The correlation with the visual awareness scale, for example, was 0.769 p < 0.01, although in some respects our patients do not show a developmental pattern.

Work continues on these scales, particularly with the reliability and validity. We are of the opinion that these assessments will prove to be of considerable importance in clinical practice as there is at present no adequately validated measure for monitoring small changes in the progress of functional behavior. Such changes are likely to be missed unless they are being looked for in a structured manner. This failure to observe can result in staff becoming poorly motivated because they think the patient is not progressing, and can also lead to inadequate patient care that fails to match progress in functioning.

REFERENCES

Albert, M. L. (1973). A simple test of visual neglect. *Neurology, 23,* 658-664.

Bricolo, A., Turazzi, S., & Ferlotti, G. (1980). Prolonged post-traumatic unconsciousness: Therapeutic assets and liabilities. *Journal of Neurosurgery, 52,* 625-634.

Caplan, B. (1987). Assessment of unilateral neglect: A new reading test. *Journal of Clinical and Experimental Neuropsychology, 9,* 359-364.

Costa, L. D., Vaughan, H. G., Horwitz, M., & Ritter, W. (1969). Patterns of behavioral deficit associated with visual spatial neglect. *Cortex, 5,* 242-263.

Denes, F., Semenza, C., Stoppa, E., & Lis, A. (1982). Unilateral spatial neglect and recovery from hemiplegia: A follow up study. *Brain, 105,* 543-552.

Diller, L., & Gordon, W. A. (1981). Rehabilitation and clinical neuropsychology. In S. B. Filskov & T. J. Boll (Eds.), *Handbook of clinical neuropsychology* (pp. 702-733). New York: Wiley.

Eson, M. E., Yen, J. R., & Bourke, R. J. (1978). Assessment of recovery from serious head injury. *Journal of Neurology Neurosurgery and Psychiatry, 41,* 1,036-1,042.

Felce, D., Jenkins, J., de Kock, U., & Mansell, J. (1983). *The Bereweeke Skill-Teaching System: Assessment Checklist.* Windsor, England: NFER-Nelson.

Hagen, C., Malkmus, D., & Durham, P. (1979). Levels of cognitive functions. In C. A. Downey (Ed.), *Rehabilitation of head injured adults: Comprehensive physical management.* Downey, CA: Professional Staff Association of Ranchos Los Amigos Hospital, Inc.

Halligan, P., Cockburn, J., & Wilson, B. A. (1991). The behavioral assessment of visual neglect. *Neuropsychological Rehabilitation, 1,* 5-32.

Hart, T., & Hayden, M. E. (1986). The ecological validity of neuropsychological assessment and remediation. In B. Uzzell & Y. Gross (Eds.), *Clinical neuropsychology of intervention* (pp. 21-50). Boston: Martinus Nijhoff.

Heilman, K. M., Watson, R. T., & Valenstein, E. (1985). Neglect and related disorders. In K. M. Heilman & E. Valenstein (Eds.), *Clinical neuropsychology* (2nd ed.) (pp. 243-250). Oxford University Press.

Holland, A. L. (1980). *Communicative abilities in daily living.* Baltimore: University Park Press.

Horn, S., Watson, M., Wilson, B. A., & McLellan, D. L. (1992). The development of new techniques in the assessment and monitoring of recovery from severe head injury: A preliminary report and case study. *Brain Injury, 6,* 321-325.

Jennett, B., & Bond, M. (1975). Assessment of outcome after severe brain damage. *Lancet, 1,* 480-484.

Jennett, B., & Teasdale, G. (1977). Aspects of comas after severe head injury. *Lancet, 1,* 878-881.

Jones, H. G. (1970). Principles of psychological assessment. In P. Mittler (Ed.), *The psychological assessment of mental and physical handicaps* (pp. 1-25). London: Tavistock Publications.

Kinsella, G., & Ford, B. (1985). Hemi-inattention and the recovery patterns of stroke patients. *International Rehabilitation Medicine, 7,* 102-106.

Kotler-Cope, S. (1990). *Memory impairment in older adults: The interrelationships between objective and subjective clinical and everyday memory assessment.* Paper presented at the Annual Meeting of the Southern Society for Philosophy and Psychology, Louisville, KY.

Levin, H. S., Grossman, R. G., Rose, J. E., & Teasdale, G. (1979). Long term neuropsychological outcome of closed head injury. *Journal of Neurosurgery, 50,* 412-422.

Levin, H. S., High, W. M., Goethe, K. E., Sisson, R. A., Overall, J. E., Rhoades, H. M., Eisenberg, H. M., Kalisky, Z., & Gary, H. E. (1987). The neurobehavioural rating scale: Assessment of the behavioral sequelae of head injury by the physician. *Journal of Neurology, Neurosurgery and Psychiatry, 50,* 183-193.

Lezak, M. D. (1983). *Neuropsychological assessment* (2nd ed.). New York: Oxford University Press.

Randt, C. T., Brown, E. R., & Osborne, D. P. (1980). A memory test for longitudinal measurement of mild to moderate deficits. *Clinical Neuropsychiatry, 2,* 184-194.

Rappaport, M., Hall, K., Hopkins, K., Belleza, T., & Cope, N. (1982). Disability rating scale for severe head trauma: Coma to community. *Archives of Physical Medicine and Rehabilitation, 63,* 118-123.

Saxton, J., McGonigle, K. L., Swihart, A. A., & Boller, F. (1993). *The Severe Impairment Battery*. Flempton, Suffolk, England: Thames Valley Test Company.

Schwartz, A. F., & Macmillan, T. (1989). Assessment of everyday memory after severe head injury. *Cortex, 25,* 665-671.

Shackleton-Bailey, M., & Piddock, P. (1982). *HALO: An introduction to the Hampshire assessment for living with others*. Obtainable from Hampshire Social Services Dept., Trafalgar House, The Castle, Winchester SO23 8UQ, England.

Shearer, D., Billingsley, J., Froman, A., Hilliart, J., Johnson, F., & Shearer, M. (1972). *The Portage guide to early education*. Portage, WI: CESA.

Shiel, A. (1990). *An investigation of the relationship between unilateral neglect and ADL dependency in right hemisphere stroke patients*. Unpublished Masters' Thesis, Southampton University Medical School, England.

Stover, S. L., & Zeiger, H. E. (1976). Head injury in children and teenagers: Functional recovery correlated with duration of coma. *Archives of Physical Medicine and Rehabilitation, 57,* 201-205.

Sunderland, A., Harris, J. E., & Baddeley, A. D. (1983). Do laboratory tests predict everyday memory? A neuropsychological study. *Journal of Verbal Learning and Verbal Behavior, 22,* 341-357.

Teasdale, G., Murray, G., Parker, L., & Jennett, B. (1979). Adding up the Glasgow Coma score. *Acta Neurochir. Supp. 28*, pp. 13-16.

Teasdale, G., & Jennett, B. (1974). Assessment of coma and impaired consciousness: A practical scale. *Lancet, 2,* 81-84.

Wang, P. L., & Ennis, K. E. (1986). Competency assessment in clinical populations: An introduction to the cognitive competency test. In B. P. Uzzell & Y. Gross (Eds.), *Clinical neuropsychology of intervention*. Boston: Martinus Nijhoff.

Warrington, E. K. (1984). *The Recognition Memory Test*. Windsor, England: NFERNelson.

Watson, M., & Horn, S. (1991). The ten-pound note test: Suggestions for eliciting improved responses in the severely brain injured patients. *Brain Injury,* in press.

Watson, M., Horn, S., & Curl, J. (1992). Searching for signs of revival: Uses and abuses of the Glasgow Coma Scale (or the GCS revisited). *Professional Nurse, 7,* 670-674.

Wechsler, D. (1945). A standardized memory scale for clinical use. *Journal of Psychology, 19,* 87-95.

Wechsler, D. (1987). *The Wechsler Memory Scale - Revised*. San Antonio, TX: The Psychological Corporation.

Whiting, S., & Lincoln, N. (1980). An ADL assessment for stroke patients. *British Journal of Occupational Therapy 43,* 44-46.

Wilson, B. A. (1985). Adapting "Portage" for neurological patients. *International Rehabilitation Medicine, 7,* 6-8.

Wilson, B. A. (1987). *Rehabilitation of memory*. New York: Guilford Press.

Wilson, B. A. (1988). Future directions in the rehabilitation of brain injured people. In A. L. Christensen & B. P. Uzzell (Eds.), *Neuropsychological Rehabilitation*. Boston: Kluwer.

Wilson, B. A. (1989). Designing memory therapy programs. In L. Poon, D. Rubin, & B. A. Wilson (Eds.), *Everyday cognition in adulthood and later life* (pp. 615-638). New York: Cambridge University Press.

Wilson, B. A. (199la). Behavior therapy in the treatment of neurologically impaired adults. In P. R. Martin (Ed.), *Handbook of behavior therapy and psychological science: An integrative approach* (pp. 227-252). New York: Pergamon Press.

Wilson, B. A. (1991b). Long term prognosis of patients with severe memory disorders. *Neuropsychological Rehabilitation.*

Wilson, B., Cockburn, J., & Baddeley, A. D. (1985). *The Rivermead Behavioural Memory Test manual.* Flempton, Bury St. Edmunds, Suffolk, England: Thames Valley Test Company.

Wilson, B. A., Cockburn, J., Baddeley, A. D., & Hiorns, R. (1989). The development and validation of a test battery for detecting and monitoring everyday memory problems. *Journal of Clinical and Experimental Neuropsychology, 11,* 855-870.

Wilson, B,. A., Cockburn, J., & Halligan, P. (1987). *The Behavioural Inattention Test.* Flempton, Bury St. Edmunds, Suffolk, England: Thames Valley Test Company.

APPENDIX A

NEUROBEHAVIORAL ASSESSMENT FORMAT

CONTENTS OF APPENDIX A

IDENTIFYING DATA

I. IDENTIFYING INFORMATION

Patient's Name_____ **Age**_____D.O.B._____

Gender _____ Social Security Number_____-_____-_____
Next of Kin_____(Guardian)_____
   Address_____ Telephone(_____)_____
Patient's Address_____ Telephone(_____)_____

Highest Education Level Attained by Patient_____
Academic Affiliation_____
Address of School_____

Occupation_____
Job Title and Employer_____
Date of Beginning and Terminating Position_____

Financial Assistance/Disability Insurance_____
Address of Agency_____

Annual Income_____

Marital Status_____

Socioeconomic Information
   Patient's Ethnic Background_____

Father: Occupation_____
             Educational Level_____
             Income_____
             Ethnic Background_____
Mother: Occupation_____
             Educational Level_____
             Income_____
             Ethnic Background_____

II. HEALTH INSURANCE AND METHOD OF PAYMENT
FOR SERVICES

Person Responsible for Payment_____
    Billing Address_____

Health Insurance Policies Held_____
    Policy Number(s) _____
    Name of Insurance Company_____
    Address_____

Eligibility for Veterans' Benefits_____

III. LANGUAGE AND HANDEDNESS BACKGROUND

A.   **Language Background**_____
     Place of Birth_____
     Languages Spoken (List Order Learned) _____
     Language Spoken in Patient's Home_____

B.   **Hand Preference**
     Which hand does the Patient use to do each of the following?
     Sign his/her name?   Right___   LEFT___   EITHER___
     Throw a ball to hit a target?   Right___   LEFT___   EITHER___
     Cut with scissors?   Right___   LEFT___   EITHER___
     Left-handed as a child?   no   dk   YES
     Switched to using the right?   no   dk   YES
     Parents left-handed?   Mother___   Father___   Both___
     Left-handed brothers and sisters?   no   dk   YES
     Left-handed children?   has none__   no   dk   YES

IV. EXAMINER'S CREDENTIALS

Examiner's Credentials: Student___   Intern___   Resident___   Post-Doctoral___
                              M.A.___   Ph.D.___   M.D.____
                              Specialty Boards _____
                              M.A./M.S. (Specify Discipline)_____
                              M.S.W._____
                              Nursing R.N., B.S.N., M.S.N., Ph.D._____

Supervisor's Credentials:_____

REFERRAL ISSUES

Patient: _____   **Referral Source:** _____

Name: _____   Name: _____

Address:_____Zip:_____   Address:_____Zip:_____

Telephone: (____)_____   Telephone: (____)_____

                                      Specialization:_____

Date of Referral: _____

CASE STATUS

List	(Check One)		
	Suspected	Identified	Confirmed
1. Neurological Illness			
_____	_____	_____	_____
2. Psychopathology			
_____	_____	_____	_____
3. Cognitive Deficits			
_____	_____	_____	_____

REFERRAL ISSUES

	Rule Out	Describe	Document
1. Neurological Illness	_____	_____	_____
2. Psychopathology	_____	_____	_____
3. Cognitive Deficits	_____	_____	_____
a. Global	_____	_____	_____
b. Selective	_____	_____	_____
I. Orientation/Awareness/Attention	_____	_____	_____
II. Perceptual	_____	_____	_____
III. Motoric/Practice/Sequencing/ Executive Functioning	_____	_____	_____
IV. a. Expressive Language	_____	_____	_____
1.) Speech	_____	_____	_____
2.) Writing	_____	_____	_____
b. Receptive Language	_____	_____	_____
1.) Speech	_____	_____	_____
2.) Reading	_____	_____	_____
V. Conceptual/Calculational	_____	_____	_____
VI. Memory	_____	_____	_____

PURPOSE OF NEUROBEHAVIORAL ASSESSMENT

DOCUMENT COURSE OF ILLNESS _____

ASSESS TREATMENT RESPONSE _____

GENERATE NEUROBEHAVIORAL DIAGNOSTIC FORMULATION _____

GENERATE MANAGEMENT PLAN _____

GENERATE REHABILITATION PLAN _____

DOCUMENT DISABILITY FOR FORENSIC/MEDICOLEGAL APPLICATION _____

PRESENTING COMPLAINT

a. **Presenting Complaint (Verbatim Description):**_____

_____

_____

b. For any sensory, perceptual, motoric, cutaneous, cephalic, or somatic complaints, follow patient's description with,

    "What area(s) is effected?" "What parts of the body?"_____

    "Where do you see it, hear it, feel it, etc.?"_____

    "Which side?"   L___R___B___

c. First happened?_____

d. How long did it last?_____

e. **Happened since then?**   Yes___ No___

    How often?_____

    Always the same?   Yes___ No___

        How does it change?_____

    Happen more often or less often than when you first noticed it?

        More___ Less___ Same___

f. **Other changes or symptoms before, during or after (the problem)?**   Yes___ No___

    Describe_____

    _____

g. **Anything which caused (the problem)?**   Yes___ No___

    Describe_____

    _____

h. **Anything which makes (the problem) better?**   Yes___ No___

                 Medication___ Alcohol___ Drugs___

    Describe_____

    _____

i. **Anything which makes (the problem) worse?**   Yes___ No___

                 Medication___ Alcohol___ Drugs___

    Describe_____

    _____

j. **Does (the problem) cause any other difficulties for you?**   Yes___ No___

    Describe_____

    _____

k. **Does (the problem) upset you?**   Yes___ No___

Repeat a-k for each symptom reported spontaneously by the patient.

SYMPTOM INQUIRY CODING SHEET

Presenting Complaint
History of the Present Illness
Review of Systems

PATIENT_____SYMPTOM_____

a. **DESCRIPTION:**_____

_____

b. **LOCUS:**_____
1. Corporeal Space:
    L Face___L Torso___LUE___LLE   R Face___R Torso___RUE___RLE
2. Extra Corporeal Space
    Right Hemifield____Left Hemifield____Both Sides
3. Non-localized____
4. Difficulty Specifying Locus____

c. **ONSET:** Age_____Date:_____
1. Mode: Abrupt_____Gradual____
2. Prodroma_____
3. Precipitus_____

d. **DURATION:** Symptom_____ Syndrome_____

e. **RECURRENCE:** Yes ___ No ___
    Frequency_____

f. **ASSOCIATED SYMPTOMS:**_____

g. **COURSE:**
1. <u>Clinical</u>:   Static___   Cyclic___   Episodic___   Isolated___
2. <u>Changes</u>:
    <u>Direction of Change Over Time:</u>   <u>Velocity of Change:</u>
    Static ___ Progressive___ Resolving___   Rapid___ Moderate___   Slow___
    Stereotypy: Yes___   No_____

    In Severity_____
    In Frequency_____
    In Associated Symptoms_____

h. **TERMINATION:**   Abrupt____   Gradual____

i. **PALLIATIVES:** Yes___ No___

j. **IRRITANTS:** Yes___ No___

k. **RELATED PROBLEMS:**   Yes___ No___

l. **AFFECTIVE RESPONSE:**
   Fear____ Depression____ Anger____ Guilt____ Euphoria____ Apathy____ Other_____

m. **PATIENT'S SUBJECTIVE EXPLANATION:**   Yes___ No___
_____

n. **PHARMACOLOGICAL ISSUES:**   Yes___ No___
   Medication_____
   Drugs_____
   Alcohol_____

HISTORY OF PRESENT ILLNESS

A. Age of onset:_____   Date of onset:_____

B. Prodroma: _____
_____

C. Course of Illness:
    1. Direction of Change in Syndrome
        Static_____Progressive_____Resolving_____
    2. Variations in Clinical Course:
        Periods of Exacerbation (dates and descriptions):_____
_____
        Periods of Remission (dates and descriptions):_____
_____
        Cyclic_____Episodic_____
        Precipitating Factors:_____
_____

    3. Velocity: Rapid   Slow____

D. Ameliorating Factors:_____
_____

E. Exacerbating Factors: _____
_____

F. Treatments and Consultations: _____
_____
    1. Current:_____
_____
    2. Past:_____
_____

G. Current Medications: _____
_____

MEDICAL HISTORY

A. Have you ever been hospitalized?   YES____ no____ DK____
B. Have you ever received medical treatment for any of
   the following conditions?
   1. Heart disease   YES____ no____ DK____
     a. Poor circulation   YES____ no____ DK____
     b. High blood pressure   YES____ no____ DK____
     c. Low blood pressure   YES____ no____ DK____
     d. Anemia or other blood disease   YES____ no____ DK____
   2. Lung disease   YES____ no____ DK____
   3. Liver disease   YES____ no____ DK____
   4. Intestinal disorders (chronic or severe)   YES____ no____ DK____
   5. Thyroid, adrenal, or other hormonal disorders   YES____ no____ DK____
     a. Diabetes   YES____ no____ DK____
   6. Kidney disease   YES____ no____ DK____
   7. Deformities   YES____ no____ DK____
   8. Infectious illness (severe, chronic or recurrent):   YES____ no____ DK____
     a. Meningitis   YES____ no____ DK____
     b. Encephalitis   YES____ no____ DK____
     c. High fevers   YES____ no____ DK____
     d. High fevers in infancy   YES____ no____ DK____
     e. Cold sores   YES____ no____ DK____
     f. Venereal disease   YES____ no____ DK____
     g. Ear infections   YES____ no____ DK____
   9. Neurological disorders   YES____ no____ DK____
     a. Seizures   YES____ no____ DK____
     b. Head injury with loss of consciousness or
       significant aftereffects   YES____ no____ DK____
  10. Allergic reactions   YES____ no____ DK____
     a. Poisoning or overdose   YES____ no____ DK____
     b. Drug or alcohol problems   YES____ no____ DK____
     c. Vitamin deficiency   YES____ no____ DK____
  11. Psychiatric Illness   YES____ no____ DK____
     a. Medications for nerves/sleep   YES____ no____ DK____
     b. Treatment by psychological, psychiatric or
       mental health professional   YES____ no____ DK____
     c. Hospitalized for psychiatric illness   YES____ no____ DK____

Treated for_____   Dates of Treatment_____
By: Dr._____   _____

Release of information form signed and obtained   Yes___ No___

Treated for_____   Dates of Treatment_____
By: Dr._____   _____

Release of information form signed and obtained   Yes___ No___

Treated for_____   Dates of Treatment_____
By: Dr._____   _____

Release of information form signed and obtained   Yes___ No___

Hospitalized at_____Hospitalized for_____
Address or City_____

Hospitalized at_____Hospitalized for_____
Address or City_____

Hospitalized at_____Hospitalized for_____
Address or City_____

DEVELOPMENTAL HISTORY

RECORDS

Check the information sources which were used:

<u>Reliability Rating:</u>   1 = Reliable   2 = Questionable

Patient   _____

Relatives(s)   _____
Mother   _____
Father   _____
Sibs   _____
Spouse   _____
Children   _____

Other   _____

Baby books   _____
Old Photos   _____
Home movies   _____

Attorney   _____
Obstetrician   _____
Gynecologist   _____
Pediatrician   _____
Psychiatrist   _____
Hospital Records   _____
Neuropsychologist   _____
Psychologist   _____
Audiologist   _____
Speech Pathologist   _____
Teacher   _____
School Transcripts   _____
  Other _____

PRE-, PERI-, AND POST-NATAL EPOCHS

I. PREGNANCY

A. Maternal Health And General Condition

1. Mother's age at time of patient's birth?		age_____	
2. First pregnancy?	no	dk	YES
3. a. Prior difficulty becoming pregnant?	no	dk	YES
b. Prior miscarriage?	no	dk	YES
c. Prior abortions?	no	dk	YES
d. Prior stillbirths?	no	dk	YES
4. Incompatible blood types (Rh negative)?	no	dk	YES
5. Regularly seen by doctor during first four months of this pregnancy?	no	dk	YES
6. Significant emotional stress during pregnancy?	no	dk	YES
a. Cause of stress:		_____	
b. Reactions and duration:		_____	
c. Mother pleased with pregnancy?	no	dk	YES
d. Family pleased?	no	dk	YES
7. Deprived of adequate nutrition?	no	dk	YES

B. Illnesses

8. Illnesses during the pregnancy with the patient?	no	dk	YES
a. Diabetes	no	dk	YES
b. Hypertension	no	dk	YES
c. German measles	no	dk	YES
d. Flu	no	dk	YES
e. Other	no	dk	YES

C. Surgery

9. Surgery during this pregnancy?	no	dk	YES
a. Describe:		_____	
b. General anesthetic?		_____	

D. Medications

10. Prescribed medications?	no	dk	YES
a. List		_____	
b. Medications were taken?	no	dk	YES
c. Regularly?	no	dk	YES

E. Toxins

11. Smoked more than two packs?	no	dk	YES
12. a. Drank alcohol?	no	dk	YES
b. What?		_____	
c. How much?		_____	
13. a. Unprescribed drug use?	no	dk	YES
b. List:		_____	
14. Exposed to X-rays/other radiation?	no	dk	YES
15. Area of body X-rayed? Head__ Foot__ Back__ Chest__			
Other	no	dk	YES

16. a. Exposed to organic pesticides (DDT, DDE, or Dioxin)?   no   dk   YES
    b. Exposed to mercury?*
    *(Work with fungicides, batteries, thermometers; dental
    hygienists, photographers, wood preservatives.)   no   dk   YES
    c. Exposed to lead?*
    *(Work in ceramics, enamel, rubber and glass manufacture.
    Painters, plumbers, solderers, and battery manufacturers.
    Workers working with gasoline additives and smelter workers)   no   dk   YES

17. a. Toxemia during pregnancy?

    b. Toxemic convulsions?   swollen ankles____
    c. Toxemic coma?   high blood pressure____
                           excessive vomiting____
                                no   dk   YES
                                no   dk   YES

II. BIRTH INFORMATION
A. Date And Place Of Birth
1. Patient's date of birth?   _____
2. a. Hospital?   _____
    b. Attending physician?   _____
3. Adopted?   no   DK   YES
4. Biological mother and father married at time of conception?   NO   DK   yes

B. Labor
1. a. Length of labor?   Hours_____
    b. Induced labor?   no   dk   YES
    c. Reason: Complication of pregnancy_____
         List:_____
         Convenience_____

C. Delivery
1. Membranes ruptured prior to delivery?   no   dk   YES
2. Gestational age?   _____
    a. Prematurity (less than 9 months)?   no   dk   YES
    b. Postmaturity (more than 10 months)?   no   dk   YES
3. Birth weight?   lbs. _____ oz.___
    a. Weighed less than 5 pounds?   no   dk   YES
    b. Birth weight as compared to mother's other children?   _____
4. In what position was baby born?   Specify_____
    a. Born head first?   no   dk   YES
5. a. Caesarean section performed?   no   dk   YES
    b. Reason   _____
6. a. Multiple birth (twins)?   no   dk   YES
    b. How many babies?   _____
    c. How many babies survived?   _____
    d. Birth order of patient (first, second, etc.)   _____
7. Forceps?   no   dk   YES
8. General anesthetic?   no   dk   YES
9. a. Cord knotted at birth?   no   dk   YES
    b. Cord wrapped around baby's neck at birth?   no   dk   YES
10. Cyanosis (born blue)?   no   dk   YES
11. a. Required incubator?   no   dk   YES
    b. How long?   _____

III. NEONATAL EPOCH
A. Activity And Responsiveness

1. Weak cry?	no	dk	YES
2. Slept more than other babies?	no	dk	YES
3. Less active than other babies?	no	dk	YES
4. More irritable than other babies?	no	dk	YES
5. Enjoyed being touched/comforted less than other babies?	no	dk	YES
6. Less cuddly than other babies?	no	dk	YES
7. Less responsive than other babies?	no	dk	YES
8. Reactivity to being held?			
a. Patient molded to mother's body when being held?	no	dk	YES
b. Felt limp?	no	dk	YES
c. Cried more when held than when left alone?	no	dk	YES

B. Feeding

1. Feeding disturbances?	List_____		
a. Colic?	no	dk	YES
b. Difficulty sucking?	no	dk	YES
c. Tongue thrust?	no	dk	YES
d. "Weak feeder" showed little interest in feeding, sucked weakly?	no	dk	YES
e. 1.) Excessive vomiting?	no	dk	YES
2.) Ate food which was just vomited?	no	dk	YES
2. Weight loss?	no	dk	YES
a. Amount lost?	_____		

C. Illnesses

1. a. Infectious illnesses?	no	dk	YES
b. List	_____		
Medications taken?	no	dk	YES
	_____		
2. a. Other Illnesses?	no	dk	YES
b. List	_____		
Medications taken?	no	dk	YES
	_____		
3. Difficulty breathing?	no	dk	YES
4. Jaundice?	no	dk	YES
Transfusions required?	How many?____		
Phototherapy required?	How long?_____		

D. Hospitalizations

1. a. Returned to hospital overnight?	no	dk	YES
b. Reason	_____		
c. Length of absence from mother/primary care person?	dk Days__ Weeks__ Months__		

E. Surgery
1. Required surgery?   Reason/Procedures_____

I. SOMATIC DEVELOPMENT

A. Physical Development

Neonate - 5 yrs.

Height

1. Small for age (one month to three years)?   no   dk   YES
2. Height 30"/weight 30 lbs. by age 3?   no   dk   YES
3. Height 40"/weight 40 lbs. by age 4?   no   dk   YES

Deformities

4. a. Physical deformities?   no   dk   YES
   b. Describe deformity   _____
   c. Age deformity appeared?   _____

Weight

5. a. Unusual or excessive weight gains/losses   no   dk   YES
      (lasting more than 3-4 months)?
   b. How much weight was gained/lost?   Gains___Losses___ lbs___.

6 - 13 yrs.

Height and Growth

1. Height (compared with other children of same age)? short___average___tall___
2. Excessive/unusual growth spurts
   (compared with other children)?   no   dk   YES   Age___
3. Periods during which patient failed to grow as fast as
   other children?   no   dk   YES
4. a. Physical deformities present?   no   dk   YES
   b. Describe abnormality (club foot, cleft palate, etc.)   _____
   c. Age deformity appeared (include disfiguring injuries,
      paralysis, etc.)   _____

Weight

5. a. Periods of excessive weight gain/loss   no   dk   YES
      (weight gain/loss lasting more than 3-4 months)?
   b. Amount of weight gain/loss-----lbs.
   c. Duration of gain/loss   _____
   d. Pattern recurred before age 13?   no   dk   YES
6. a. Worried excessively about becoming fat?   no   dk   YES
   b. complained of "feeling fat" when actually of average
      or below weight?   no   dk   YES
7. Binge eating (often ate very large amounts of food?   no   dk   YES

Sexual Development

8. Sexual development (pubescence) relative
   to peers: a. earlier___ b. average___ c. later___
9. **Female:** Signs of sexual maturity (puberty) appeared at age?
   a. Menstruation   _____
   b. Breast development   _____
10. **Male:** Signs of sexual maturity (puberty) appeared at age?
    a. Voice change   _____
    b. Facial hair first noticeable   _____

B. Motoric
1. <u>Gross Motor</u>
   Neonate - 5 yrs
   a. Crawled by 9 months?   no   dk   YES age_____
   b. Cruised (hung on to objects going from object
      to object, e.g., chairs and other furniture) when
      learning to walk?   no   dk   YES age_____
   c. Sat up alone by 6 months of age?   no   dk   YES age_____
   d. Walked unsupported by one year?   no   dk   YES age_____
   e. Walked on toes after 1-1/2 years?   no   dk   YES age stopped___
   f. Drooled after 2-1/2 years: no   dk   YES age stopped___
   g. Clumsy or poorly
      coordinated?   no   dk   YES   age began___   age stopped_____
   h. 1. Original hand preference?   NEITHER   dk   R   L
      2. Age preference appeared?   dk   age_____
      3. Trained to use right hand?   dk   age_____
   6 - 13 yrs.
   a. Coordination: Clumsy/poorly coordinated_____
                                                             Average_____
                                                   Well coordinated_____

   b. Enjoyed or excelled at sports?   no   dk   YES
      1. Favorite sports?   Team_____
                                                       Individual_____

                                                             Ball_____
                                                       Swimming_____
                                                          Track_____

      2. Sports liked least?   Team_____
                                                       Individual_____

                                                             Ball_____
                                                       Swimming_____
                                                          Track_____
   c. Learned to ride bicycle?   Never___
                                                   With difficulty___
                                                Without difficulty___
                                                     Age learned?_____
   d. Picked for teams?   Last__ Middle___ First___
   e. Difficulty in playing games which involved
      following commands?
      (Simon Says, Mother May I, etc.)   no   dk   YES

2. **Fine Motor**
   Neonate - 5 yrs.
   a. Problems cutting paper, tying shoes, using buttons,
      stringing beads (fine motor coordination)   no   dk   YES
   6 - 13 yrs.
   b. good with hands, sewing, crafts, making models, playing
      marbles, pitching pennies   NO   dk   yes

3. **Graphomotor**
   Neonate - 5 yrs.
   a. Trouble with writing?   no   dk   YES age____
   b. Trouble with drawing?   no   dk   YES age____
   6-13 yrs.
   a. Trouble with writing?   no   dk   YES age____
   b. Trouble with drawing?   no   dk   YES age____

4. **Movement Abnormalities**
   Neonate - 5 yrs.
   6-13 yrs.
   a. 1. Abnormalities of movement or muscle development   no   dk
         Paralysis   YES age____ frequency____   duration____
                                                                  RUE RLE LUE LLE
         Limpness   YES age____ frequency____   duration____
         Undeveloped muscles YES age____ frequency____   duration____
         Difficulty walking YES age____ frequency____   duration____
         Stiffness of muscles YES age____ frequency____   duration____
         Shaking/trembling   YES age____ frequency____   duration____
         Awkward, twisting/
          writhing movements YES age____ frequency____   duration____
         Odd/peculiar hand or
         finger movements   YES age____ frequency____   duration____
      2. Marked slowing of bodily
         activity (when not
         physically ill)   YES age____ frequency____   duration____
      3. Involuntary jerky
         movements (tics)   YES age____ frequency____   duration____
      4. Presence of purposeless movements:
         Rocking   YES age____ frequency____   duration____
         Headbang   YES age____ frequency____   duration____
         Handflap   YES age____ frequency____   duration____
         Other _____   YES age____ frequency____   duration____

C. Sensory
   1. Vision
   Neonate - 5 yrs.
   6 - 13 yrs.
       a. Problems with eyes or vision other than requiring eyeglasses
            (eyes turning in, strabismus, lazy eyes, etc.)?   no   dk   YES age____-____
                                                                               L_____ R_____

                                                                 Describe_____

       b. Saw things that other people did not
           (illusions, hallucinations, visions)?   no   dk   YES age____
                                                                               L_____ R_____

       c. Describe patient's sensitivity to light: Underresponsive____
                                                                 Average ____
                                                                 Overresponsive____
       d. Wore eyeglasses?   no   dk   YES   age____
   2. Auditory
   Neonate - 5 yrs.
   6 - 13 yrs.
       a. Hearing problems?   no   dk   YES   age____
                                                                 Describe_____
       b. Wore a hearing aid?   no   dk   YES   age____
       c. Hearing tested?   no   dk   YES   age____
       d. Recurrent ear infections?   no   dk   YES   age_____
                                                                               L___ R___
       e. Complained of distortions of sounds?   no   dk   YES   age____
                                                                               L___ R___
       f. Heard things others did not (voices, strange
           sounds, hallucinations)?   no   dk   YES   age____
                                                                               L___ R___
       g. Describe sensitivity to sound as: Underresponsive____
                                                                 Average____
                                                                 Overresponsive_____

 3. Olfactory
   Neonate - 5 yrs.
   6 - 13 yrs.
       a. Unable to smell (not due to congestion)?   no   dk   YES   age____-____
       b. Unusually sensitive to smells?   no   dk   YES   age____-____
       c. Smelled things that others did not (hallucinations)? no   dk   YES   age____-____
                                                                               Pleasant ____
                                                                            Unpleasant ____
                                                                      Emanating from self ____
                                                                    Emanating from envir. ____
 4. Gustatory
   Neonate - 5 yrs.
   6 - 13 yrs.
       a. Unable to taste (not due to congestion)?   no   dk   YES   age____-____
       b. Unusually sensitive to food tastes?   no   dk   YES   age____-____
       c. Tasted things that others did not (hallucinations)? no   dk   YES   age____-____

5. **Tactile**

    Neonate - 5 yrs.

    a. Baby felt stiff when held rather than cuddly?   no   dk   YES

    b. Disliked being touched (infancy and childhood)?   no   dk   YES

    c. Unusually sensitive skin (infancy and childhood)?   no   dk   YES

    6-13 yrs.

    a. Disliked being touched?   no   dk   YES

    b. Unusually sensitive skin?   no   dk   YES

    c. Described unusual feelings on skin (numbness,

      tingling, or other unusual sensations)?   no   dk   YES

                         Describe_____

                         L FACE___ L TORSO___LUE___ LLE___

                         R FACE___ R TORSO___ RUE___ RLE___

    d. Sensitivity to pain: Underresponsive___

                         Average___

                         Overresponsive___

                         Describe_____

D. **Vegetative**
   1. **Sleep and Arousal**
     Neonate - 5 yrs.

a. Persistent sleep problems?	no	dk	YES	age__-__
	Describe_____			
b. Difficulty in falling asleep?	no	dk	YES	age__-__
c. Sleepwalking?	no	dk	YES	age__-__
d. Toothgrinding?	no	dk	YES	age__-__
e. Frequent bad dreams?	no	dk	YES	age__-__
f. Night terrors (woke up screaming without recall of dream)?	no	dk	YES	age__-__
g. Restless sleeper (moved around a great deal during sleep)?	no	dk	YES	age__-__
h. Went to bed earlier and rose earlier than other family members (after age 4)?	no	dk	YES	age__-__

     6-13 yrs.

a. Persistent sleep problems?	no	dk	YES	age__-__
	Describe_____			
b. Difficulty in falling asleep?	no	dk	YES	age__-__
c. Easily tired or fatigued?	no	dk	YES	age__-__
d. Went to bed earlier and rose earlier than other family members (after age 6)?				
e.. Toothgrinding?	no	dk	YES	age__-__
f. Frequent bad dreams?	no	dk	YES	age__-__
g. Sleepwalking	no	dk	YES	age__-__
h. Night terrors (woke up screaming without recall of dream)?	no	dk	YES	age__-__
i. Restless sleeper (moved around a great deal during sleep)?	no	dk	YES	age__-__
j. Wet bed after age 8?	no	dk	YES	age__-__
k. Lost bowel control while asleep after age 6 (not caused by physical illness)?	no	dk	YES	age__-__
l. Fainted frequently?	no	dk	YES	age__-__

   2. **Activity and Arousal**
     Neonate - 5 yrs.
     6 - 13 yrs.

a. Activity compared to peers?	Less Active__	As Active__	More Active__	
b. Wore out clothes more frequently?	no	dk	YES	age__-__
c. Marked difficulty sitting still/fidgety?	no	dk	YES	age__-__
d. Always on the go/driven like motor?	no	dk	YES	age__-__
e. Difficulty paying attention?	no	dk	YES	age__-__
f. Easily distracted?	no	dk	YES	age__-__
g. Ran and climbed constantly?	no	dk	YES	age__-__

     Episodic Phenomena

h. Lost track of conversations?	no	dk	YES	age__-__
i. Became unresponsive for periods?	no	dk	YES	age__-__
j. Daydreamed more than other children?	no	dk	YES	age__-__
k. Had seizures, fits, or convulsions?	no	dk	YES	age__-__
	Describe_____			

       1. Was there more than one?   no   dk   YES   age__-___

       2. If so, how frequently did the patient
          have seizures?   _____

       3. Until what age?   _____

3. Feeding

Neonate - 5 yrs. (Patient's first month of life.)

    a. Feeding problems during infancy?   no   dk   YES   age__-__

    b. Sensitivity to particular foods?   no   dk   YES   age__-__

    c. Tongue thrust?   no   dk   YES   age__-__

    d. Problem eater?   no   dk   YES   age__-__

    e. Frequent colic?   no   dk   YES   age__-__

    f. Frequent projectile vomiting?   no   dk   YES   age__-__

Neonate - 5 yrs. (First month through age 13.)

    g. Feeding problems?   no   dk   YES   age__-__

    h. Problem eater?   no   dk   YES   age__-__

    i. Sensitivity to particular foods?   no   dk   YES   age__-__

    j. Frequent projectile vomiting?   no   dk   YES   age__-__

    k. Food fads?   no   dk   YES   age__-__

    l. Pica (ate inedible objects)?   no   dk   YES   age__-__

    m. Binge eater?   no   dk   YES   age__-__

    n. Drank unusually large quantities of liquids?   no   dk   YES   age__-__

    o. Frequent stomachaches?   no   dk   YES   age__-__

      School mornings only?   no   dk   YES

4. Evacuative

Neonate - 5 yrs.

6 - 13 yrs.

<u>Bowel</u>

    a. Toilet trained by age 3 years?   no   dk   YES   age__-__

    b. 1. Bowel control problems after age 3?   no   dk   YES   age__-__

         2. Frequency?   _____

    c. Frequent diarrhea?   no   dk   YES   age__-__

    d. Frequent constipation?   no   dk   YES   age__-__

<u>Bladder</u>

e. 1. Bladder control problems after age 3?   no   dk   YES   age__-__
   2. Frequency   _____

f. Urinated unusually frequently?   no   dk   YES   age__-__

g. Bladder control frequently lost (daytime after
   the age of 3 years)?   no   dk   YES   age__-__

h. Difficulty urinating?   no   dk   YES   age__-__

5. **Respiratory**
   Neonate to 5 yrs.
   6 - 13 yrs.
   a. Breath-holding spells?   no   dk   YES   age__
   b. Hyperventilation (forced overbreathing)? no   dk   YES   age__
   c. Irregular/difficult breathing?   no   dk   YES   age__
   d. Asthma?   no   dk   YES   age__
   e. Sleep apnea?   no   dk   YES   age__
   f. Other respiratory difficulties?   no   dk   YES   age__
                                               Describe_____

   g. Shortness of breath when frightened or nervous? no dk YES age__
   h. 1. Allergies?   no   dk   YES   age__
      2. Food?   no   dk   YES   age__
                                               Specify Allergen_____
                                               Describe Reaction____

      3. Medicines?   no   dk   YES   age__
                                               Specify Allergen_____
                                               Describe Reaction____

      4. Airborne matter (pollen, hay fever,
         dust, animals)?   no   dk   YES   age__
                                               Specify Allergen_____
                                               Describe Reaction____

6. **Cardiovascular**
   Neonate - 5 yrs.
   6 - 13 yrs.
   a. High blood pressure/hypertension?   no   dk   YES   age__-__

II. COGNITIVE DEVELOPMENT

A. General Intellectual Level

Neonate - 5 yrs.

1. Describe patient's intelligence in relation to other children?
   Retarded___Slow learner___Average___Above Average ___Superior very bright___
   Genius___

2. a. Retardation suspected?   no   dk   YES   age__
   b. Mental retardation diagnosed?   no   dk   YES   age__

6 - 13 yrs.

1. Describe patient's intelligence in relation to other children?
   Retarded___Slow learner___Average___Above Average ___Superior very bright___
   Genius___

2. a. Retardation suspected?   no   dk   YES   age__
   b. Mental retardation diagnosed?   no   dk   YES   age__

3. a. Learning disability suspected?   no   dk   YES   age__
   b. Mental retardation diagnosed?   no   dk   YES   age__

4. Favorite activities during childhood?   List_____

	Liked	Disliked
a. Drawing, painting or sculpting	_____	_____
b. Collecting (stamps, coins, dolls, etc.)	_____	_____
c. Model building	_____	_____
d. Dolls	_____	_____
e. Dress-up	_____	_____
f. Reading	_____	_____
g. Cooking, sewing	_____	_____
h. Playing musical instrument	_____	_____
i. Fishing, hunting	_____	_____
j. Board games	_____	_____
k. Sports	_____	_____
l. Dramatics	_____	_____
m. Dancing	_____	_____
n. Puzzles	_____	_____
o. Animals	_____	_____
p. Science	_____	_____
q. Mechanics	_____	_____
r. Other	Specify_____	

5. What did he/she excel at most?   _____

B. Language

    1. Expressive Language

        Neonate - 5 yrs.

a. Single words by age 1-1/2 years?	NO	dk	yes
b. Complete, three-word sentences by age three years?	NO	dk	yes
c. Difficulty understanding patient's speech more than that of other children (ages 3-5)?	no	dk	YES
d. Speech difficulties (stuttering or stammering)?	no	dk	YES

        6 - 13 yrs.

a. More difficulty understanding patient's speech than children of same age?	no	dk	YES
b. Baby talk persisted late?	no	dk	YES
c. Patient expressed ideas in speech in full sentences that followed in a logical order by age 5?	NO	dk	YES

          d. Speech problems present?

	Present	Age
1. Drooling	_____	_____
2. Confusion pronoun	_____	_____
3. Stuttering/stammering	_____	_____
4. Any other articulation disorder	_____	_____
5. Speech block (after third grade)	_____	_____
6. Lisping	_____	_____
7. Difficulty saying "l" or "r"	_____	_____

e. Repeated meaningless things frequently?	no	dk	YES	age__
f. Difficulty finding words to express him/herself?	no	dk	YES	age__
g. "Lost voice" or became unable to speak (for several weeks)?	no	dk	YES	age__
h. Refused to speak to anyone (prolonged periods of over several weeks)?	no	dk	YES	age__

    2. Receptive Language

        Neonate - 5 yrs.

a. Difficulty understanding what was said?	no	dk	YES	age__

        6-13 yrs.

a. Difficulty understanding what was said?	no	dk	YES	age__
b. Difficulty following directions?	no	dk	YES	age__

C. Visuospatial
6 - 13 yrs.
<u>Difficulty</u>

1. Finding way to new places	no	dk	YES
2. Telling time	no	dk	YES
3. Tying shoes	no	dk	YES
4. Reading music	no	dk	YES
5. Puzzles	no	dk	YES
6. Reading maps	no	dk	YES
7. Using written instructions	no	dk	YES
8. Talked out loud when doing any of the above tasks?	no	dk	YES

D. Memory
6 - 13 yrs.

1. Forgetful?	no	dk	YES	age__
2. Difficulty memorizing information for school (poems, pledge of allegiance, words of songs, times tables, etc.)?	no	dk	YES	age__
3. Relied on notes to remember to do things?	no	dk	YES	age__
4. Needed a tape recorder to "take notes" in class?	no	dk	YES	age__
5. Difficulty learning or following rules of games?	no	dk	YES	age__

E. Judgement
6 - 13 yrs.

1. Got into trouble often?	no	dk	YES	age__
2. Accident prone?	no	dk	YES	age__
3. Acted impulsively often?	no	dk	YES	age__
4. Unable to work alone independently?	no	dk	YES	age__
5. Failed to finish projects?	no	dk	YES	age__
6. Did not seem to listen to what others said?	no	dk	YES	age__
7. Failed to respond to disciplinary actions of parents?	no	dk	YES	age__
8. Blamed others frequently?	no	dk	YES	age__

F. School

6 - 13 yrs.

1. Elected offices in school? no dk YES
   List_____

2. Prizes won/school honors? no dk YES
   List_____

3. Skipped grades? no dk YES
   Specify 1 2 3 4 5 6 7 8 9 10 11 12

4. Failed or repeated grades? no dk YES
   Specify 1 2 3 4 5 6 7 8 9 10 11 12

5. Ungraded or special classes? no dk YES
   Specify English/Reading __
   Spelling __
   Math __
   Science __
   Social Studies __
   Art/Shop __
   Gym __

6. Special education/tutoring help provided? no dk YES
   Specify English/Reading __
   Spelling __
   Math __
   Science __
   Social Studies __
   Art/Shop __
   Gym __

7. Truancy
   (not going to school and going to places other
   than home during school hours)? no dk YES age__

8. Wanted to stay out of school to remain at home
   with parent(s) (periods of more than several weeks)? no dk YES age__

9. Physical complaints on school days only
   (e.g., headache, stomachache, nausea) (periods of more
   than several weeks)? no dk YES age__

10.a. Teachers complained about child's behavior
    in class (more than one teacher)? no dk YES age__

   b. Complaints regarding any of the following:
      1. Failed to complete homework no dk YES age__
      2. Wouldn't listen no dk YES age__ /
      3. Talked or called out in class no dk YES age__
      4. Would not respond to discipline no dk YES age__
      5. Fought in class no dk YES age__
      6. Failed subjects no dk YES age__

11. Student average:_____   Poor___   Average___   Good___
12. a. Did about equally well in all subjects   NO   dk   yes
    b. Favorite subjects   A'S-B'S   B'S-C'S   C'S-D'S   F'S
       1. English/Reading   _____   _____   _____   _____
       2. Spelling   _____   _____   _____   _____
       3. Math   _____   _____   _____   _____
       4. Science   _____   _____   _____   _____
       5. Social Studies   _____   _____   _____   _____
       6. Art/Shop   _____   _____   _____   _____
       7. Gym   _____   _____   _____   _____
    c. Worst subjects
       1. English/Reading   _____   _____   _____   _____
       2. Spelling   _____   _____   _____   _____
       3. Math   _____   _____   _____   _____
       4. Science   _____   _____   _____   _____
       5. Social Studies   _____   _____   _____   _____
       6. Art/Shop   _____   _____   _____   _____
       7. Gym   _____   _____   _____   _____
13. Slow learner at everything?   no   dk   YES   Began at age___   Ended___
14. Learning difficulties?
    a. English/Reading   no   dk   YES   Began at age___   Ended___
    b. Spelling   no   dk   YES   Began at age___   Ended___
    c. Math   no   dk   YES   Began at age___   Ended___
    d. Science   no   dk   YES   Began at age___   Ended___
    e. Social Studies   no   dk   YES   Began at age___   Ended___
    f. Art/Shop   no   dk   YES   Began at age___   Ended___
    g. Gym   no   dk   YES   Began at age___   Ended___
15. Behavior problems?   no   dk   YES   Began at Age___   Ended___
    a. Fighting?   no   dk   YES   Began at Age___   Ended___
    b. Clowning?   no   dk   YES   Began at Age___   Ended___
    c. Getting into trouble?   no   dk   YES   Began at Age___   Ended___
    d. Calling out in class
       out of turn?   no   dk   YES   Began at Age___   Ended___
16 Suspended from school?   no   dk   YES   Began at age___   Ended___

G. Unusual Thoughts

Neonate - 5 yrs.

6 - 13 yrs.

1. Strange or unusual thoughts?   no dk YES

                                 Religious   _____

                                 Supernatural Beings   _____

                                 Monsters   _____

                                 Machines   _____

                                 Computer Controlled   _____

                                 Preoccupied with Death   _____

                                 Felt People Were Out to Get Him/Her _____

                                 Other   _____

2. Others besides patient's parents expressed concern
over patient's strange or unusual thoughts?   no   dk   YES   age__-__

3. Strange or unusual behaviors?   no   dk   YES   age__-__

                                              Describe_____

4. Unpleasant/disturbing thoughts that
he/she could not stop thinking about
(for a period of at least several months, or which
recurred often)?   no   dk   YES   age__-__

5. Performed acts over and over again (washing hands
many times a day, checking light switched, etc.)
lasting several months   no   dk   YES   age__-__

III. INTERPERSONAL
A. General
Neonate - 5 yrs.

6 - 13 yrs.

1. Maturity of actions relative to peers: More Mature__ As Mature__ Less Mature__
2. Patient wanted to be_____ when he/she grew up? Describe_____

   6-13 yrs.
3. Self-confidence:

   a. Confident and sure of him/herself?   **NO** dk yes

   b. Needing constant attention and reassurance?   no dk **YES**

   c. Easily embarrassed?   no dk **YES**

   d. Odd, different from other children same age?   no dk **YES**
4. Patient's heroes as a child?   _____

B. Parents
Neonate - 5 yrs.

6 - 13 yrs.

1. Favorite times/activities spent with father during childhood?   List_____
2. Favorite times/activities spent with mother during childhood?   List_____
3. Parent's nickname for patient?   Specify_____
4. Mother's absence (periods longer than 1 month)?

   Reason: no dk   **YES** age__-__

                                          a. Divorce   _____

                                          b. Separation   _____

                                          c. Physical illness   _____

                                          d. Psychiatric illness   _____

                                          e. Military Service   _____

                                          f. Other   _____
5. Father's absence (periods longer than 1 months)?   no dk   **YES** age__-__

   Reason: a. Divorce   _____

                                            b. Separation   _____

                                          c. Physical illness   _____

                                          d. Psychiatric illness   _____

                                          e. Military Service   _____

                                          f. Other   _____

Conflicts

6. a. Significant tensions or conflicts between either

       parent and patient?   no dk   **YES** Age__-__

   b. Focus of conflicts:

Neonate - 5 yrs.

    1. Toilet Training   no dk   **YES** age__-__

    2. Food/feeding   no dk   **YES** age__-__

    3. Behavior   no dk   **YES** age__-__

    4. Sleeping/bedtime/curfew   no dk   **YES** age__-__

6-13 yrs.

    5. School   no dk   **YES** age__-__

    6. Responsibilities around the home   no dk   **YES** age__-__

    7. Drugs   no dk   **YES** age__-__

    8. Smoking   no dk   **YES** age__-__

9. Bedtime/curfew/sleeping	no	dk	YES age__-__
10. Sex	no	dk	YES age__-__
11. Religion	no	dk	YES age__-__
12. Values or morals	no	dk	YES age__-__

7. Patient's reactions to tensions/conflicts:

a. Angrily	no	dk	YES age__-__
b. Overly obedient (always "giving in")	no	dk	YES age__-__
c. Staying cool and aloof	no	dk	YES age__-__
d. Disobedient, stubborn	no	dk	YES age__-__
e. Becoming suspicious	no	dk	YES age__-__
f. Crying	no	dk	YES age__-__
g. Blaming others	no	dk	YES age__-__
h. Manipulating other people, trying to get other people to do things for him/her	no	dk	YES age__-__
i. Argues	no	dk	YES age__-__
j. Withdraws	no	dk	YES age__-__
k. Does things that make parents angry	no	dk	YES age__-__
l. Often complained of feeling sick or being in pain	no	dk	YES age__-__
m. Difficult to control	no	dk	YES age__-__

8. Patient's reactions were very unpredictable? — no dk YES age__-__

9. Severe physical punishment by either or both parents? — no dk YES age__-__

10. a. Parents were worried that there was something wrong with, or different about, the child? — no dk YES age__-__

　　b. Parent's concerns:

1. Physical development	no	dk	YES age__
2. Physical health/illness	no	dk	YES age__
3. Mental illness	no	dk	YES age__
4. School academics	no	dk	YES age__
5. Social	no	dk	YES age__
6. Behavior/conduct	no	dk	YES age__

11. Very noticeable changes in the way patient acted/felt toward parents (for any periods of at least several months)? — no dk YES age__

　　a. Describe　　　　　_____

　　b. Until what age　　　_____

　　c. What caused the change　_____

　　d. Did patient return to usual self_____ — no dk YES age__

12. Clung to parent(s) and followed them around constantly? — no dk YES age__

13. Avoided sleeping away from home (going to camp staying overnight with friends, relatives)? — no dk YES age__

14. Refused to sleep alone/came into parent's bedroom at night? — no dk YES age__

15. Temper tantrums/became very upset when separated from parents? — no dk YES age__

16. Often expressed a desire to live away from home or with someone else? — no dk YES age__

C. **Siblings**
   Neonate - 5 yrs.
   6 - 13 yrs.
   1. How many siblings lived with patient
      (including biological, adopted, and foster siblings)?   _____
   2. How many of the children were older than the patient?   _____
   3. Siblings typical reaction to patient:
      a. Got along well, friendly with patient   no   dk   YES   age____
      b. Usually played happily together   no   dk   YES   age____
      c. Ignored patient   no   dk   YES   age____
      d. Blamed patient and used as scapegoat   no   dk   YES   age____
      e. Treated patient as favorite   no   dk   YES   age____
      f. "Babied" and protected patient   no   dk   YES   age____
      g. Patient "followed" older siblings   no   dk   YES   age____
      h. Intense competition and rivalry between
         siblings   no   dk   YES   age____
   4. a. Siblings left home while patient was under the
         age of 5 years (for periods of more than 3 months)?   no   dk   YES   age____
      b. Patient visibly upset or depressed by separation?   no   dk   YES   age____
   5. Very noticeable changes in the way patient
      acted/felt toward siblings (for any periods of at
      least several months)?   no   dk   YES   age____
                              a. Describe   _____
                              b. What caused the change?   _____
                              c. Did patient return to usual   no   dk   YES   age____

D. Peers

Neonate - 5 yrs.

1. Age patient began to actively play with other children? _____

2. Friends before 5 years of age?   no   dk   YES   age__-___

3. Attended nursery school, camp, or any type of
organized pre-school activity   no   dk   YES   age__-___
   a. Enjoyed?   no   dk   YES   age__-___
   b. Successful at tasks?   no   dk   YES   age__-___
   c. Made friends?   no   dk   YES   age__-___

Neonate - 5 yrs.

6 - 13 yrs.

4. Patient's interest in other children:
   a. Interested in other children?   no   dk   YES   age__-___
   b. Approached other children to engage them
      in play?   no   dk   YES   age__-___
   c. Sough after as a playmate by other children?   no   dk   YES   age__-___
   d. A loner or withdrawn?   no   dk   YES   age__-___
   e. Fearful of meeting new children?   no   dk   YES   age__-___
   f. Shy with other children?   no   dk   YES   age__-___
   g. A bully?   no   dk   YES   age__-___
   h. A leader?   no   dk   YES   age__-___
   i. A follower?   no   dk   YES   age__-___
   j. Suspicious of other children?   no   dk   YES   age__-___
   k. Manipulative with other children?   no   dk   YES   age__-___
   l. Teased or picked on by other children?   no   dk   YES   age__-___
   m. Fought frequently with other children?   no   dk   YES   age__-___
                                                                     Describe_____

5. age of children patient usually played with: dk__ Younger___ Same___ Older___

6. Had imaginary or make-believe friends?   no   dk   YES   age__-___

7. Very noticeable changes in the way patient acted/
felt toward other children (for any periods of at least
several months)?   no   dk   YES
   a. age of patient at the time?   _____
   b. Describe changes   _____
   c. Until what age?   _____
   d. What caused change?   _____
   e. Did patient return to usual self?   no   dk   YES

6 - 13 yrs.

8. Typically went out of way to help friends or do
favors for them?   NO   dk   yes   age__-___

9. a. Typically was sought after by other children
      to play at team sports?   no   dk   YES   age__-___
   b. First to be chosen for teams?   LAST__ Middle__ First__

10. Was patient more interested in friends than in family
by age 10?   no   dk   YES   age__

11. Had a "best friend" between the ages of 8 to 11
years old?   no   dk   YES   age__
                                                                                       Same sex___
                                                                                       Opposite sex___

12. Member of a clique or gang during childhood?   no   dk   YES   age__

13. Member of clubs during childhood?   NO   dk   yes   age__
                                                                     List _____

E. Significant Others, Pets And Inanimate Objects
   Neonate - 5 yrs.
   6 - 13 yrs.
  1. Adults, other than patient's parents, with whom
     he/she was especially close during first five years?   no   dk   YES age___-___

     a. Uncle   ____
        Aunt   ____
        Grandparent   ____
        Nurse   ____
        Housekeeper   ____
        Boarder   ____
        Other   _____
     b. Person died, moved away or lost contact during
        first five years?   no   dk   YES age___-___
  2. Very frightened by the presence of new people or
     strangers (crying after age 2)?   no   dk   YES age___-___
  3. Stuffed animal, toy or blanket or other object
     which was always held?   no   dk   YES age___-___
  4. Pets during the first five years of life?   no   dk   YES age___-___
     a. Took care of pet?   no   dk   YES age___-___
     b. Played with pet?   no   dk   YES age___-___
     c. Injured pet seriously?   no   dk   YES age___-___

F. Community
   6 - 13 yrs. (only)
  1. Belonged to any organizations/clubs outside of
     school?   no   dk   YES age___-___
  2. Patient repeatedly became involved in delinquent
     acts?   no   dk   YES age___-___
     a. Vandalized property   no   dk   YES age___-___
     b. Lied repeatedly   no   dk   YES age___-___
     c. Stole outside of the home   no   dk   YES age___-___
     d. Ran away from home overnight   no   dk   YES age___-___
     e. Frequently broke rules at home (curfew, bedtime,
        smoking, taking things without permission)   no   dk   YES age___-___
  3. Patient felt guilty after doing wrong?   no   dk   YES age___-___
  4. Intentionally did serious physical harm to someone?   no dk YES
     a.Ages ____,____,____,____
  5. Threatened suicide?   no   dk   YES age___-___
  6. Attempted suicide?   no   dk   YES age___-___
  7. What did patient use to attempt to do this
     (pills, razor blade, etc.)   no   dk   YES age___-___
  8. Substance use (between the ages of 6-13)?   no   dk   YES age___-___
     a. Tobacco   no   dk   YES age___-___
     b. Alcohol   no   dk   YES age___-___
     c. Marijuana, hashish, pot   no   dk   YES age___-___
     d. Barbiturates, "downers," quaaludes, "reds," etc.   no   dk   YES age___-___
     e. "Speed," amphetamine, dexadrine, etc.   no   dk   YES age___-___
     f. Hallucinogens, LSD, PCP, mescaline   no   dk   YES age___-___
     g. Opiates, heroin, methodone, opium   no   dk   YES age___-___
     h. Cocaine   no   dk   YES age___-___
     i. Other   _____

IV. PSYCHOSEXUAL

Neonate - 5 yrs.

A. Persistent thumb sucker after age 3 years?	no	dk	YES	age__-___
B. Fecal incontinence after age 3?	no	dk	YES	age__-___
C. Smeared feces?	no	dk	YES	age__-___

Neonate - 5 yrs.
6 - 13 yrs.

D. Unusually shy about undressing in front of others?	no	dk	YES	age__-___
E. Unusual pleasure undressing in front of others?	no	dk	YES	age__-___
F. Masturbated more openly or more often than other children?	no	dk	YES	age__-___
G. Gender confusion:	no	dk	YES	age__-___
1. Enjoyed dressing up in clothes of opposite sex?	no	dk	YES	age__-___
2. Preferred playing games usually preferred by children of opposite sex?	no	dk	YES	age__-___
3. Expressed desire to be of opposite sex?	no	dk	YES	age__-___

6 - 13 yrs.

H. Liked by member of the opposite sex?	NO	dk	yes	age__-___
I. Age began dating or going to parties with boys and girls present?				_____
J. Ever had a "crush"?	NO	dk	yes	age__-___
K. First boyfriend/girlfriend of opposite sex?	NO	dk	yes	age__-___
L. Source of first information about sex, reproduction, "facts of life"?				

Friends	_____
Parents	_____
School classes (health, etc.)	_____
Sex partner	_____
Other	_____

Neonate - 5 yrs.
6 - 13 yrs.

M. Voluntary sexual experiences (6-13)?				
N. Sexually abused, assaulted, or molested against will?	no	dk	YES	age__-___
O. Often attempted to secretly watch people while they were undressed?	no	dk	YES	age__-___
P. Gestures, mannerisms, and interests more like those of children of opposite sex?	no	dk	YES	age__-___
Q. Concerned about homosexuality	no	dk	YES	age__-___

V. AFFECTIVE

Neonate - 5 yrs.

6 - 13 yrs.

A. What brought patient the greatest happiness?   N-5_____

        6-13_____

B. Most stressful event?   N-5_____

        6-13_____

C. Noticeable emotional changes (periods of at

    least several months)?   no   dk   YES age__-__

    1. Sadder, more depressed   no   dk   YES age__-__

    2. More fearful, anxious   no   dk   YES age__-__

    3. More angry than usual   no   dk   YES age__-__

    4. More moody and irritable   no   dk   YES age__-__

    5. More easygoing, happy   no   dk   YES age__-__

6 - 13 yrs.

D. Patient's emotions best described as:

    1. Easygoing   no   dk   YES age__-__

    2. Exceptionally unemotional, hard to tell

        how patient felt toward people   no   dk   YES age__-__

    3. Very unpredictable, would change rapidly   no   dk   YES age__-__

    4. Feelings seemed to be very strong   no   dk   YES age__-__

    5. Good sport when things did not go his/her way?   no   dk   YES age__-__

Fear

Neonate - 5 yrs.

6 - 13 yrs.

E. More fearful or frightened than other children?   no dk YES

    Avoidance Y ___ N ____

    Object of Fear _____

    age ___-___

F. Worried often about being hurt, killed or kidnapped?   no   dk   YES

    avoidance Y ___ N ____

    irrational Y ___ N ____

    age ___-___

G. Persistent nightmares that parents or child might

    have been hurt, killed or taken away?   no   dk   YES avoidance irrational___

    age ___-___

6 - 13 yrs.

H. Specific fears:

    1. Being alone   no dk YES avoidance ___ irrational ___ ages ___

    2. Public places   no dk YES avoidance ___ irrational ___ ages ___

    3. Crowds   no dk YES avoidance ___ irrational ___ ages ___

    4. Animals   no dk YES avoidance ___ irrational ___ ages ___

    5. Germs   no dk YES avoidance ___ irrational ___ ages ___

    6. Death   no dk YES avoidance ___ irrational ___ ages ___

    Describe _____

I. Usually tense and unable to "unwind" or relax?   no dk YES age ___-___

J. "Worrier" (worried about things that might happen

    or could go wrong)?   no dk YES age ___-___

K. Worried a great deal about what other people

    thought of him/her?   no dk YES age ___-___

L. Avoided new people?   no dk YES age ___-___

<u>Rage</u>
  Neonate - 5 yrs.
  6 - 13 yrs.
  M. Easily angered?   no   dk   YES age ___-___
  N. Frequent tantrums/outbursts (after age 4)?   no   dk   YES age ___-___
  6 - 13 yrs.
  O. Threw things?   no   dk   YES age ___-___
  P. Fights?   no   dk   YES age ___-___
  Q. Violence using weapon?   no   dk   YES age ___-___
<u>Depression</u>
  Neonate - 5 yrs.
  6 - 13 yrs.
  R. Sad, blue?   no   dk   YES age ___-___
  S. Withdrawn?   no   dk   YES age ___-___
  T. Cried often?   no   dk   YES age ___-___
  U. Complained frequently?   no   dk   YES age ___-___
  V. Hard to get interested in things?   no   dk   YES age ___-___
  6 - 13 yrs.
  W. Hopeless?   no   dk   YES age ___-___
  X. Guilty ruminations/self blame?   no   dk   YES age ___-___
  Y. Looked sad most of the time?   no   dk   YES age ___-___
<u>**Mood Swings and Elation**</u>
  Neonate - 5 yrs.
  6 - 13 yrs.
  Z. Rapid changes in mood?   no   dk   YES age ___-___
     Unprecipitated changes in mood?   no   dk   YES age ___-___
     Periods of elation without discernible precipitant?   no   dk   YES age ___-___

SOCIAL HISTORY

PATIENT _____   DATE _____

I. FAMILY MEDICAL HISTORY

A. Physical Health

I. Does anyone in your family have the same problem
(as presenting problem)?   Yes _____ No _____

II. Has anyone in the family ever had or been treated for:

<u>Specify Relation</u>

1. Heart disease   _____
       a. Poor circulation   _____
       b. High blood pressure   _____
       c. Low blood pressure   _____
       d. Anemia or other blood disease   _____
2. Lung disease   _____
3. Liver disease   _____
4. Intestinal disorders (chronic or severe)   _____
5. Endocrine or hormone problems   _____
       a. Diabetes   _____
       b. Thyroid   _____
       c. Adrenal   _____
       d. Parathyroid   _____
       e. Pituitary   _____
6. Kidney disease   _____
7. Deformities   _____
8. Infectious illness (severe, chronic, or recurrent):   _____
       a. Meningitis   _____
       b. Encephalitis   _____
       c. High fevers   _____
       d. High fevers in infancy   _____
       e. Cold sores   _____
       f. Venereal disease   _____
       g. Ear infections   _____
9. Neurologic disorders   _____
10. Seizures   _____
11. Head injury with loss of consciousness
    or significant after effects   _____
        a. Loss of memory or intellect (dementia)   _____
        b. Movement disorders   _____
        c. Muscle disorders   _____
        d. Strokes   _____
        e. Other diseases of brain or nervous system   _____

12. Allergic reactions   _____
    a. Poisoning or overdose   _____
    b. Drug or alcohol problems   _____
    c. Vitamin deficiency   _____
13. Psychiatric illness   _____
    a. Medications for nerves/sleep
    b. Treatment by psychological, psychiatric or
       mental health professional   _____
    c. Hospitalized for psychiatric illness   _____

B. Family Neurological Illness

   I. Does anyone in your family have or have they ever had problems with:

<u>Specify Relation</u>

     1. Learning Disabilities
       a. Reading   _____
       b. Arithmetic   _____
       c. Writing   _____
       d. Fainting, blackouts or loss of consciousness   _____
       e. Seizures   _____
       f. Movement, balance, coordination
          problems   _____
       g. Headaches   _____
     2. Sensory Impairments
       a. Sight   _____
       b. Smell   _____
       c. Taste   _____
       d. Hearing   _____
       e. Touch   _____

C. Family Psychiatric Illness

     1. Psychiatric hospitalization   _____
     2. Psychiatric treatment   _____
     3. Mental retardation   _____
     4. Arrests
       a. Specify what for: _____
     5. Bad temper   _____
     6. Violence   _____
     7. Alcoholism   _____
     8. Drug use
       a. Which drugs?   _____
       b. How much use?   _____
     9. Use of prescription drugs for sleep, calming
       down, or pepping up   _____

II. PEER RELATIONS

1. Do you have friends?   Yes ___   No ___
2. Any close friends?   Yes ___   No ___
3. How long have you known your friends?   _____
4. What kinds of things do you do together?   _____
5. Make new friends easily?   Yes ___   No ___
6. Do things go wrong with people once you've
    made friends with them?   Yes ___   No ___
    a. What goes wrong?   _____

III. SEXUAL HISTORY

1. Are you sexually active?   Yes ___   No ___
    a. Have you ever been sexually active?   Yes ___   No ___
    b. Nature of first sexual experience   Age ___
                                                            Reactions _____
    c. Pleased about it?   Yes ___   No ___

    d. Childhood sexual experiencs?   Yes ___   No ___
                                                            Describe _____
2. Age at puberty   _____
    (FEMALES)
    a. Age first menstruation   _____
                                                            Reactions _____
    b. Age breast development   _____
    (MALES)
    a. Age facial hair   _____
    b. Age voice-breaking   _____
3. Were you ever concerned or worried about:
    a. Genitals   Age & Describe _____
    b. Masturbation   Yes ___   No ___
    c. Homosexuality   Yes ___   No ___
    d. Sexual enjoyment   Yes ___   No ___
4. Frightening or overwhelming sexual experiences?   Age & Describe _____

IV. WORK HISTORY
A. Career
1. Setbacks? _____
2. Changes? _____
3. Difficulties? _____
4. Forte? _____

B. Current Position
1. Nature of work? _____
2. Job title? _____
3. Actual duties? _____
4. Salary? _____
5. Starting date? _____
6. Promotions?   Yes ___ No ___
7. Demotions?   Yes ___ No ___

C. List All Previous Positions Chronologically On Separate Page(s), Including Notable Features, As Above.

V. MILITARY EXPERIENCE
1. Were you in the service?   Yes ___ No ___
(If "NO," skip this section)
   a. Branch of service? _____
   b. Nationality of service? _____
   c. Starting date? _____
   d. Discharge date? _____
     1. Nature of discharge? _____
   e. Highest rank? _____
   f. Demotions?   Yes ___ No ___
     1. Reason? _____
2. Actual duties? _____
3. Combat duty?   Yes ___ No ___
   a. Injuries?   Yes ___ No ___
   b. Describe _____
   c. Any lasting effects   Yes ___ No ___
4. Receiving any VA benefits?   Yes ___ No ___
   Describe _____
5. Where were you stationed? _____

VI. SCHOOL HISTORY

A. Did you attend junior high school?   Yes ___ NO ___
(If "NO," go to next section)
    1. School?   _____
    2. Dates attended?   _____
        a. Leave school for any period of time?   YES ___ no ___
            1. Why?   _____
            2. How long?   _____
    3. Major subject?   _____
    4. Best subject?   _____
    5. Worst subject?   _____
    6. Average?   _____
    7. Extracurricular activities?   _____
    8. Disciplinary actions?   _____
    9. Honors or awards?   _____
   10. Source of income in school?   _____
   11. Degree?   _____

B. High school education?   Yes ___ NO ___
(If "NO," go to next section)
    1. School?   _____
    2. Dates attended?   _____
        a. Leave school for any period of time?   Yes ___ no ___
            1. Why?   _____
            2. How long?   _____
    3. Major subject?   _____
    4. Best subject?   _____
    5. Worst subject?   _____
    6. Average?   _____
    7. Extracurricular activities?   _____
    8. Disciplinary actions?   _____
    9. Honors or awards?   _____
   10. Source of income in school?   _____
   11. Degree?   Yes ___ No ___

C. College education?   Yes ___ No ___
(If "NO," go to next section)
    1. School?   _____
    2. Dates attended?   _____
        a. Leave school for any period of time?   Yes ___ No ___
            1. Why?   _____
             2. How long?   _____
    3. Major subject?   _____
    4. Best subject?   _____
    5. Worst subject?   _____
    6. Average?   _____
    7. Extracurricular activities?   _____
    8. Disciplinary actions?   _____
    9. Honors or awards?   _____
   10. Source of income in school?   _____
   11. Degree?   Yes ___ No ___

D. Graduate education?   Yes ___ No ___

(If "NO," go to next section)
1. School? _____
2. Dates attended? _____
   a. Leave school for any period of time? Yes ___ No ___
      1. Why? _____
      2. How long? _____
3. Major subject? _____
4. Best subject? _____
5. Worst subject? _____
6. Average? _____
7. Extracurricular activities? _____
8. Disciplinary actions? _____
9. Honors or awards? _____
10. Source of income in school? _____
11. Degree? _____

E. Vocational education Yes ___ No ___
(If "NO," go to next section)
1. School? _____
2. Dates attended? _____
   a. Leave school for any period of time? Yes ___ No ___
      1. Why? _____
      2. How long? _____
3. Skills studied? _____
4. Difficulties in vocational training? Yes ___ No ___
5. Disciplinary actions? Yes ___ No ___
6. Source of income in school? _____
7. Certificate or diploma? _____

VII. LIVING SITUATION
   A. **Current residence**
      1. Address?_____
      2. Kind of residence (i.e., house, farm, apt.)?_____
      3. Dates of residence?_____
      4. Anyone living with you?   Yes ____ No ____
         a. How many?   _____
         b. Relationship?   _____
         c. Occupation?   _____
         d. Age?   _____
         e. Gender?   M ____   F ____
         f. Combined income?   _____
      5. Who manages the money?   _____
         a. Can you plan and budget?   Yes ____ No ____
         b. Do you balance your own checkbook?   Yes ____ No ____
         c. Does the statement reconcile?   Yes ____ No ____
         d. Are you in debt?   Yes ____ No ____
  B. **Previous residence(s): List addresses on separate sheet, including type and dates of residence.**

VIII. SOCIAL INVOLVEMENT

1. Community activities?   Yes ___ No ___
2. Organization membership?   Yes ___ No ___
3. Assisted by any organization?   Yes ___ No ___
4. Cultural/ethnic background?   _____
5. Family's cultural/ethnic background?   _____
6. More than one language at home?   Yes ___ No ___
   a. Which is spoken most?   _____
7. Discriminated against?   Yes ___ No ___
8. Neighborhood changing?   Yes ___ No ___

IX. LEGAL INVOLVEMENTS

1. Court appearances?   Yes ___ No ___
2. Family Court?   Yes ___ No ___
3. Other agencies?   Yes ___ No ___
4. Arrests?   Yes ___ No ___
5. Lawsuits?   Yes ___ No ___
6. Bankruptcy?   Yes ___ No ___
7. Tax Liens?   Yes ___ No ___

X. PERSONAL AND FAMILY GOALS, VALUES, RELIGION

1. What would you like to be doing in five years? _____
2. Three wishes?   _____
3. Three most admired people?   _____
4. What did your family want you to be like?   _____
   a. How do they feel about you now?   _____
   b. How do you feel about them?   _____
5. Your religion?   _____
   a. Practicing?   Yes ___ No ___
   b. Change from your family's religion?   Yes ___ No ___

XI. DESCRIPTION OF A TYPICAL DAY
A. Patient's Categorical Descriptors
1. With whom do you usually spend your time? _____
2. What do you usually do? _____
3. Hobbies or interests? _____
4. How do you spend your leisure time? _____
5. How much time alone? _____
6. How do you get around? _____
   a. Difficulties?   Yes ____ No ____

B. Hourly Chronology Of Patient's Typical Day

_____ _____ _____
_____ _____ _____
_____ _____ _____
_____ _____ _____
_____ _____ _____
_____ _____ _____
_____ _____ _____
_____ _____ _____

REVIEW OF SYSTEMS

I. MENTAL STATUS
A. Negative Cognitive Symptoms

	No	YES	Queried
1. AWARENESS			
a. Difficulty concentrating?	___	___	___
b. Thoughts slowed?	___	___	___
c. Thoughts blocked? Loose thoughts?	___	___	___
d. Confused about?	___	___	___
1. Where you were?	___	___	___
2. How you got there?	___	___	___
3. What was happening?	___	___	___
e. Unable to account for a period of time?	___	___	___
2. VISUOPERCEPTUAL SYMPTOMS			
a. Reading maps?	___	___	___
b. Finding your way around?	___	___	___
c. Telling left from right?	___	___	___
d. Do you get lost?	___	___	___
e. Telling what things are when you look at them?	___	___	___

3. DYSPRACTIC SYMPTOMS

a. Difficulty in doing ay tasks with your hands?   RUE ____   LUE ___

	No	YES	Queried
b. Difficulty using utensils or working with tools?	___	___	___
c. Difficulty putting your clothes on?	___	___	___
d. Any of your limbs do things by itself; do things that you don't tell it to do?	___	___	___

RUE __   RLE __   LUE __ LLE __

	No	YES	Queried
e. Speech slurred?	___	___	___
f. Difficulty using your lips or tongue?	___	___	___
g. Mouth or tongue move uncontrollably?	___	___	___

4. LINGUISTIC SYMPTOMS

<u>Expressive Language</u>

Difficulty:

	No	YES	Queried
a. Speaking?	___	___	___
b. Finding the right word?	___	___	___
c. Pronouncing words?	___	___	___
d. Spelling?	___	___	___
e. Writing?	___	___	___

<u>Receptive Language</u>

Difficulty:

	No	YES	Queried
f. Understanding what was said to you?	___	___	___
g. Reading out loud?	___	___	___

5. CONCEPTUAL AND SYMBOLIC SYMPTOMS

	No	YES	Queried
a. Difficulty working with numbers?	___	___	___
b. Surprised at others' reactions?	___	___	___
c. How good is your judgement?	___	___	___
d. People criticize you for no good reason?	___	___	___

     e. Made big plans that did not work out? ____ ____ ____

     f. Got into trouble or jams? ____ ____ ____

  6. **MEMORY SYMPTOMS**

     a. Forgetful or absentminded? ____ ____

     b. Trouble remembering? ____ ____

        1. Words? ____ ____ ____

        2. Names? ____ ____ ____

        3. Faces? ____ ____ ____

        4. Numbers? ____ ____ ____

B. Positive Cognitive Symptoms

  1. **AWARENESS**

     a. Thoughts race? ____ ____ ____

     b. Things seem strangely brilliant, clear,
        or vivid to you? ____ ____ ____

  2. **FAMILIARITY**

	No	Yes	Queried
a. Things that you see/hear ever seem strangely familiar to you as though you had seen or heard them before?	____	____	____
b. Things which you have seen/heard before ever seem strangely unfamiliar?	____	____	____

  3. **MATERIALITY**

     a. Feel as though you are no longer inside
        your body standing outside yourself? ____ ____ ____

     b. Felt as though everything around you seemed
        unreal, flat as on TV? ____ ____ ____

     c. Seem as though there is more than one person
        inside of you? ____ ____ ____

  4. **CORPOREALITY**

     a. Very concerned about your health? ____ ____ ____

     b. Often worried about illness which doctors said
        you did not have? ____ ____ ____

     c. Ever felt doctors do not take your problems
        seriously? ____ ____ ____

     d. Used any special diets, exercises, vitamins
        in order to keep from becoming ill? ____ ____ ____

     e. Very concerned that you were overweight? ____ ____ ____

     f. Anything seriously wrong with your body? ____ ____ ____

        1. Any parts missing or eaten away? ____ ____ ____

        2. Any body parts there that should not be there? ____ ____ ____

     g. See or feel parts of your body changing size or
        shape, looking unusual or floating away? ____ ____ ____

     h. See yourself in the wrong place? ____ ____ ____

  5. **TEMPORALITY**

     a. Worry about things that may happen in
        the future? ____ ____ ____

     b. Thing a lot about things that have gone
        wrong in the past, disappointments, losses,
        things that you feel were wrong? ____ ____ ____

6. **VOLITION**
    a. Difficulty making decisions?   ____   ____   ____
    b. Felt helpless, problems so big that nothing
        would fix things?   ____   ____   ____
    c. Made impulsive decisions you later regretted?   ____   ____   ____
    d. Spent much more money that you could afford?   ____   ____   ____
    e. Acted much more freely in your sex life than
        you would have liked?   ____   ____   ____
    f. Times when you have made big plans or started
        projects that did not work out?   ____   ____   ____
    g. Had thoughts or music that you could not get
        out of your head?   ____   ____   ____
    h. Could not resist doing the same thing over
        and over?   ____   ____   ____
    i. Any things you feel that you have to do exactly
        the same way each time?   ____   ____   ____
    k. Felt that you had to check and recheck things
        to make sure that they were "just right"?   ____   ____   ____
    l. Perfectionist?   ____   ____   ____

7. **CAUSALITY**
    a. Believed you could do things that other
        people could not?   ____   ____   ____
    b. Especially religious?   ____   ____   ____
    c. Especially interested in philosophy?   ____   ____   ____
    d. Thought a lot about life or why things happen?   ____   ____   ____
    e. Felt anyone or anything was out to hurt you or
        do you wrong?   ____   ____   ____
    f. Felt anyone against you?   ____   ____   ____
    g. Troubled by jealousy?   ____   ____   ____
    h. Felt someone or something outside of yourself
        was making you:
        1. Think things?   ____   ____   ____
        2. Feel things?   ____   ____   ____
        3. Want to do things?   ____   ____   ____
    i. Felt that you were sending your thoughts to
        anyone?   ____   ____   ____
    j. Felt as though someone had put thoughts into
        your head?   ____   ____   ____
    k. Felt as though someone had taken the thoughts
        out of you head or stolen them?   ____   ____   ____

C. Affective Symptoms

	No	Yes	Queried
1. FEAR			
a. Any things or situations so frightening that you would go to great lengths to avoid them?	___	___	___
b. Troubled by feelings of "nervousness," fear, or anxiety?	___	___	___
c. More nervous than most people?	___	___	___
d. Feel nervous more often than most people?	___	___	___
e. Suddenly felt so terrified you thought you were going to lose your mind or die?	___	___	___
2. ANGER			
a. Felt irritable/easy to annoy?	___	___	___
b. Is getting angry a problem?	___	___	___
c. Get more angry than most people?	___	___	___
d. Ever hurt someone?	___	___	___
1. Gotten into trouble as a result of getting angry?	___	___	___
2. Recently thought about hurting someone?	___	___	___
e. Ever thought about hurting or killing yourself?	___	___	___
1. Thought about killing yourself recently?	___	___	___
2. Do you have a plan/how would you do it?	___	___	___
3. Anyone with whom you have been close with died around this time or year?	___	___	___
4. Anyone you have know committed suicide?	___	___	___
3. DEPRESSION			
a. Felt sad, depressed, blue, down-in-the-dumps?	___	___	___
b. Felt worthless, no good or inadequate?	___	___	___
c. Times when you cried a lot?	___	___	___
e. Felt hopeless, unable to change things for the better?	___	___	___
4. ELATION			
a. Times when you have felt high, full of energy, like you could to just about anything?	___	___	___
b. Times when your mood changed for no apparent reason?	___	___	___

II SPECIAL SENSES

A. Visual Symptoms

1. **Trouble with your eyes or eyesight?** ___ ___ ___
   a. Vision problem completely corrected by
      eyeglasses? ___ ___ ___
      1. Age glasses were first prescribed?   Age___
      2. Nearsighted? ___ ___ ___
      3. Farsighted? ___ ___ ___
      4. Astigmatic? ___ ___ ___
   b. Color blind? ___ ___ ___
      1. What colors do you confuse?   Colors _____
   c. Glaucoma? ___ ___ ___
   d. Cataracts? ___ ___ ___
   e. Trouble seeing out of one eye? ___ ___ ___
      1. Which eye?   L___ R___
      2. Lazy eye?   L___ R___
   f. Trouble with your eye(s) begin following
      an injury? ___ ___ ___
   g. Pain in your eye(s) ___ ___ ___
   h. Bump into things? ___ ___ ___
      1. On which side?   L___ R___ B___

2. **Distortions of vision? Do things ever look
   peculiar or different?** ___ ___ ___
   a. Ordinary objects ever look unusal or distorted? ___ ___ ___
      (e.g., bent, stretched, torn, strangely colored)
   b. Objects ever seem to change size? ___ ___ ___
      1. Seem smaller? ___ ___ ___
      2. Larger: ___ ___ ___
      3. Both? ___ ___ ___
   c. Objects ever seem to be at a different distance
      than you expect them to be? ___ ___ ___
      1. Nearer? ___ ___ ___
      2. Farther? ___ ___ ___

3. **Unusual visual experiences?** ___ ___ ___
   a. Seen things that other people could not? ___ ___ ___
      1. Spots? ___ ___ ___
      2. Flashing lights? ___ ___ ___

4. **Seen things that are not actually present
   (e.g, faces or people)?** ___ ___ ___
   1. Images move by themselves? ___ ___ ___
   2. Move when you move your eyes? ___ ___ ___
   3. On which side do you see them?   L___ R___ B___
   a. Seen things that are really there but which other
      people do not see (e.g., people or faces)? ___ ___ ___
      1. Images move by themselves? ___ ___ ___
      2. Move when you move your eyes? ___ ___ ___
      3. On which side do you see them?   L___ R___ B___

5. **Ever had double vision?** ____ ____ ____

   a. Objects look blurry even with your glasses on? ____ ____ ____

   b. Objects seem to move or shimmer when
you look at them? ____ ____ ____

   c. Objects appear double, or do you see more than
two images? ____ ____ ____

      1. When one eye is closed? ____ ____ ____

      2. Images side by side? ____ ____ ____

      3. Which image is the real image? ____ ____ ____

      4. Images seem more separated when you look to
the right? to the left? Up? Down?   L__ R__

        Up__ Down__

B. **Auditory Symptoms**
   1. **Trouble hearing?** ___ ___ ___
      a. Improved with a hearing aid? ___ ___ ___
      b. Which ear affected?   Both ___ L ___ R ___
      c. At what age did your hearing loss begin?   Age ___
      d. Did hearing get worse? ___ ___ ___
      e. Hearing loss temporary? ___ ___ ___
         Hearing returned to normal? ___ ___ ___
      f. Trouble understanding what people say? ___ ___ ___
         1. Other sounds (non-speech) seem distorted
            also? ___ ___ ___
         2. Trouble telling where sounds are coming from? ___ ___ ___
   2. **Heard noises or other unusual sounds (e.g.,
      hissing, clicking, music)?** ___ ___ ___
      a. Did the sound beat like a pulse? ___ ___ ___
      b. Did you hear the sound come from: ___ ___ ___
         1. Inside your head? ___ ___ ___
         2. Outside your head? ___ ___ ___
      c. In which ear?   Both ___ L ___ R ___
   3. **Heard other unusual sounds (e.g., music,
      voices)?** ___ ___ ___
      a. From which side does it come?   Both ___ L ___ R ___
         1. From inside your head? ___ ___ ___
         2. From outside your head? ___ ___ ___
         3. From your ears? ___ ___ ___
            a. Which ear?   Both ___ L ___ R ___
      b. Do sounds or voices seem usual, strange, or
         distorted? ___ ___ ___
      c. Do sounds or voices seem as thought they are
         too close or too far away? ___ ___ ___
   4. **Heard voices?** ___ ___ ___
      a. Voices really there? ___ ___ ___
         1. Which side do you hear them on?   Both ___ L ___ R ___
      b. Just seem as though they are really there? ___ ___ ___
      c. Whose voice(s)? _____
      d. More than one voice? ___ ___ ___
         1. Voices talk to each other? ___ ___ ___
         2. Talk about you? ___ ___ ___
         3. Voices say bad or offensive things about you? ___ ___ ___
      e. What did the voice(s) say? _____
      f. Voice(s) tell you to do anything? ___ ___ ___
         1. What did the voice(s) tell you to do? _____
         2. Ever carried out the instructions? ___ ___ ___
         3. Do you think you would do what the
            voice(s) told you to do? ___ ___ ___

C. **Olfactory Symptoms**
  1. **Lost your ability to smell?**   _____   _____   _____
    a. Has it affected your sense of taste?   _____   _____   _____
  2. **Strange or unusual odors?**   _____   _____   _____
    a. Times when things do not smell the way
       they are supposed to?   _____   _____   _____
    b. Noticed strange or unusual odors, odors that
       other people do not smell?   _____   _____   _____
      1. Come from one direction?   L___ R___ B___
      2. Come from outside yourself?   _____   _____   _____
      3. Come from your own body?   _____   _____   _____

D. **Gustatory Symptoms**   No   Yes   Queried
  1. **Loss of taste?**   _____   _____   _____
  2. **Strange or unusual tastes?**   _____   _____   _____
    a. Times when things do not taste the way they
       are supposed to?   _____   _____   _____
    b. Noticed any strange or unusual tastes,
       tastes other people do not taste?   _____   _____   _____

E. Somatosensory Symptoms
1. Loss of sensation or numbness?   ____   ____   ____
2. Strange or unusual sensations in your body or
    on your skin?   ____   ____   ____
    a. Tingling?   ____   ____   ____
    b. Itching?   ____   ____   ____
    c. Buzzing?   ____   ____   ____
    d. Burning?   ____   ____   ____
    e. Pins and needles?   ____   ____   ____
    f. Wetness?   ____   ____   ____
    g. Things crawling?   ____   ____   ____
    h. Felt like someone touched you?   ____   ____   ____

R Face____   L Face____
R Neck____   L Neck__
RUE____   LUE____
R Torso____   L Torso____
RLE___   LLE___

III. MOTOR   No   Yes   Queried

   1. **Loss of balance when you stand still?**   ____   ____   ____

      a. Tend to fall more in one direction?   ____   ____   ____

         1. Which direction?   L___ R___ Forward___ Backward ___

      b. Balance worse:

         1. When you first stand up?   ____   ____   ____

         2. With eyes closed?   ____   ____   ____

         3. In the dark?   ____   ____   ____

   2. **Difficulty in walking?**   ____   ____   ____

      a. Trouble more with one leg than the other?   L___ R___

      b. Legs get weak or stiff?   ____   ____   ____

      c. Trip a great deal?   ____   ____   ____

      d. Stagger when you walk?   ____   ____   ____

      e. Veer or drift more to one side?   ____   ____   ____

         1. Which side?   L___ R___

      f. Step backward or step in place before starting to walk?   ____   ____   ____

   3. **Weakness or loss of strength in any part of your body?**   ____   ____   ____

      a. All parts of the body affected equally?   ____   ____   ____

         1. Which are weakest?   _____

      b. All parts of the limbs equally weak?   ____   ____   ____

         1. Weakness more in the hips and shoulders or in the hands and feet?   Hips/Shoulders   Hands/Feet

                                                L__R__/L__ R__   L_R__/L_R__

      c. Loss of muscle bulk?   ____   ____   ____

      d. Weakness more noticeable:

         1. After physical labor?   ____   ____   ____

         2. In the evening?   ____   ____   ____

         3. In the morning?   ____   ____   ____

   4. **Clumsy or lost coordination:**   ____   ____   ____

      a. Whole body affected?   ____   ____   ____

      b. Limbs most affected?   RUE___ LUE___ RLE___ LLE___

   5. **Unusual or uncontrolled movements?**   ____   ____   ____

      a. Movements continuous or almost always present? ____   ____   ____

      b. Occur at regular intervals?   ____   ____   ____

      c. Movements rhythmic?   ____   ____   ____

      d. Parts of the body most involved?   _____

                                            R Face___   L Face___

                                          R Neck___   L Neck__

                                          RUE___   LUE___

                                          R Torso___   L Torso___

                                          RLE___   LLE___

      e. How far do they move?   _____

      f. Body movements slowed?   ____   ____   ____

      g. Stiffness in your arms and legs?   ____   ____   ____

      h. Change in posture?   ____   ____   ____

IV. VISCERAL

A. Eating And Digestive Dysfunction

1. Appetite changed?   Lost____   Increased____
2. Weight change (>10lbs.) over 6-month period? ____ ____ ____
3. Diarrhea? ____ ____ ____
4. Constipation? ____ ____ ____
5. Lost bowel control? ____ ____ ____
6. Strange or unusual sensations in your stomach? ____ ____ ____
7. Felt that stomach was going up toward your throat? ____ ____ ____

B. Sleep And Arousal Disturbances

1. How many hours do you usually sleep each night? _____
2. Difficulty falling asleep? ____ ____ ____
3. Keep waking up during the night? If yes-what
   wakens you? ____ ____ ____
   a. To go to the bathroom? ____ ____ ____
   b. Bad dreams? ____ ____ ____
   c. Waken for no reason? ____ ____ ____
4. Wake up too early in the morning and unable
   to go back to sleep? ____ ____ ____
5. Still feel tired in the morning when you wake up? ____ ____ ____
6. Fatigued or low on energy at any particular time
   of the day? ____ ____ ____
   a. Morning? ____ ____ ____
   b. Afternoon? ____ ____ ____
   c. Evening? ____ ____ ____
7. Fall asleep suddenly or unexpectedly, at times when
   you do not want to sleep? ____ ____ ____
8. Times when you have not needed as much sleep
   as usual? ____ ____ ____
9. Strange or frightening dreams that waken you? ____ ____ ____
10. Remember any of your recent dreams? ____ ____ ____
11. What do you dream about? _____
12. Do they recur? ____ ____ ____
13. Sleep getting better or worse?   Better__   Worse__ Same__

C. Sexual Dysfunction
1. Concerns or problems regarding sex?   ___   ___   ___
2. Times when you lost interest in sex?   ___   ___   ___
3. Times when you did not enjoy sex as
   much as usual?   ___   ___   ___
4. Times when you felt unusually interested in sex?   ___   ___   ___
5. Times when you were much more sexually
   active than usual?   ___   ___   ___
6. Change in what interested you sexually?   ___   ___   ___
7. Difficulty in reaching orgasm?   ___   ___   ___

FOR WOMEN:
8. Pain or unusual sensations during intercourse?   ___   ___   ___
9. Painful menstrual periods?   ___   ___   ___
10. Excessive bleeding during your periods?   ___   ___   ___
11. Periods been irregular?   ___   ___   ___
12. Missed menstrual periods?   ___   ___   ___

FOR MEN:
13. Difficulty in having or maintaining an erection?   ___   ___   ___
14. Reached orgasm too soon?   ___   ___   ___

D. General Arousal Symptoms
1. **Bladder**
   a. Felt you had to urinate more often than usual?   ___   ___   ___
   b. Felt you had to urinate more urgently than usual? ___   ___   ___
   c. Lost control of your bladder?   ___   ___   ___
      1. When awake or asleep?   Awake___ Asleep___
2. **Cutaneous**
   a. Rashes on your skin?   ___   ___   ___
   b. Skin felt cold?   ___   ___   ___
   c. Excessive sweating?   ___   ___   ___
   d. Sweat more on one side your body?   ___   ___   ___
      1. Which side?   L___   R___
   e. Mouth felt dry?   ___   ___   ___
3. **Cardiovascular**
   a. Fingers or toes ever become pale or blue? ___   ___   ___
   b. Felt your heart going too fast?   ___   ___   ___
   c. Chest pains?   ___   ___   ___
   d. Pains in your hands or feet?   ___   ___   ___
4. **Respiratory**
   a. Trouble breathing?   ___   ___   ___
   b. Catching your breath?   ___   ___   ___
   c. Choking or smothering feeling?   ___   ___   ___
   d. Difficulty breathing during sleep?   ___   ___   ___

V. PAROXYSMAL

	No	Yes	Queried
1. a. Headaches?	___	___	___
1. Steady?	___	___	___
2. Throbbing?	___	___	___
3. Pounding?	___	___	___
4. Stabbing?	___	___	___
b. Does it get better if you change position?	___	___	___
c. Does it waken you from sleep?	___	___	___
2. Dizzy?	___	___	___
a. Confused afterwards?	___	___	___
3. Felt as though either you or the room was spinning?	___	___	___
a. Fallen or felt like falling?	___	___	___

1. To which side?   L__   R__   Front__   Back__

	No	Yes	Queried
b. Walked like you were drunk?	___	___	___
c. Confused afterwards?	___	___	___
4. Blacked out?	___	___	___
5. Fainted?	___	___	___
6. Lost consciousness for any reason?	___	___	___
a. Know what had happened when you came to?	___	___	___
b. Confused afterwards?	___	___	___
1. How long?	_____		
c. Bite your tongue?	___	___	___
d. Lose control of your bladder or bowels?	___	___	___

  e. Weak afterwards?   RUE__   LUE__   RLE__   LLE__
                               Face__   Neck__   Body__

	No	Yes	Queried
f. Experience any unusual sensations?	___	___	___
g. Know it was coming?	___	___	___
h. Remember any feelings you had before blacking out?	___	___	___

ROS: SYMPTOM INQUIRY FORMAT

a. Complaint (Verbatim Description):_____
_____
_____

b. For any sensory, perceptual, motoric, cutaneous, cephalic, or somatic complaints, follow
   patient's description with, **"What area(s) is effected?"** **"What parts of the body?"**_____
   "Where do you see it, hear it, feel it, etc.?"_____
   "Which side?"   L___ R___ B___

c. First happened?_____

d. How long did it last?_____

e. **Happened since then?**
                                                                      Yes___ No___
   How often?_____
   Always the same?   Yes___ No___
       How does it change?_____
   Happen more often or less often than when you first noticed it?
                                                     More___ Less___ Same___

f. **Other changes or symptoms before, during or after (the problem)?**   Yes___ No___
       Describe_____
_____

g. **Anything which caused (the problem)?**   Yes___ No___
       Describe_____
_____

h. **Anything which makes (the problem) better?**   Yes___ No___
                                             Medication___ Alcohol___ Drugs___
       Describe_____
_____

i. **Anything which makes (the problem) worse?**   Yes___ No___
                                             Medication___ Alcohol___ Drugs___
       Describe_____
_____

j. **Does (the problem) cause any other difficulties for you?**   Yes___ No___
       Describe_____
_____

k. **Does (the problem) upset you?**   Yes___ No___

SYMPTOM INQUIRY CODING SHEET
REVIEW OF SYSTEMS

PATIENT_____SYMPTOM_____

a. DESCRIPTION:_____

_____

b. LOCUS:_____

    1. Corporeal Space:

        Right   Left

        RFace___RTorso___RUE___RLE   LFace___LTorso___LUE___LLE

    2. Extra Corporeal Space

        Right Hemifield____Left Hemifield____Both Sides

    3. Non Localized____

c. ONSET: Age_____   Date:_____

    1. Mode: Abrupt   Gradual____

    2. Prodroma_____

    3. Precipitus_____

d. DURATION: Symptom_____   Syndrome_____

e. RECURRENCE: Yes ___ No ___

    Frequency_____

f. ASSOCIATED SYMPTOMS:_____

g. COURSE:

    1. <u>Clinical</u>:   Static___   Cyclic___   Episodic___   Isolated___

    2. <u>Changes</u>:

        <u>Direction of Change</u>   <u>Velocity of Change:</u>

        Over Time: Static ___ Progressive___ Resolving___   Rapid___ Moderate___

                                                        Slow___

        Stereotypy: Yes___   No_____

        In Severity_____

        In Frequency_____

        In Associated Symptoms_____

h. TERMINATION: Abrupt____   Gradual____

i. PALLIATIVES: Yes___ No___

j. IRRITANTS: Yes___ No___

k. RELATED PROBLEMS: Yes___ No___

l. AFFECTIVE RESPONSE:
Fear____   Depression____   Anger____   Guilt____   Euphoria____   Apathy____
Other_____

m. PATIENT'S SUBJECTIVE EXPLANATION: Yes____ No____

_____

n. PHARMACOLOGICAL ISSUES: Yes____ No____
Medication_____
Drugs _____
Alcohol_____

OBSERVATIONS OF THE PATIENT
NARRATIVE RECORDING SYSTEM

A. General Appearance
  1. Physical Appearance
     a. skin
     b. hair
     c. nails
     d. odor, sweating
  2. Dress/Grooming
  3. Height
  4. Weight
  5. Somatotype, Physical Condition
  6. Attitude, Demeanor

B. Facial Appearance
  1. Craniofacial Anomalies
  2. Maturity of Faces/Features
  3. Affective Expressions
     a. quality
        • anger
        • fear
        • sadness
        • elation
        • confusion
        • blunting
     b. quantity (facial mobility)
        • blunted, inanimate, mask-like
        • within normal limits
        • hyperanimated

C. Motor Behavior
  1. Psychomotor Activity
     a. retardation/bradykinesia
        • paralysis
        • paresis
     b. hypermotility/hyperkinesia
     c. dyskinesias
        • chorea
        • athetosis
        • hemiballismus
  2. Psychomotor Reactivity
  3. Postural, Gait, Carriage Anomalies
     a. ataxia
     b. wide-based gait
     c. shuffling gait
     d. anergic posture

    e. limitations of posture
- assistance
- sitting

    f. standing

    g. bizarre posture

    h. rocking

    i.   head banging

4. Tremor
5. Other Adventitious Movements

D. **Respiration**
   1. Assistance Level
   2. Rate
   3. Rhythm
   4. Depth
   5. Anomalies
      a. sighing
      b. breath holding
      c. hyperventilation

E. **Communicative Functions**
   1. **Expressive Speech and Language**
      a. voice
      b. articulation
      c. prosody
      d. rhythm
      e. rate
      f. length of utterance/phrase
      g. speech content, aphasic phenomena
         - anomia
         - circumlocution
         - semantic paraphasia
         - phonemic paraphasia
         - neologism:
            - meaningful
            - meaningless
         - echolalia
         - palalaia
         - empty speech
         - paucity of spontaneous output
   2. **Receptive Speech and Language**
         - impaired speech/language comprehension
         - phoneme/word level
         - propositional/syntactic level

F. **Thought Organization**
   1. Orientation and Consciousness
   2. Perceptual Functions
      a. visual
      b. auditory
      c. olfactory
      d. gustatory
      e. tactile
   3. Behavioral Programming, Praxis, and Sequencing
   4. Language
   5. Conceptual and Calculations
      a. concreteness
      b. blocking

    c. slogia
    d. loosening of associations
    e. viscosity
    f. circumstantially/obsessionalism
    g. tangentiality
    h. flight of ideas
    i. clanging

6. Memory
- memory dysfunction
- forgetfulness
  - names
  - dates
  - events
  - faces
  - immediate
  - short-term
  - long-term

G. Thought Content
1. Poverty of Associations
2. Grandiose/Expansive Thought
3. Somatic Concerns
   - illness
   - weight
   - personal appearance (cosmetic)
4. Somatic Delusions
5. Worries/Anxieties About Reasonable Future Events
6. Guilty Ruminations/Self-Accusatory Notions
7. Concerns
   - compulsions
   - rituals
   - perfectionisms
8. Religious Themes
9. Philosophical Themes
10. Persecutory Ideation
11. Observed Responses to:
    - made feelings
    - made impulses
    - made actions
    - thought broadcasting
    - thought insertion
    - thought withdrawal
12. Expressed Concerns
    a. fear
       - specified objects/situations
       - unspecified objects/situations
       - panic attacks
    b. anger
       - irritability
       - rage dyscontrol
       - homicidal intent
    c. suicidal ideation
    d. depressive ideation

H. Perception
   1. Observed responses to:

	sight	sound	taste	smell	touch
dimunition					
illusion					
hallucination					

I. Observed Affect

    1. **Tonic**

        a. warmth

        b. fear

        c. anger

        d. sadness

        e. elation

        f. Witzelsucht/giddiness

        g. blunting/indifference

    2. Phasic (reactions/rate)

        a. response to

            • reassurance

            • manipulation

        b. precipitous/reactive

        c. recalled

        d. ego dystonic/syntonic

        e. accompanied by associated symptoms

        f. duration

J. Examiner's Affective State

    1. Warmth

    2. Empathy

    3. Anger

    4. Anxiety

    5. Depression

    6. Sexual Arousal

    7. Praecox Feel

    8. Other

OBSERVATIONS OF THE PATIENT
CHECKLIST RECORDING SYSTEM

Physical Appearance
  Skin
    fever signs
    - sweats
    - dry, cracked lips
      general color/pigmentation
    - flushing
    - pallor
    - jaundiced
      - skin
      - conjunctiva
    - sallow
    - silver tinge
    - red/purple Malar flush
    localized color/pigmentation
    - strawberry marks
    - shagreen patches
    - cafe au lait spots
    - port wine spots
    - purpura
    - petechia
    - blue/slate gray spots
    structural anomalies
    - cachectic face
    - mask-like butterfly
    - xanthelasma
    - telangectasis
    - corrugation in forehead
    - agryia
    - cauliflower ears
    - scars/keloids
    - linear scars at hairline
    - cutaneous tubers in butterfly
      distribution
    - pedunclular polyps
    - periorbital edema
    - cold sores
    - crinkly appearance at edge of eyes
    - tortuosity of blood vessels

Hair
    amount/distribution
    - hirsutism
    - baldness
    - excessive hair on back of neck
    - low forehead
    texture
    - dry/broken
    - tightly coiled, broken
    color
    - pale blond
    - prematurely graying

Nails
    - clubbing
    - cynanosis
    - horizontal ridges
    - biting

Odor/Sweating
    - musty
    - body odor
    - feces
    - urine
    - alcohol

Dress/Grooming (neglect)
    unilateral
    - left side
    - right side
    bilateral

Height

Weight

Somatotype/Physical Condition
    emaciation
    cachexia
    structural abnormalities
    pregnancy
    flexion
    posture
    - erect
    - military
    - bent

Facial Appearance
Craniofacial Anomalies

Faces
- hemiatrophy
- hypertelorism
- brows meeting in the middle
- depressions
- enlarged frontal bossae
- tumefactions
- acromegaly
- racitic deformities
- mask-like

Head
- hydrocephaly
- macrocephaly
- microcephaly
- oxycephaly

Maturity of Faces/Features

Affective Expressions

quality
- anger
- fear
- sadness
- elation
- confusion
- blunting

Non-Affective Facial Mobility
- tics
- mouthings
- grimacing
- fluttering eyelids
- spontaneous oral movements

Eyes
- squint
- disconjugate gaze
- palpebral fissures
- ptosis
- pupils

Perception

Observed Responses to <u>V</u>　<u>A</u>　<u>O</u>　<u>G</u>　　<u>SS</u>
　　impairment of　　__ __ __ __　　__
　　distortions of　　__ __ __ __　　__
　　hallucinations of　__ __ __ __　　__

Motor Behavior
Psychomotor Activity
　retardation/bradykinesia
- paralysis
- paresis
　hypermotility/hyperkinesis
　dyskinesias
- chorea
- athetosis
- hemiballusmus
- tics

Psychomotor Reactivity

Postural, Gait, Carriage, Anomalies

　negative
- foot drop
- absence of associated arm movements
- shuffling gait
- exaggerated arm movements
- unilateral
- bilateral
- Marche a petit pas

　wide-based gait
　shuffling gait
　anergic posture
　limitations of posture
- assistance
- sitting
- standing
　bizarre posture
　rocking
　head banging

Tremor

Other adventitious movements

Hypoactivity

Hyperactivity

Communicative Function
Expressive Speech and Language
    voice
    articulation
    prosody
    rhythm
    rate
    length of utterance/phrase
    speech content: aphasic phenomena
      • anomia
      • circumlocution
      • semantic paraphasia
      • phonemic paraphasia
      • neologism:
          • meaningful
          • meaningless
    echolalia
    palalaia
    empty speech
    paucity of spontaneous output

Receptive Speech and Language
    impaired speech/language
    comprehension
        phoneme/work level
        propositional/syntactic level
        pragmatic awareness

Thought Content
Poverty of Associations
Grandiose/Expansive Thought
Somatic Concerns
    • illness
    • weight
·   • personal appearance
Somatic Delusions
Worries/Anxieties About Reasonable
Future Events
Guilty/Self-Accusatory Notions

Concerns
    • compulsions
    • rituals
    • perfectionism
Religious Themes
Philosophical Themes
Persecutory Ideation
Observed Responses to
    made feelings
    made impulses
    made actions
    thought broadcasting
    thought insertion
    thought withdrawal

Thought Organization
Alogia
Blocking
Loosening of Associations
Concreteness
Viscosity
Tangentiality
Circumstantially/Obsessionalism
Short Attention Span
Distractibility
Perseveration
Clanging
Flight of Ideas

Memory dysfunction
    • names
    • dates
    • events
    • faces
      forgetfulness/incidental memory
      compulsive rechecking
      omissions
      approximate answers
      confabulations
      contaminations

Observed Affect
Tonic (overall tone)
    warmth
    fear
    anger
    sadness
    elation
    Witzelsucht/giddiness
    blunting/indifference

Phasic (reactions/rate)
    response to
- reassurance
- manipulation

    precipitous/reactive
    recalled
    ego dystonic/syntonic
    accompanied by associated symptoms
    duration

Examiner's Affective State
    Warmth
    Empathy
    Anger
    Anxiety
    Depression
    Sexual Arousal
    Praecox Feel
    Other

Respiration
    Assistance Level
    Rate
    Rhythm
    Depth
    Anomalies
- sighing
- breath holding
- hyperventilation
- labored breathing upon minimal exertion

INDEX

A

acting-out dyscontrol, 60-61

Activation Level, Input Source, and Modes of Processing (AIM) Model - See AIM Model

Activities of Daily Living (ADL), 12, 82-83,85,109,135, 138, 140, 162

Adaptive Psychodynamics, 56, 57

AIM Model, 61

Alzheimer's disease (AD), 243-258, 263, 276

Americans with Disabilities Act (ADA), 378

aphasia, 243-258

Aphasia Screening Test, 245

appetitive functions, 45, 50, 54

arousal, 50

assessment of children, 301-310

attention/awareness, 49, 147-167

Attention Capacity Test, 158

Auditory Comprehension Test, 212

auditory functions, 212

auditory perception, 205

B

Beck Depression Inventory, 276-344

Behavior Change Inventory, (BCI) 346

behavior theory, 76-77

Behavioral Assessment of Vocational Skills (BAVS), 401

Behavioral Evaluation of Frontal Functions (BEFF), 401

Behavioral Inattention Test (BIT), 417-419

behavioral programming, 49

Bender-Gestalt, 209-210

Bender Visual Motor Gestalt Test, 306

D

E

F

K

L

M